Nasal Reconstruction

Guest Editor

DANIEL G. BECKER, MD

FACIAL PLASTIC SURGERY CLINICS OF NORTH AMERICA

www.facialplastic.theclinics.com

February 2011 • Volume 19 • Number 1

SAUNDERS an imprint of ELSEVIER, Inc.

W.B. SAUNDERS COMPANY
A Division of Elsevier Inc.

1600 John F. Kennedy Blvd., Suite 1800, Philadelphia, PA 19103-2899

http://www.theclinics.com

FACIAL PLASTIC SURGERY CLINICS OF NORTH AMERICA Volume 19, Number 1
February 2011 ISSN 1064-7406, ISBN 978-1-4557-0442-2

Editor: Joanne Husovski
Developmental Editor: Donald Mumford

Facial Plastic Surgery Clinics of North America (ISSN 1064-7406) is published quarterly by Elsevier Inc., 360 Park Avenue South, New York, NY 10010-1710. Months of issue are February, May, August, and November. Business and Editorial Offices: 1600 John F. Kennedy Blvd., Suite 1800, Philadelphia, PA 19103-2899. Periodicals postage paid at New York, NY, and additional mailing offices. Subscription prices are $329.00 per year (US individuals), $459.00 per year (US institutions), $375.00 per year (Canadian individuals), $550.00 per year (Canadian institutions), $449.00 per year (foreign individuals), $550.00 per year (foreign institutions), $156.00 per year (US students), and $217.00 per year (foreign students). Foreign air speed delivery is included in all *Clinics* subscription prices. All prices are subject to change without notice. POSTMASTER: Send address changes to *Facial Plastic Surgery Clinics*, Elsevier Health Sciences Division, Subscription Customer Service, 3251 Riverport Lane, Maryland Heights, MO 63043. **Customer service: 1-800-654-2452 (US and Canada); 1-314-447-8871 (outside US and Canada); Fax: 314-447-8029; E-mail:journalscustomerservice-usa@elsevier.com (for print support); journalsonline support-usa@elsevier.com (for online support).**

Reprints. For copies of 100 or more of articles in this publication, please contact the Commercial Reprints Department, Elsevier Inc., 360 Park Avenue South, New York, NY 10010-1710. Tel.: 212-633-3812; Fax: 212-462-1935; E-mail: reprints@elsevier.com.

Facial Plastic Surgery Clinics of North America is covered in *MEDLINE/PubMed* (*Index Medicus*).

Printed and bound by CPI Group (UK) Ltd, Croydon, CR0 4YY

Transferred to Digital Print 2011

Contributors

CONSULTING EDITOR

J. REGAN THOMAS, MD, FACS
Professor and Chairman, Department
of Otolaryngology, University of Illinois
at Chicago, Chicago, Illinois

EDITORIAL BOARD

SHAN R. BAKER, MD
Professor and Chief, Section of Plastic and
Reconstructive Surgery, University of
Michigan, Ann Arbor, Michigan

ROBERT KELLMAN, MD
Professor and Chairman, Department of
Otolaryngology, State University of New York
Upstate Medical University, Syracuse, New York

RUSSELL W.H. KRIDEL, MD
Clinical Associate Professor, Department of
Otolaryngology–Head and Neck Surgery,
Division of Facial Plastic Surgery, University of
Texas Health Science Center, Houston, Texas

STEPHEN W. PERKINS, MD
Private Practitioner, Perkins Facial Plastic
Surgery, Indianapolis, Indiana

ANTHONY P. SCLAFANI, MD, FACS
Director of Facial Plastic Surgery, The New
York Eye and Ear Infirmary, New York, New
York; and Professor of Otolaryngology–Head
and Neck Surgery, New York Medical College,
Valhalla, New York

GUEST EDITOR

DANIEL G. BECKER, MD, FACS
Clinical Associate Professor, Department of
Otolaryngology–Head and Neck Surgery,
University of Pennsylvania, Philadelphia,
Pennsylvania; Becker Nose and Sinus Center,
Sewell, New Jersey

AUTHORS

MARCELO B. ANTUNES, MD
Resident, Department of
Otorhinolaryngology–Head and
Neck Surgery, University of Pennsylvania
Health System, Philadelphia,
Pennsylvania

DAVID J. ARCHIBALD, MD
Department of Otorhinolaryngology–Head
and Neck Surgery, Mayo Clinic College of
Medicine, Rochester, Minnesota

SHAN R. BAKER, MD
Section of Facial Plastic and Reconstructive
Surgery, Department of Otolaryngology–Head
and Neck Surgery, University of Michigan,
Ann Arbor, Michigan

DANIEL G. BECKER, MD, FACS
Clinical Associate Professor, Department of
Otolaryngology–Head and Neck Surgery,
University of Pennsylvania, Philadelphia,
Pennsylvania; Becker Nose and Sinus Center,
Sewell, New Jersey

AMIT D. BHRANY, MD
Facial Plastic and Reconstructive Surgery,
Department of Otolaryngology–Head and
Neck Surgery, University of Washington,
Seattle, Washington

JASON D. BLOOM, MD
Fellow, Division of Facial Plastic and
Reconstructive Surgery, Department
of Otolaryngology, New York University
Medical Center, New York, New York

ARA A. CHALIAN, MD
Associate Professor and Chief, Division
of Facial Plastics and Reconstructive
Surgery, Department of Otorhinolaryngology–
Head and Neck Surgery, University
of Pennsylvania, Philadelphia, Pennsylvania

MICHAEL W. CHU, MD
Resident Physician, Department of
Otolaryngology–Head and Neck Surgery,
Eastern Virginia Medical School,
Norfolk, Virginia

MINAS CONSTANTINIDES, MD
Assistant Professor, Division of Facial
Plastic and Reconstructive Surgery,
Department of Otolaryngology, New York
University School of Medicine,
New York, New York

ERIC J. DOBRATZ, MD
Director of Facial Plastic and Reconstructive
Surgery; Assistant Professor, Department
of Otolaryngology–Head and Neck Surgery,
Eastern Virginia Medical School,
Norfolk, Virginia

CALLUM FARIS, MBBS, MRCS, DOHNS
Department of Otolaryngology, Southampton
University Hospitals, Southampton,
United Kingdom

OREN FRIEDMAN, MD
Director, Facial Plastic and Reconstructive
Surgery, Associate Professor,
Otorhinolaryngology, Department of
Otorhinolaryngology–Head and Neck Surgery,
Mayo Clinic College of Medicine, Rochester,
Minnesota

WILLEM P. GODEFROY, MD, PhD
Department of Otolaryngology–Head and Neck
Surgery, Center for Facial Plastic
Reconstructive Surgery, Diakonessen Hospital
Zeist/Utrecht, Zeist, The Netherlands

SARA IMMERMAN, MD
Department of Otolaryngology, New York
University School of Medicine, New York,
New York

CODY A. KOCH, MD, PhD
Department of Otorhinolaryngology–Head
and Neck Surgery, Mayo Clinic College
of Medicine, Rochester, Minnesota

PETER J.F.M. LOHUIS, MD, PhD
Department of Head and Neck Oncology
and Surgery, The Netherlands Cancer
Institute, Antoni van Leeuwenhoek Hospital,
Amsterdam; Department of Otolaryngology–
Head and Neck Surgery, Center for Facial
Plastic Reconstructive Surgery,
Diakonessen Hospital Zeist/Utrecht,
Zeist, The Netherlands

FREDERICK J. MENICK, MD
Private Practice; Chief, Division of Plastic
Surgery, St Joseph's Hospital, Tucson,
Arizona

CHRISTOPHER J. MILLER, MD
Assistant Professor and Director, Division of
Dermatologic Surgery, Department of
Dermatology, Perelman Center for Advanced
Medicine, University of Pennsylvania Health
System, Philadelphia, Pennsylvania

AJANI NUGENT, MD
Resident, Department of Otolaryngology–Head
and Neck Surgery, Emory Healthcare, Emory
University, Atlanta, Georgia

KENNETH K.K. OO, MBBS, MSc
Fellow, Department of Otolaryngology–Head
and Neck Surgery, University of Virginia
Health System, Charlottesville, Virginia

STEPHEN S. PARK, MD, FACS
Professor and Vice-Chair, Department
of Otolaryngology–Head and Neck Surgery;
Director, Division of Facial Plastic and
Reconstructive Surgery, University
of Virginia Health System, Charlottesville,
Virginia

EVAN R. RANSOM, MD
Resident, Department of Otorhinolaryngology–
Head and Neck Surgery, University
of Pennsylvania Health System, Philadelphia,
Pennsylvania

JACOB D. STEIGER, MD
Steiger Facial Plastic Surgery, Boca Raton, Florida

ABEL-JAN TASMAN, MD
Section of Facial Plastic and Reconstructive Surgery, Department of Otolaryngology–Head and Neck Surgery, Cantonal Hospital, St Gallen, Switzerland

HADE D. VUYK, MD, PhD
Department of Otolaryngology and Facial Plastic Reconstructive Surgery, Tergooi Hospitals, Blaricum, The Netherlands

TOM D. WANG, MD
Professor, Division of Facial Plastic and Reconstructive Surgery, Department of Otolaryngology–Head and Neck Surgery, Oregon Health and Science University, Portland, Oregon

STEPHEN M. WEBER, MD, PhD
Assistant Professor, Division of Facial Plastic and Reconstructive Surgery, Department of Otolaryngology–Head and Neck Surgery, Oregon Health and Science University, Portland, Oregon

W. MATTHEW WHITE, MD
Assistant Professor, Division of Facial Plastic and Reconstructive Surgery, Department of Otolaryngology, New York University School of Medicine, New York, New York

SETH A. YELLIN, MD
Chief, Division of Facial Plastic Surgery, Department of Otolaryngology–Head and Neck Surgery, Emory Healthcare; Assistant Professor, Emory University School of Medicine; Director, Emory Facial Center, Atlanta, Georgia

Contents

Nasal reconstruction provides a challenging task for any facial plastic surgeon. In performing reconstructive surgery on the nose, one must balance both the functional aspects of the nasal airway with the aesthetic responsibilities of being the central fixture of the face. Before performing surgery, the surgeon must grasp the importance of the anatomic nasal relationships and subunits, the physiology of the skin, the flaps or grafts used to reconstruct these areas, and the basic steps in wound healing. Accurate preoperative planning and analysis of the nasal defect are also vital to producing both an aesthetic and functional nose.

Defects of the nasal dorsum or sidewall can result from trauma, congenital lesions, extirpation of neoplasms, or iatrogenic injuries. Simple techniques are often used to reconstruct defects in this area with excellent outcomes. Complex defects require more sophisticated techniques including multilayer closures using pedicled flaps or free tissue transfer. This review discusses key anatomic and functional principles and techniques to assist in planning for reconstruction of nasal dorsum and sidewall defects from any cause.

Reconstruction of nasal tip and columella defects is demanding area with a range of reconstructive options, varying in complexity depending on requirements from simple skin grafting to multiple stage reconstruction with regional flaps. A framework is suggested to aid the reader in choice of reconstruction by classifying the defect based on size and the requirements of one to three layer (full thickness) reconstruction.

With its complex symmetric contours and central facial location, the nose plays a key role in characterizing the face. Among the cosmetic subunits of the nose, the delicate nasal ala has a particularly marked influence on breathing and cosmetic appearance. Therefore, reconstruction of defects of the nasal ala requires careful attention to preserve and restore function and cosmesis. Reconstructive surgeons have a wide variety of options and techniques to repair specific defects of the nasal ala. Attention to detail, knowledge of the nasal anatomy, and precise surgical techniques allows for the optimum results with the lowest risk of complications.

the workhorse for major nasal resurfacing today. Contemporary nasal reconstruction with forehead flaps uses the well-established concept of facial and nasal subunits, restoring the three-dimensional morphology by replacing missing tissue with like tissue. This article covers the history of forehead flap surgery, current concepts in flap design, surgical steps, potential complications, defect analysis, lining, framework, and cover as a means of restoring the three-dimensional nasal morphology.

Microvascular reconstruction of nasal defects is a complex procedure and must consider 3 nasal components: skin, osteocartilaginous framework, and intranasal lining. These layers can be reconstructed with various flaps and grafts. The commonly used flaps are the first dorsal metacarpal flap, dorsalis pedis flap, auricular helical rim flap, and radial forearm and prelaminated flaps. These flaps can be composed of skin and cartilage or skin and bone. The decision is based on the patient's needs taking into consideration the extent of the defect and presence or absence of nasal septum and columella.

Nasal reconstruction has been refined to the point that its goals should include full restoration of form and function in addition to providing an aesthetically-pleasing result. Contemporary facial plastic surgeons have all the tools available in their armamentarium to repair the complex composite structure of nasal lining, structure, and skin cover. Nasal defects most often result from oncologic surgery or, less commonly, nasal trauma. While defects of nasal cover are more prominent, the impact of unrepaired nasal lining defects should not be underestimated. Meticulous repair of lining, structure and cover are all required for functional, stable and aesthetic nasal reconstruction.

Nasal reconstruction after resection for cutaneous malignancies poses a unique challenge to facial plastic surgeons. The nose, a unique 3-D structure, not only must remain functional but also be aesthetically pleasing to patients. A complete understanding of all the layers of the nose and knowledge of available cartilage grafting material is necessary. Autogenous material, namely septal, auricular, and costal cartilage, is the most favored material in a free cartilage graft or a composite cartilage graft. All types of material have advantages and disadvantages that should guide the most appropriate selection to maximize the functional and cosmetic outcomes for patients.

Reconstruction of complex full-thickness nasal defects requires the reconstitution of the mucous internal nasal lining, the cartilaginous framework, and the aesthetic contour of the cutaneous nasal covering. Goals of reconstruction include restoration of a functional nasal airway and redefinition of the contours of the nose as well as its relationship to the cheek and lip with the least amount of morbidity to the patient. This article details a multistaged approach to repairing such a defect using an ipsilateral septal mucoperichondrial flap, multiple cartilage grafts, a paramedian forehead flap, and a cheek flap in a woman who had undergone Mohs surgery.

A woman presents after Mohs excision of a basal cell carcinoma within the right alar. A composite defect of her right upper lip, cheek, and ala is present. Although distressed, her concerns are somewhat alleviated by the prior successful reconstruction of a full-thickness defect of her left ala, some years previously. This content presents the principles of the repair, the surgical plan, and details of the multiple procedures performed for successful reconstruction.

Facial Plastic Surgery Clinics of North America

THE CLINICS ARE NOW AVAILABLE ONLINE!

Access your subscription at:
www.theclinics.com

Reconstruction of Nasal Defects for Head and Neck Surgeons, Facial Plastic Surgeons, and Plastic Surgeons

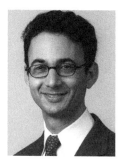

Daniel G. Becker, MD
Guest Editor

With skin cancers on the rise, otolaryngologist–head and neck surgeons and facial plastic and reconstructive surgeons face an increasing number of patients with facial defects requiring reconstruction after cancer excision. In this issue of *Facial Plastic Surgical Clinics of North America*, we focus on nasal reconstruction. Experts on surgical reconstruction of nasal deformities address the range of abnormalities encountered and describe in detail surgical methods available to treat these problems.

After a review of the anatomy, physiology, and general concepts in nasal reconstruction, specific focus is given to each of the nasal "subunits" and treatment options for defects in these areas. Another important way to think about nasal reconstruction is in terms of the specific reconstructive flaps, and individual, detailed, and well-illustrated articles are devoted to the most commonly employed flaps. When reconstructing a nasal defect, consideration must be given not only to the external surface but also to the internal lining and to structural support. Important articles on these subjects can be found in this issue. Finally, two complex case studies bring together many of the important concepts and surgical techniques covered in the issue.

It has been a great privilege and honor to serve as guest editor of this issue of *Facial Plastic Surgery Clinics*. I would like to thank and to congratulate the authors for their hard work. It is our hope that this issue of *Facial Plastic Surgery Clinics* will improve the otolaryngologist–head and neck surgeons' and facial plastic surgeons' understanding of the surgical treatment of nasal deformities.

Daniel G. Becker, MD
Department of Otolaryngology–Head
and Neck Surgery
University of Pennsylvania
3400 Spruce Street, 5 Silverstein
Philadelphia, PA 19104

Becker Nose and Sinus Center
400 Medical Center Drive, Suite B
Sewell, NJ 08080

E-mail address:
drbecker@therhinoplastycenter.com

Facial Plast Surg Clin N Am 19 (2011) xiii
doi:10.1016/j.fsc.2010.10.015
1064-7406/11/$ — see front matter © 2011 Elsevier Inc. All rights reserved.

Anatomy, Physiology, and General Concepts in Nasal Reconstruction

Jason D. Bloom, MD[a], Marcelo B. Antunes, MD[b],
Daniel G. Becker, MD[b,*]

KEYWORDS

- Nasal reconstruction • Nasal anatomy • Skin physiology
- Wound healing • Facial lines

ANATOMY, PHYSIOLOGY, AND GENERAL CONCEPTS IN NASAL RECONSTRUCTION

Nasal reconstruction has made great strides in the last 50 years. Nasal reconstructive surgeons have gotten away from the idea of "filling the hole" and now have multiple options, which enable them to achieve an aesthetically pleasing nose and good functional results.[1] As the central and often the most noticeable feature of the face, the nose is also one of the most difficult to reconstruct. Nasal reconstruction requires a thorough understanding of this complex, 3-dimensional structural and topographic anatomy. Also, key to this type of surgery is the relationship of the nose to the surrounding tissues of the face and how these tissues can be used for a reconstruction that is cosmetically normal for the patient and enables them to breathe properly.

The first step in nasal reconstructive surgery is an understanding of the nasal anatomy. The facial plastic surgeon must understand the intimate relationships between the underlying nasal support structures, the cover of the external skin, the function of the nasal lining, and the unique aspects of the location and contours of the nose.

Nasal Anatomy

Skin

The skin thickness varies depending on the different locations of the nose. In fact, this variation is what originally determined the nasal subunits when described by Gonzalez-Ulloa and colleagues.[2] The thickest area is the caudal portion of the nose, on the nasal tip and ala, with its skin rich in sebaceous glands. This nasal skin progressively gets thinner until it reaches the rhinion, where it is the thinnest,[3] and again as it transitions from the tip to the columella and the alar rim.[4,5]

Soft-tissue envelope

The soft-tissue envelope is composed of 4 layers: the superficial fatty layer, the fibromuscular layer, the deep fatty layer, and the perichondrial/periosteal layer.[4] The superficial fatty layer is intimately connected to the dermis. Immediately deep to this layer is the fibromuscular layer. This construction is called the nasal superficial musculoaponeurotic system (SMAS) and is in continuity with the rest of the SMAS overlying the face. The mimetic muscles of the nose are within this layer. The next layer is the deep fatty layer, which encases the neurovascular system, supplying the skin-soft-tissue envelope.[6] Between this layer and the perichondrium/periosteum lies the avascular plane that is used to deglove the nose during rhinoplasty.

As mentioned previously, part of the soft-tissue envelope is composed of a muscular layer. The mimetic muscles of the nose are usually divided into 4 groups.[6,7] The elevator muscles shorten the nose and dilate the nostrils. They are the

[a] Division of Facial Plastic and Reconstructive Surgery, Department of Otolaryngology, New York University Langone Medical Center, 550 First Avenue, NBV Suite 5E5, New York, NY 10016, USA
[b] Department of Otorhinolaryngology—Head and Neck Surgery, University of Pennsylvania Health System, 3400 Spruce Street, 5 Silverstein, Philadelphia, PA 19104, USA
* Corresponding author. Becker Nose and Sinus Center, 400 Medical Center Drive, Suite B, Sewell, NJ 08080.
E-mail address: beckermailbox@aol.com

Facial Plast Surg Clin N Am 19 (2011) 1–11
doi:10.1016/j.fsc.2010.10.001

procerus, levator labii superioris alaeque nasi and anomalous nasi. The depressor muscles, which lengthen the nose and dilate the nostrils, consist of the alar nasalis and depressor septi nasi. The compressor muscles lengthen the nose and narrow the nostrils. They are the transverse nasalis and compressor narium minor. Finally, the minor dilator muscle, the dilator naris anterior, widens the nostrils.

Lining
The nasal vestibule is lined by a strip of thin skin (stratified squamous keratinized epithelium). This epithelium loses its keratinizing nature and transitions into the nasal mucosa (pseudostratified columnar ciliated epithelium) as it moves further into the nose. This epithelium, called the respiratory epithelium, lines the sinonasal cavity with the exception of the area covered by the olfactory epithelium. The nasal mucosa has a rich vascular supply, which makes it an attractive option for flaps in reconstructing the inner lining of full-thickness nasal defects.[8]

Blood supply
The blood supply to the nose comes from branches of both the external carotid artery (through the facial artery and the infraorbital artery) and internal carotid artery (through the ophthalmic and anterior ethmoidal artery) (**Fig. 1**).[4]

In the external carotid artery system, the facial artery has 2 terminal branches, the angular artery and the superior labial artery. The former passes in a deep groove between the nasal alae and the cheek, deep to the levator labii-superioris alaeque nasi muscle, and gives off the lateral nasal branch, which provides the blood supply to the lateral portion of the caudal nose. The angular artery then continues, following the rim of the pyriform aperture, giving off about 7 to 14 branches that perforate through the soft-tissue envelope to supply the nasal skin.[9] The superior labial artery courses medially to the columella, where it gives off septal branches to supply the anterior portion of the nasal septal mucosa, and it terminates as the columellar artery, which runs between the medial crus of the lower lateral cartilage (LLC) and is frequently transected during the transcolumellar approach for an open rhinoplasty. The infraorbital artery arises from the infraorbital foramen with the infraorbital nerve and supplements the blood supply with branches that give rise to the lateral nasal artery and the dorsal nasal artery.

The internal carotid system also gives rise to an extensive vascular network that supplies the nose. The ophthalmic artery has both ocular and orbital branches. One of the orbital branches is the anterior ethmoidal artery, which provides the blood supply for the anterosuperior portion of the nasal cavity. After running in the skull base between the frontal sinus and the anterior ethmoid sinuses, it emerges between the cephalic edge of the upper lateral cartilage (ULC) and the caudal edge of the nasal bone, providing part of the blood supply to

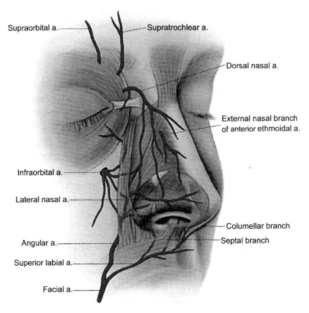

Fig. 1. Blood supply to the external nose. (*From* Jewett BS. Anatomic considerations. In: Baker SR, Naficy S. Principles of nasal reconstruction. St Louis (MO): Mosby; 2002. p. 19; with permission.)

the nasal tip, along with the lateral nasal artery. The ophthalmic artery finally gives rise to 2 terminal branches: the frontal artery and the dorsal nasal artery. The latter pierces the orbital septum and exits the orbit just superiorly to the medial canthal ligament and runs down to anastomose with the lateral nasal artery, creating a rich, axial arterial network.

Sensory nerve supply

The skin overlying the nose is innervated by the ophthalmic (V_1) and maxillary (V_2) branches of the trigeminal nerve (**Fig. 2**). The cutaneous branches of the ophthalmic nerve are the supratrochlear, the infratrochlear, and the external nasal nerves. The supratrochlear branch exits at the supraorbital foramen, and the infratrochlear branch exits the orbit just superior to the medial canthus. They provide sensory supply to the skin of the nasion, radix, and rhinion and the cephalic portion of the lateral nasal sidewall. The external nasal branch comes from the anterior ethmoid nerve and emerges between the ULC and the nasal bone, accompanied by the anterior ethmoidal artery. This branch innervates the skin of the caudal nasal dorsum and nasal tip.

The branches of the maxillary nerve are the infraorbital nerve and the nasopalatine nerve. The infraorbital branch courses on the roof of the maxillary sinus and exits the cranium at the infraorbital foramen. It innervates the skin of the caudal portion of the lateral nasal sidewall, ala, and nasal vestibule. The nasopalatine branch enters the nose through the incisive foramen and innervates the nasal septal mucosa.

Bone and cartilaginous framework

The bony framework is a pyramidal structure that consists of the paired nasal bones and the ascending process of the maxilla on either side. The cephalic portion articulates with the frontal bone superiorly and caudally, forming the cranial portion of the pyriform aperture (**Fig. 3**). The nasal bones are thicker superiorly and progressively become thinner until their free edge inferiorly.[10] The nasal bones are, on average, 25 mm, but their length can vary significantly. They fuse at the midline and give an internal projection that supports the perpendicular plate of the ethmoid bone. Inferiorly, the nasal bones articulate with the overlapped cephalic portion of the ULC, which are fused medially with the cartilage of the nasal septum. This area of confluence between the nasal bones, perpendicular plate of the ethmoid bone, ULCs, and cartilage of the nasal septum is connected by a dense fibrous tissue and is called the "keystone area."[11,12] This region provides critical support to the midvault of the nose.

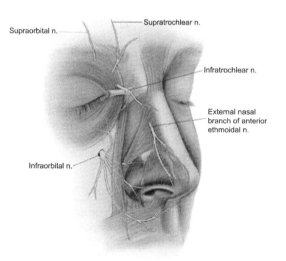

Fig. 2. The sensory nervous innervation to the external nose. (*From* Jewett BS. Anatomic considerations. In: Baker SR, Naficy S. Principles of nasal reconstruction. St Louis (MO): Mosby; 2002. p. 19; with permission.)

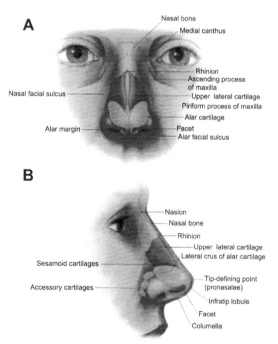

Fig. 3. (*A, B*) The bony and cartilaginous framework of the nasal skeleton. (*From* Jewett BS. Anatomic considerations. In: Baker SR, Naficy S. Principles of nasal reconstruction. St Louis (MO): Mosby; 2002. p. 19; with permission.)

The upper cartilaginous vault is made by the ULCs and the fused cartilaginous nasal septum. The cephalic two-thirds of the ULCs are fused with the nasal septum, and as they extend inferiorly, the ULC gradually separates and flares laterally from the septum.[13] The lateral portion of the ULC does not have any skeletal support because it does not articulate with the pyriform aperture but ends in an area called the external lateral triangle. This area is bordered by the pyriform aperture, the ULC, and the cephalic border of the lateral aspect of the LLC. It is covered by the transverse nasalis muscle and may contain one or more sesamoid cartilages. The most caudal aspect of the LLC ideally forms an angle with the nasal septum at the area of the internal nasal valve, which is described in more detail later in the article.

The lower cartilaginous framework is formed by the LLC. This paired cartilage morphology is made of 3 portions: the medial, middle, and lateral crura. The medial crus has 2 components: the footplate and the columellar portion. These segments rotate in 2 angles: the angle of cephalic rotation and the angle of footplate diversion. The medial crus has its configuration in 3 anatomic variations: the asymmetric parallel, flared symmetric, and straight symmetric.[14] Anteriorly, the medial crus transitions to the middle crus in the columellar breakpoint. The middle crus is made up of the lobular and the domal segments. The lobular segment is usually camouflaged by the overlying soft-tissue envelope. On the other hand, the domal segment is often visible and is critical in determining the tip-defining points. Its external expression depends on its angulation, the divergence of the 2 defining points, and the thickness of the overlying soft tissue. The middle crus is connected to the opposite side by the interdomal ligament. Superiorly, the LLC curves and transitions into the lateral crus. This portion of the LLC plays a major role in determining the shape of the alar region. It articulates superiorly with the caudal edge of the ULC in the "scroll area" where there is usually some degree of overlap, most commonly with the LLC coming externally to the ULC.[7] The LLC varies in shape and size,[15] and the longitudinal axis of the lateral crus approaches 45°.[3] This angle turns the LLC to a more cephalic position as it projects laterally, away from the alar rim, and that is the reason why the LLC provides support only to the medial half of the nasal ala.[16,17]

Nasal valves

The nasal valves are the portion of the nose that regulates airflow, because they have the narrowest cross-sectional area of the entire airway.[18] They are usually described individually as the external and internal nasal valves. The resistance in the nasal airway can be divided between the nasal vestibule, internal nasal valve, and the turbinated cavity of the nasal passage. Whereas the nasal vestibule contributes only about one-third of the nasal resistance and the nasal passage with its turbinates contribute only minimally, the nasal valves comprise the major areas of resistance in the nasal cavity.[19]

The internal nasal valve corresponds to the area between the head of the inferior turbinate, the nasal septum, and the ULC.[20] A key portion of this valve is the angle between the nasal septum and the ULC, the normal range of which is 10° to 15°.[18] The internal nasal valve area is the flow-limiting segment of the nasal airway and comprises about 50% of the total airway resistance from the nasal vestibule to the alveoli.[21] Nasal resistance functions according to Poiseuille's law; it is inversely proportional to the fourth power of the radius of the nasal passages (resistance = [viscosity × length]/radius⁴).[22,23] This means that small changes in the size of the nasal valve can have exponential effects on the airflow resistance. As mentioned earlier, Bernoulli principle plays a key role in the physiology of the nasal valve. As the air flows across the narrowed nasal valve, the velocity increases and pressure decreases. This negative pressure in the valve area causes further nasal valve collapse.[24] Not only the internal nasal valve but also the external nasal valve or nasal ala may collapse from the increased negative pressures developed from inspiration.

The external nasal valve is formed by the nasal ala and its supporting structures. It consists of the columella (fixed portion) medially and the lateral crura of the LLC (mobile portion). This mobile portion tends to collapse with inspiratory flow by the Bernoulli effect, but this collapse is resisted by the action of the dilator nares and the levator labii alaeque muscles along with the intrinsic strength of the LLC. The flow in the external nasal valve is primarily determined by the position of the cartilage and is minimally influenced by the degree of mucosal engorgement.[25]

Subunit Approach to Cutaneous Anatomy

In the early days of facial reconstruction, the main goal was to provide tissue coverage to the defect without significant concern with the cosmetic appearance. This concept started to change in the 1950s when surgeons started to advocate the use of "like tissue" to replace "like tissue." They noted that, by giving the reconstructed defect an appropriate contour and color match, the viewing eye would more likely perceive the area as normal. As described earlier, the initial work for improving facial reconstruction was made by Gonzalez-Ulloa and colleagues,[2] when they observed that the face had distinct units with transition lines between them. They postulated that these units would be determined by differences in the underlying histologic characteristics between the adjacent areas. The skin characteristics include thickness, amount of subcutaneous fat, color, texture, and presence of hair. The transition lines, or aesthetic borders, include the anterior hairline, mental crease, melolabial crease, orbital rim, preauricular crease, and nasofacial groove. The investigators determined that the main aesthetic units of the face are the forehead, eyelids, cheeks, lips, mentum, auricles, and nose. Placing incisions along those transition lines would camouflage the reconstruction. Millard[26,27] expanded the concept, advocating that not only the incisions should be transition lines but also the entire unit should be reconstructed.

Building on those previous concepts, Burget and Menick[28] further developed this philosophy, dividing the nose into subunits (**Fig. 4**). In a landmark article, they identified the specific topographic subunits as the dorsum, tip, columella and the paired ala, sidewalls, and soft triangles. They suggested that when reconstructing nasal defects, replacing entire subunits generally provided better aesthetic results. Their results were supported by data from perceptive psychology.[29] They also described the "50% rule," advocating that, in patients in whom more than 50% of the involved subunit was removed, the reconstruction should encompass the entire subunit, which would include removing healthy skin from the surrounding area. For defects that were less than 50% of the subunit, the reconstruction should provide adequate contour and color match, without removing healthy tissue.

The human eye usually focuses on the unexpected and glosses over the expected, taking it for normal appearance. The subunit principle was proposed with the goal of making the reconstruction look as close to normal as possible, so that the human eye would just gloss over and not be caught, like it might when the repair was by simply filling the defect. Observing the contralateral subunit would also aid in the reconstruction by providing information about the size and contour to achieve symmetry.

The actual point of transition between the nasal subunits is more subjective than with other facial units. The lines of transition are determined by the underlying structural framework rather than histologic difference. They are highlighted when an incident light is directed on the nasal surface, creating shadows on the borders of adjacent subunits. The nasal tip subunit is determined by the domal portion of the LLCs. Inferiorly it transitions to the columella, which extends inferiorly to the upper lip. Superiorly, the tip transitions to the nasal dorsum at the supratip depression, where the LLCs raise the skin. The dorsum extends superiorly to the nasion, where it transitions to the forehead unit. The lateral border of the dorsum is defined by the ULC and the junction of the nasal bones with the frontal process of the maxilla. This border creates a shadow that determines the subunit of the nasal sidewalls, which extends to the junction between the nose and cheek. Inferiorly, the sidewall ends at the alar crease where the nasal ala subunit starts, which is a smooth convexity that is supported by fibrofatty tissue without cartilaginous support. Between the nasal tip and the ala, there are the soft tissue facets that are defined by the shadow from the nasal tip.

Although the principle of nasal subunits is critical when planning nasal reconstruction, other factors should also be taken into consideration. These factors are skin color match, texture, contour, actinic damage, and the patient's comorbidities. The bilobed flap and the nasal dorsum rotation advancement flap are popular and useful techniques that innately violate the boundaries of the subunit principle. Recently, some investigators described modifications on nasal reconstruction with regard to the subunit principle. One study advocated that defects that include the nasal

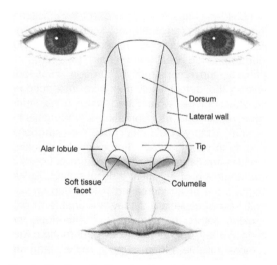

Fig. 4. The 9 aesthetic subunits of the nose consisting of the dorsum, tip, columella and the paired ala, sidewalls, and soft triangles. (*From* Baker SR. Flap classification and design. In: Baker SR, editor. Local flaps in facial reconstruction. Philadelphia: Elsevier Health Sciences; 2007. p. 76; with permission.)

dorsum and tip consistently have better cosmetic results than defects isolated to the nasal tip or dorsum.[30] Another study by Singh and Bartlett[31] proposed that other factors would prevail over nasal subunits in certain conditions such as in patients with Fitzpatrick skin types I and II, prominent sebaceous glands on the nasal skin, and the presence of actinic damage.

Defect Analysis

To accurately reconstruct a nasal defect, the surgeon must have a clear understanding of the layers of the nasal tissues and obstacles that can pose a threat to achieving an excellent aesthetic and functional reconstructive repair. One of the first aspects to consider is that in analyzing the defect to be repaired, the surgeon must evaluate and determine the layers of the nose that are involved in the defect and which are missing. Before beginning any surgery, especially complex nasal reconstructions, the surgeon must have a plan to execute and express to the patient so that the patient knows what to expect during the procedure and recovery period. Manson and colleagues[32] described nasal reconstruction as a 3-part approach, that is, the overlying skin, structural framework, and internal lining should each be evaluated individually before the final repair decisions are made.

When analyzing the defect in reference to the nasal skin, the surgeon must consider the location of the defect on the nose. For instance, defects found on the nasal dorsum may be reconstructed with a simple vertical closure, whereas others involving the nasal tip, ala, or free nostril margin may require more complex repairs and even multistage procedures. Along those same lines, certain areas of the nose, such as the supra-alar groove and alar-facial sulcus, have unique contours that are extremely difficult to reconstruct. Not respecting these borders can lead to a conspicuous and noticeable repair.

Defect size is also extremely important to evaluate before the surgeon chooses a reconstructive option. Defects smaller than 1 cm may be repaired with local flaps from within the same subunit or even with more basic options such as a primary closure or full-thickness skin graft (FTSG), whereas larger defects may require local tissue to be transferred from areas where it is more abundant, such as the cheek. The surgeon may also use multistage flaps to reconstruct the defect.

Other vital details of the nasal skin can affect how the reconstruction will eventually turn out. These aspects of the skin include color, contour, and type or texture. The surgeon must take into account that different parts of the nose differ in skin texture. The rhinion has the thinnest skin of the nose, with minimal sebaceous units, whereas the skin of the ala is thick with abundant adnexal structures. This detail is important in deciding the location from which to borrow the local skin for reconstruction. For example, a flap using the cheek skin would have a better texture match with the thicker skin of the nasal ala than it would with the thin-skinned nasal dorsum.

Color should also be matched when considering reconstructive options. It may be that the patient has erythematous nasal skin from a condition like rosacea, in which case a defect of the nasal supratip may be better reconstructed with a local bilobe flap, which uses skin of similar color, than with a paramedian forehead flap, which would likely not hide the borders of the flap because of the stark differences in skin color.

Assessing the underlying nasal framework and structure is also critical before outlining a plan for surgical repair. The surgeon must accurately analyze whether the defect interferes with the cartilaginous or bony framework of the nasal scaffold. If the LLCs are resected or altered, additional support for the nasal ala must be provided with grafts that are braced laterally on the pyriform aperture. Tip support mechanisms should always be evaluated and augmented when needed.

The mucosal lining of the nasal cavity must also be recreated when deficient. Failure to restore the nasal lining in the area of the defect can lead to severe wound contraction, adhesions, and significant distortion of the nose.[33] It is therefore critical to rebuild the nasal lining to prevent these issues. There are multiple techniques, such as flaps and grafts, which are beyond the scope of this article, used to provide nasal lining repair.

Finally, the reconstructive surgeon must look beyond the defect itself and take into account the status of the wound bed when considering nasal repair options. Sometimes, the patient's medical history can influence the surgeon's choices in wound repair. For example, smoking provides the largest challenge to the successful reconstruction of a patient's nasal defect. Active smokers are at an increased risk of flap or skin graft failure, especially if they are unable to quit smoking before the surgery.[34–36] Therefore, the surgeon may opt for an axial pattern flap with a more reliable blood supply rather than an FTSG, to repair the nasal defect. Similarly, a patient who has received previous head and neck irradiation may have a compromised blood supply to the face or nose. In these cases, similar to the case of a smoker, a more robust vascularized pedicle flap may be appropriately chosen. Besides the choice of flap, the surgeon may also decide to delay the flap or wait a prolonged period of time between the flap transfer and the pedicle division with insetting. This procedure allows the vascular supply from the surrounding wound site to have more time for neovascularization. Prior facial or nasal surgery may have previously used tissue for reconstructions and altered the vascular supply to some of the flap choices that could be selected. Accordingly, it is vital to elicit this surgical history from the patient and examine the patient's skin and scars to see what type of reconstruction or surgery was performed during the first operation.

Skin Flap Physiology and Skin Biomechanics

Skin has 3 biomechanical properties that describe how it moves and heals: nonlinearity, viscoelasticity, and anisotropy.[37]

Nonlinearity
This mechanical skin property means that skin stretch differs depending on how much force is applied; the more the skin is stretched, increasing amounts of pressure are required to further deform the skin.[38] Also, there is an asymptote or point at which the skin cannot be stretched anymore. These concepts are related to the amount of collagen, elastin, and ground substance that composes the skin. This nonlinear relationship is demonstrated with the stress-strain curve (**Fig. 5**). Stress is defined as force per unit of cross-sectional area, and strain is the change in skin length divided by its original length.[38,39] This curve can be broken down into 3 sections. The first section of the curve is flat, explaining that a small stress leads to a large skin strain or stretch, which is the result of deformity of the skin elastin network. The second section of the curve, sometimes called the transition section, shows that as more force is applied to the skin, it becomes harder to stretch it further. This difficulty could be because of the change in the collagen fiber orientation that occurs at this point. The third section of this graph demonstrates that once the skin has been stretched or strained a significant amount, a large force is required to even achieve a small amount of additional stretch. At this point, the recruitment of additional collagen fibers to shoulder the increased stress and the orientation of the fibers in the direction of the applied force create a detrimental situation of tension and poor wound healing.[39,40] Of note, the skin properties change further with age and sun damage. With these problems, the skin begins to lose both its collagen and elastin fibers, shifting the curve to the right.[40,41]

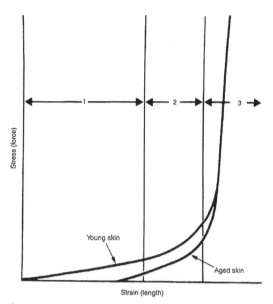

Fig. 5. Stress-strain curve demonstrating the relationship between the amount of force or stress needed to strain or deform young and aged skin. (*From* Larrabee WF Jr. Immediate repair of facial defects. Dermatol Clin 1989;7:662; with permission.)

Viscoelasticity
One of the viscoelastic skin properties is stress relaxation. If a constant force is applied over a period to stretch the skin to a given length and then maintained at that length, there is a subsequent decrease in skin tension.[42]

Another viscoelastic property of the skin is creep. This phenomenon occurs when an increase in skin length is noted over time, when a certain tension is applied to a segment of skin. Skin creep has been attributed to the parallel alignment of collagen fibers, fragmented elastin, and a displacement of extracellular fluid from within the dermis. The process of tissue expansion uses skin creep, not to create new skin but to recruit skin that is adjacent to the defect, allowing it to be closed with minimal tension.[39,40,43] Creep can also be subcategorized into biologic and mechanical types. Biologic creep refers to skin expansion from the slow application of a subcutaneous force, whereas mechanical creep occurs when the skin stretches beyond its normal extensibility in a shorter amount of time. It is the latter type that is commonly seen when using a tissue expander to recruit more skin.

Anisotropy
This term refers to the fact that the mechanical properties of the skin vary with direction.[39,40] There may be tension on the skin when a defect is attempted to be closed in one direction,

whereas closing in a different direction might allow that same area of skin to be closed without tension. This property comes into play largely when surgeons are thinking about the placement of their incisions for defect closures.

There is wide variation in facial skin tension among the different anatomic units. For example, the skin on the eyelids and cheek has much lower tension than that on the forehead and the nose. However, at any given point, the skin is under tension in every direction. This tension is present constantly and is modified by muscle action (it could increase or decrease the tension). This tension is the force responsible to separate the edges of a wound. Originally described by Borges and Alexander,[44] the relaxed skin tension lines (RSTLs) are a series of imaginary facial lines, along which the skin has the least amount of tension for closure (**Fig. 6**). These lines are usually not visible at rest, but can be seen as the furrows that form from pinching the skin together.[42,45,46] Incisions placed parallel to these lines heal without stress or tension on the wound closure.[44,47] A wound following these lines remains narrow, but if it is made perpendicular to the RSTLs, the edges

may begin to widen or gap. Borges[46] advocated that no other single factor (not even surgical technique) is as important as the direction of the wound being parallel to the RSTLs for the formation of an acceptable scar. He recommended that if an incision should be done in an antitension line, it should be done in a zigzag pattern, better following the RSTLs. RSTLs are always parallel or concentric or meet at an acute angle. Their direction does not vary significantly among individuals. Around facial apertures, such as the nares and mouth, these lines tend to be radial. Also, they are not coincident with wrinkles in the glabella, the upper portion of the crow's feet, and the mentolabial fold.

Another series of lines that are important in the planning of incisions are the lines of maximal extensibility (LME), which run perpendicular to the RSTLs. Extensibility is defined as the lengthening of the skin under tension, caused by stretching of the elastic fibers on the skin. This extensibility varies depending on the direction in which the tension is applied.[48] The tension in the wound is the least in the plane parallel to the LME, which allows for the largest amount of skin stretch at the widest area of the defect to help with closure. Both lines, RSTL and LME, are important when recruiting adjacent tissues to close wound defects. The tension on the skin flap used for reconstruction is an essential consideration because excessive tension may compromise the blood supply in the distal portion of the flap.

Furthermore, the orientation of a wound has a direct correlation to the scar appearance. The orientation of fusiform excisions should be closed in the direction of the LME, so that the scar or incision is situated in the facial RSTLs,[38,46] allowing for the most optimal tissue healing and scar outcome. At present, RSTLs provide the most acceptable orientation for the placement of surgical incisions.

Blood Supply to Local Skin Flaps

Understanding the vascular supply to the skin and soft tissue is vital to the operative planning of the reconstructive surgeon. When designing local flaps for nasal defect repair, they can be described based on the blood supply into random and axial pattern flaps. Random skin flaps receive their blood supply from musculocutaneous and septocutaneous vessels, running deep to the muscles or in the muscular fascia, respectively, and then perforate through the muscles or muscular septae to provide the blood supply for the dermalsubdermal plexus of the skin. These flaps are known as random because they are not raised in a specific direction to account for the cutaneous

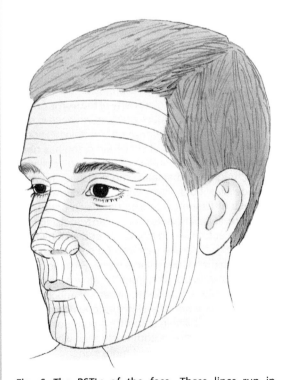

Fig. 6. The RSTLs of the face. These lines run in a perpendicular orientation to the lines of maximal extensibility. (*From* Baker SR. Flap classification and design. In: Baker SR, editor. Local flaps in facial reconstruction. Philadelphia: Elsevier Health Sciences; 2007. p. 73; with permission.)

vascular supply. The survival of these random pattern flaps is based on the perfusion pressure of the underlying vessels. Because of this requirement, the length-width ratio for flap design should maximally approach 3:1.[49] To this end, care must be taken to perform the dissection in a subcutaneous plane when raising these flaps, to preserve the subdermal blood supply.

Axial pattern flaps, on the other hand, have a blood supply that comes from direct cutaneous vessels that run in the subcutaneous tissue along the directional axis of the flap. The survival of these flaps is based on the actual axial vessel length.[40] When raising these types of flaps, they should be oriented and aligned specifically so that the long axis of the flap parallels the blood vessel of interest. Any skin territory outside of the distribution that is supplied by this artery becomes a random flap and again relies on the nourishment from the dermal-subdermal plexus. The rich and reliable vascular supply provided by this axial blood supply makes these flaps more amenable to primary thinning and contouring.

Furthermore, significant wound tension can affect the blood supply to a skin flap. Because it has been shown that the blood supply is inversely proportional to the distance from the flap base, a flap that is stretched with significant tension can suffer distal necrosis.[50] This is one reason why local skin flap closures should be reconstructed without tension on the closure.

Wound Healing Phases

Inflammatory phase (0–5 days)
The wound healing process begins immediately after tissue injury and once hemostasis has been achieved. For the blood of the wound to clot, a combination of local vessel vasoconstriction, fibrin deposition, and platelet aggregation must take place.[40,51] Fibrin deposition relies on the extrinsic coagulation pathway, and the platelets begin to deposit on the vessel walls once they have been exposed to the local collagen and tissue factors circulating in the wound bed. Once 10 to 15 minutes have elapsed, the initial vasoconstriction changes to a period of vasodilation, caused by the release of histamine, leukotrienes, and prostaglandins from the endothelium.[52]

The inflammatory phase gets its name from the infiltration of neutrophils that begin to predominate the wound bed. These cells patrol the wound and help to prevent local infection by debriding foreign particles and digesting bacteria. These cells peak between days 1 and 2 and then begin to decline as the monocytes and macrophages move into the area, peaking around days 4 to 5.

Proliferative or granulation phase (6–14 days)
The next phase in wound healing works to repair the epithelium, synthesize collagen, and promote the development of new blood vessels. It has been said that reepithelialization can occur about 12 hours after the initial wound injury. Reepithelialization occurs through the migration of the epithelial cells near the wound edges along the fibrin scaffold to again cover the wound bed.[40] In superficial wounds, the adnexal structures also participate in the reepithelialization process.

Epithelial cells play an important role in this phase, and fibroblasts, crucial to the synthesis of elastin, proteoglycans, and collagen, start to become active during this period in wound healing. Initially, fibroblasts produce collagen type III, abundant in an early wound, which is later converted to type I collagen. Fibroblasts also change into myofibroblasts, which are critical in the contraction of wounds, seen around days 7 to 14.[53]

Finally, the wound produces several angiogenic growth factors, such as vascular endothelial growth factor, which help to promote angiogenesis. It is this new blood vessel formation that is necessary to support the generation of the granulation tissue that exists in the wound bed.

Remodeling or maturation phase (15 days–1 year)
The final stage in wound healing is known as the remodeling or maturation phase. This is also the longest stage of the process and can last for up to a year. It is for this reason that many surgeons wait 1 year before attempting any surgical wound or scar revision procedure. Beginning 2 weeks after the creation of the wound, the collagen arrangement changes from the disorganized fibrils of the immature scar to the more parallel, thicker collagen fibril organization that is seen in a mature scar. In addition, the type III collagen that was originally present in the wound bed now becomes replaced by the type I collagen, which is the major component of the scar.[40] Neovascularization stops, and the erythema that was originally seen in the wound from the vasculature turns a whitish color as the vessels regress.

REFERENCES

1. Burget GC, Menick FJ. Nasal support and lining: the marriage of beauty and blood supply. Plast Reconstr Surg 1989;84:189–203.
2. Gonzalez-Ulloa M, Castillo A, Stevens E, et al. Preliminary study of the total restoration of the facial skin. Plast Reconstr Surg 1954;13(3):151–61.
3. Lessard ML, Daniel RK. Surgical anatomy of septorhinoplasty. Arch Otolaryngol 1985;111(1):25–9.

4. Oneal RM, Beil RJ. Surgical anatomy of the nose. Clin Plast Surg 2010;37(2):191–211.

5. Kim DW, Mau T. Surgical anatomy of the nose. In: Bailey BJ, Johnson JT, Newlands SD, editors. Head and neck surgery – otolaryngology. 4th edition. Philadelphia (PA): Lippincott Williams & Wilkins; 2006. p. 2511–32.

6. Letourneau A, Daniel RK. The superficial musculoaponeurotic system of the nose. Plast Reconstr Surg 1988;82(1):48–57.

7. Griesman BL. Muscles and cartilage of the nose from the standpoint of typical rhinoplasty. Arch Otolaryngol Head Neck Surg 1944;39:334.

8. Baker SR. Reconstruction of the nose. In: Baker SR, editor. Local flaps in facial reconstruction. 2nd edition. Philadelphia: Mosby; 2007.

9. Herbert DC. A subcutaneous pedicled cheek flap for reconstruction of alar defects. Br J Plast Surg 1978;31(2):79–92.

10. Wright WK. Surgery of the bony and cartilaginous dorsum. Otolaryngol Clin North Am 1975;8(3):575–98.

11. Pitanguy I. Surgical importance of a dermocartilaginous ligament in bulbous noses. Plast Reconstr Surg 1965;36:247–53.

12. Drumheller GW. Topology of the lateral nasal cartilages: the anatomical relationship of the lateral nasal to the greater alar cartilage, lateral crus. Anat Rec 1973;176(3):321–7.

13. McKinney P, Johnson P, Walloch J. Anatomy of the nasal hump. Plast Reconstr Surg 1986;77(3):404–5.

14. Daniel RK. The nasal tip: anatomy and aesthetics. Plast Reconstr Surg 1992;89(2):216–24.

15. Zelnik J, Gingrass RP. Anatomy of the alar cartilage. Plast Reconstr Surg 1979;64(5):650–3.

16. Gunter JP. Anatomical observations of the lower lateral cartilages. Arch Otolaryngol 1969;89(4):599–601.

17. Dion MC, Jafek BW, Tobin CE. The anatomy of the nose. External support. Arch Otolaryngol 1978; 104(3):145–50.

18. Kasperbauer JL, Kern EB. Nasal valve physiology. Implications in nasal surgery. Otolaryngol Clin North Am 1987;20(4):699–719.

19. Walsh WE, Kern RC. Sinonasal anatomy, function, and evaluation. In: Bailey BJ, Johnson JT, Newlands SD, editors. Head and neck surgery – otolaryngology. Philadelphia: Lippincott Williams Wilkins; 2006. p. 307–18.

20. Haight JS, Cole P. The site and function of the nasal valve. Laryngoscope 1983;93(1):49–55.

21. Cole P. Respiratory role of the upper airways. St Louis (MO): Mosby Year Book; 1993.

22. Lee J, White WM, Constantinides M. Surgical and nonsurgical treatments of the nasal valves. Otolaryngol Clin North Am 2009;42:495–511.

23. Miman MC, Deliktas H, Ozturan O, et al. Internal nasal valve: revisited with objective facts. Otolaryngol Head Neck Surg 2006;134(1):41–7.

24. Park SS, Becker SS. Repair of nasal obstruction in revision rhinoplasty. In: Becker DG, Park SS, editors. Revision rhinoplasty. New York: Thieme Medical Publishers; 2008. p. 52–68.

25. Shaida AM, Kenyon GS. The nasal valves: changes in anatomy and physiology in normal subjects. Rhinology 2000;38(1):7–12.

26. Millard DR Jr. Aesthetic aspects of reconstructive surgery. Ann Plast Surg 1978;1(6):533–41.

27. Millard DR Jr. Aesthetic reconstructive rhinoplasty. Clin Plast Surg 1981;8(2):169–75.

28. Burget GC, Menick FJ. The subunit principle in nasal reconstruction. Plast Reconstr Surg 1985;76(2): 239–47.

29. Menick FJ. Artistry in aesthetic surgery. Aesthetic perception and the subunit principle. Clin Plast Surg 1987;14(4):723–35.

30. Shumrick KA, Campbell A, Becker FF, et al. Modification of the subunit principle for reconstruction of nasal tip and dorsum defects. Arch Facial Plast Surg 1999;1(1):9–15.

31. Singh DJ, Bartlett SP. Aesthetic considerations in nasal reconstruction and the role of modified nasal subunits. Plast Reconstr Surg 2003;111(2):639–48.

32. Manson PN, Hoopes JE, Chambers RG, et al. Algorithm for nasal reconstruction. Am J Surg 1967;138: 528.

33. Weber SM, Baker SR. Management of cutaneous nasal defects. Facial Plast Surg Clin North Am 2009;17:395–417.

34. Goldminz D, Bennett RG. Cigarette smoking and flap and full-thickness graft necrosis. Arch Dermatol 1991;127:1012–5.

35. Kinsella JB, Rassekh CH, Wassmuth ZD, et al. Smoking increases facial skin flap complications. Ann Otol Rhinol Laryngol 1999;108:139–42.

36. Lawrence WT, Murphy RC, Robson MC, et al. The detrimental effect of cigarette smoking of flap survival: an experimental study in the rat. Br J Plast Surg 1984;37:216–9.

37. Rindenour BD, Larrabee WF. Biomechanics of skin flaps. In: Baker SR, editor. Local flaps in facial reconstruction. Philadelphia: Mosby; 1995. p. 31–8.

38. Sherris DA, Larrabee WF. Principles of facial reconstruction. A subunit approach to cutaneous repair. 2nd edition. New York: Thieme Medical Publishers; 2010.

39. Larrabee WF. Immediate repair of facial defects. Dermatol Clin 1989;7(4):661–76.

40. Honrado CP, Murakami CS. Wound healing and physiology of skin flaps. Facial Plast Surg Clin North Am 2005;13:203–14.

41. Daly CH, Odland GF. Age-related changes in the mechanical properties of human skin. J Invest Dermatol 1979;73:84–7.

42. Larrabee WF, Bloom DC. Biomechanics of skin flaps. In: Baker SR, editor. Local flaps in facial reconstruction. Philadelphia: Mosby; 2007. p. 31–9.

43. Jackson IT. Local flaps in head and neck reconstruction. St Louis (MO): CV Mosby; 1985.
44. Borges AF, Alexander JE. Relaxed skin tension lines, Z-plasties on scars, and fusiform excision of lesions. Br J Plast Surg 1962;15:242–54.
45. Marcus BC. Wound closure techniqes. In: Baker SR, editor. Local flaps in facial reconstruction. 2nd edition. Philadelphia: Mosby; 2007. p. 41–64.
46. Borges AF. Relaxed skin tension lines. Dermatol Clin 1989;7(1):169–77.
47. Borges AF. Relaxed skin tension lines (RSTL) versus other skin lines. Plast Reconstr Surg 1984;73(1): 144–50.
48. Larrabee WF Jr. Design of local flaps. Otolaryngol Clin North Am 1990;23:899–923.
49. Connor CD, Fosko SW. Anatomy and physiology of local skin flaps. Facial Plast Surg Clin North Am 1996;4:447–54.
50. Larrabee WF, Holloway GA, Sutton D. Wound tension and blood flow in skin flaps. Ann Otol Rhinol Laryngol 1984;93(2 Pt 1):112–5.
51. Lawrence WT. Physiology of the acute wound. Clin Plast Surg 1998;25(3):321–40.
52. Postlethwaite AE, Keski-Oja J, Ballan G, et al. Induction of fibroblast chemotaxis by fibronectin. J Exp Med 1981;153:494–9.
53. Bryant WM. Wound healing. Clin Symp 1977;29(3):1–36.

Reconstruction of the Dorsal and Sidewall Defects

Michael W. Chu, MD, Eric J. Dobratz, MD*

KEYWORDS

- Nasal dorsum sidewall defects • Mohs reconstruction
- Dorsal nasal flap

Nasal dorsal and sidewall defects are often considered the least complex for nasal reconstruction. Defects in these regions may be repaired with simple techniques to produce excellent results. However, more complex defects, including full-thickness defects and those involving adjacent tissues such as the medial canthus, require thoughtful analysis and planning. Nasal defects should be analyzed with consideration of both aesthetic and functional concerns. Optimal reconstructive plans incorporate the concept of replacing like with like and strategic scar placement. Characteristics unique to the dorsum and nasal sidewall include the transitioning thickness of skin and soft tissues from the nasal dorsum to cheek, the close proximity to adjacent facial units (medial canthus, eye, cheek, and forehead) and the osseocartilaginous junction located in this region. Simple defects can be repaired with direct advancement of adjacent tissue, local flaps, or skin grafts to achieve acceptable results in this region. More complex defects may require transposition flap, interpolated flaps, or even free tissue transfer. This article addresses the multiple issues that must be considered for nasal dorsal and sidewall defect reconstruction.

ANATOMY

Successful nasal reconstruction requires a thorough understanding of nasal anatomy, function, and cause of the defect being corrected. The nose functions to allow airflow and provide humidification and filtration of inspired air. The nose is a prominent facial feature and is integral to facial cosmesis, as it provides balance to the face because of its central location in both horizontal and vertical dimensions. The nose is divided into 3 layers, the mucosal lining, the osseocartilaginous framework, and the skin and soft-tissue coverage. Its surface is characterized by concave and convex curves and is divided into nasal subunits.[1] The boundaries of the nose are the glabella superiorly, the nasofacial sulcus laterally as it transitions to the cheek, and the nasal vestibule and columella inferiorly. The nose is divided into 9 subunits: 3 unilateral structures (the dorsum, tip, columella) and 6 bilateral structures (the sidewalls, ala, and soft-tissue triangles) (**Fig. 1**).

This discussion focuses on the nasal dorsum and sidewall units. From a frontal view, the dorsum of the ideal nose is symmetric and provides a gentle sweeping hourglass-shaped curve from the medial canthus to the nasal ala. The nasal dorsum contributes to nasal and midface projection from a lateral view. The nasofrontal angle defines the transition from nose to forehead and is ideally between 95° and 110°, but varies based on gender and facial harmony. The sidewall is located just lateral to the dorsum as the nose transitions to the cheek and the medial canthus adjacent to the eye.

It is important to understand the variations in the soft-tissue envelope characteristics that vary by individual skin types as well as by location. The soft-tissue envelope varies in thickness over the dorsum of the nose. The skin and subcutaneous tissue is thinnest at the rhinion, the osseocartilaginous junction,

Department of Otolaryngology Head and Neck Surgery, Eastern Virginia Medical School, 600 Gresham Drive, Suite 1100, River Pavilion, Norfolk, VA 23507, USA
* Corresponding author.
E-mail address: dobratej@evms.edu

Facial Plast Surg Clin N Am 19 (2011) 13–24
doi:10.1016/j.fsc.2010.10.011
1064-7406/11/$ — see front matter © 2011 Elsevier Inc. All rights reserved.

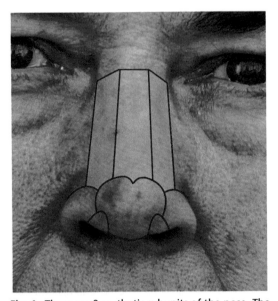

Fig. 1. There are 9 aesthetic subunits of the nose. The surgeon should consider which subunits are involved during reconstructive planning. This article focuses on the dorsal subunit (*blue*) and the paired sidewall subunits (*green*).

and is thicker more superiorly at the nasion and inferiorly at the nasal tip. The soft-tissue envelope thickens with lateral transition to the sidewall and cheek. Superiorly the tissues remain thin as the nose transitions to the adjacent medial canthus and eyelids. Reconstructive plans must consider the changing thickness of the soft-tissue envelope when repairing nasal dorsal and sidewall defects. For instance, when elevating the soft-tissue of the nose and cheek, the plane of dissection changes from below the superficial muscular aponeurotic system (sub-SMAS) plane over the nose to a subcutaneous plane over the cheek to avoid transferring thicker soft-tissue to the nose. Individual skin characteristics should be considered as well, when considering different types of closures. A classic example is the bilobe flap; thick sebaceous skin has a higher risk of developing flap necrosis, trap-door deformity, and depressed scars.

The internal nasal structure is critical and should not be neglected in planning for nasal reconstruction. Key portions of the osseocartilaginous structures of the nose are located within the nasal dorsum and sidewalls. The nasal bones, the upper lateral cartilages, and the keystone area, which is the junction of the bony cartilaginous septum and the nasal bones and upper lateral cartilages, are essential to proper nasal function. These structures provide shape to the nose and support to resist forces that collapse the nasal airway. The osseocartilagenous junction must be preserved during

reconstruction. If this junction is disrupted during ablative surgery or as a result of trauma, efforts should be made to reconstruct and reinforce the support in this area to preserve nasal function.

The blood supply to the nose is based on the dorsal nasal artery superiorly and the angular artery from the facial artery inferiorly. The internal blood supply is based largely on the sphenopalatine artery. The venous drainage includes the facial venous and pterygoid plexus. The sensory innervation is from the infraorbital nerve of the maxillary branch of the trigeminal nerve and the sphenopalatine nerve. Motor innervation of the nose is through the facial nerve and muscles of facial expression. A thorough knowledge of the anatomy will assist the surgeon during flap elevation to ensure preservation of nasal blood supply, movement, and sensation.

EVALUATION OF NASAL DEFECTS

Nasal defects can result from trauma, congenital lesions, extirpation of neoplasms, or iatrogenic injuries. Soft-tissue defects may be further classified as a wound, defect, or deformity.[2] A wound is a disruption of parts and requires repair of the disrupted parts. A defect is a loss of parts and must be addressed by bringing in new parts to the defect. A deformity, which may be congenital or iatrogenic, is a distortion of parts and requires mobilization and repositioning of parts into proper alignment and relationships. This classification provides conceptual clarity and may be applied in developing a reconstructive plan based on the cause of the defect. A nasal dorsal laceration, skin excision, or scar deformity are 3 different lesions that require different reconstructive plans for successful repair.

The size of the defect must also be considered. Park[3] describes the classification of defects greater than 1.5 cm as large defects that are less likely to be successfully closed with local flaps and often require interpolated flaps for closure. Park also advocates enlarging the defect when more than 50% of a nasal subunit is involved by resecting the remaining residual subunit to have scars camouflaged within natural creases or at borders of 2 subunits to be more inconspicuous. This concept may also be applied to defects caused by a scar deformity such as the patient shown in **Fig. 2**. This patient presented with a deformity of the alar rim causing airway obstruction after repair of a Mohs defect by a dermatologist. She also had a scar that extended into the central portion of the nasal sidewall subunit contributing to the deformity. A decision was made to resect the soft tissues of the nasal

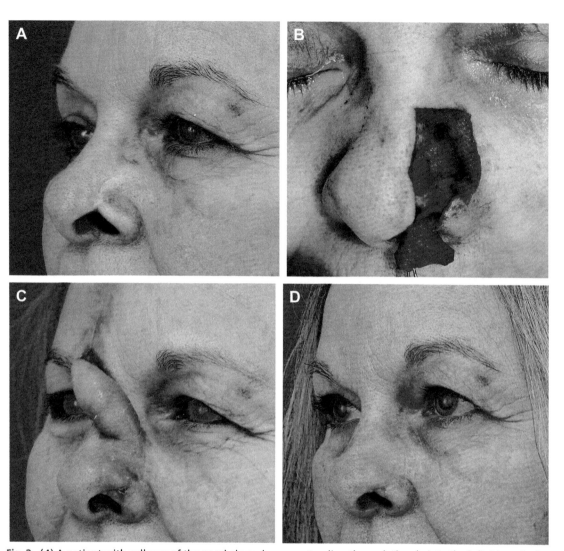

Fig. 2. (*A*) A patient with collapse of the nasal ala and a scar extending through the ala into the left sidewall after closure of a Mohs defect by a dermatologist. (*B*) Excision of a portion of the sidewall and ala with turn over for internal lining and cartilage graft for support. (*C*) Forehead flap for closure with placement of suture lines at the aesthetic borders of the sidewall subunit. (*D*) 6-month postoperative result with improvement of the alar margin but also significant improvement of the appearance of the sidewall with the scars placed at the borders of the subunit to replace the scar in the center portion of the subunit.

sidewall and place the incisions at the borders of the aesthetic subunits. A portion of the resected tissue was turned over to recreate the necessary internal lining for a full-thickness reconstruction of the contracted alar rim. The postoperative photo shows improvement at the alar rim but also a significant improvement at the sidewall where the central depressed scar was removed and less conspicuous scars are now located at the borders of the subunit.

One should also consider the reconstructive principle of replacing like with like. Depending on the size of the defect, donor tissue that adequately matches the complexity of the nose may be limited. Local tissue flaps provide similar tissue for reconstruction but may be limited by availability of sufficient tissue, donor morbidity, and scar formation. Generally, small to medium defects can be repaired by recruiting adjacent tissue. Larger defects may require a forehead or cheek flap, which tends to heal well and provide adequate tissue match. It is difficult to match tissue likeness with free tissue transfer to the external nose.

TECHNIQUES FOR NASAL DORSAL AND SIDEWALL RECONSTRUCTION

Techniques for reconstruction of the dorsal and sidewall subunits are similar and they are discussed together. As with all nasal defects, reconstructive repair varies by patient characteristics, size, depth, and location of the defect, distensibility and thickness of the surrounding tissues, patient age and health, aesthetic sensibilities of the patient, as well as the experience of the surgeon. The following is a technical description of the various reconstructive options for nasal dorsum and sidewall defects.

Secondary Intention

Healing by secondary intention is the simplest method of repair. The wound edges are not reapproximated, granulation tissue forms and epithelialization occurs from follicular appendages. This inflammatory process results in fibroblasts differentiating into myofibroblasts with wound contracture, and eventual epithelial coverage from lateral wound edge migration. Secondary intention is rarely used for nasal defects but may be used for small defects on concave surfaces such as the medial canthus or alar groove. Secondary intention is reserved for small defects (<5 mm) and poor surgical candidates. These patients must be able to perform routine wound care, cleansing, and occlusive dressing to provide coverage and prevent infection. Caution must be exercised for defects near free margins such as the nostril or eyelid. Small defects of the sidewall near the medial canthus but away from the lid margin can heal well with secondary healing.

Skin Grafts

Skin grafts are a simple, rapid, single-stage form of reconstruction indicated for large defects in high-risk patients who cannot tolerate general anesthesia for more complex procedures, and those who require close surveillance for recurrence of malignancy. Skin grafts have the disadvantage of difficulty in matching color, texture and thickness of the nose, donor site morbidity, and possible graft contracture and failure. The cephalic sidewall and dorsum of the nose are some of the best locations on the nose for skin grafts, because of the thin nature of the surrounding skin. Large areas of the nose or even total nasal defects may be reconstructed with a skin graft with a forehead flap in patients who are not fit (**Fig. 3**). In these instances, enlarging portions of the defect can be considered to allow for the suture lines to fall at the borders of the aesthetic subunits.

Skin grafts may be performed in combination with partial primary closure to reduce the size of the defect and limit donor site morbidity. In some instances the standing cone that is created during primary closure may be excised and used as a full-thickness skin graft eliminating donor site morbidity and avoiding excess tension of the primary closure (**Fig. 4**). When this technique is used to close a Mohs defect, the excess soft tissue that is beveled toward the center of the defect should be left intact, thus reducing the depth of the wound that the skin graft is placed over.

Full-thickness skin grafts are preferred for nasal reconstruction over split-thickness skin grafts as they have less contracture and are thicker allowing for better contour match. Donor sites include the supraclavicular, nasolabial fold, preauricular, and postauricular skin. Donor sites can usually be closed primarily with minimal undermining and aesthetically acceptable results.

Local Tissue Rearrangement

Primary closure/advancement flaps

Primary closure with appropriate undermining of surrounding tissues is an ideal single-stage method for closure of small to medium defects in the dorsal and sidewall subunits of the nose. The tissues surrounding the nasal defect should be widely undermined in the sub-SMAS plane before commitment to a reconstruction plan, unless a V-Y island advancement is being considered as an option for closure (undermining under the island flap disrupts the blood supply to the flap). Older patients with excess skin laxity are excellent candidates for primary closure. This method is less amenable to young patients with less skin laxity because excessive tension leads to distortion of adjacent structures and potential depression over the dorsum at the point of maximal tension.

Circular defects are common after skin cancer resection. These lesions may be made into fusiform defects to prevent standing cone deformities or dog ears. For midline defects the standing cone is excised directly caudal and cephalad to the defect creating a vertical midline scar that tends to heal favorably (**Fig. 5**).

For paramedian defects, excision of the standing cone may be offset to one side of the defect to reposition the final scar (**Fig. 6**). In this example the inferior cone was offset to create a less conspicuous midline scar at the nasal tip.

The key to primary closure is wide undermining to allow for redraping without distorting the nose, particularly the free margin of the nostril rim. The

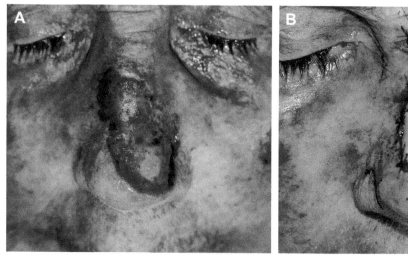
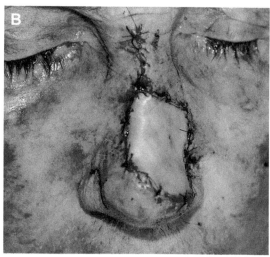
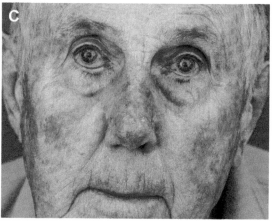

Fig. 3. (A) Elderly patient with a large defect involving the nasal dorsum, sidewall, tip, and alar subunits. He desired a simple reconstruction with a full-thickness skin graft. (B) Partial primary closure of the defect cephalad to reduce the size of the skin graft reconstruction. Portions of the remaining defect were enlarged to square off the edges of the defect and place the suture lines at aesthetic borders. (C) Postoperative result at 5 weeks.

plane of elevation should be just superficial to the perichondrium and periosteum in the sub-SMAS plane. Elevation in this plane preserves the blood supply when primary closure must be abandoned and instead a local flap must be used for closure. Efforts should be made to place resulting scars of primary closure at aesthetic borders, within existing rhytids, and parallel to relaxed skin tension lines.

Transposition flaps

Transposition flaps are rotated over an intact bridge of skin from an area of excess laxity to allow primary closure of donor site after rotation into the defect. Transposition flaps are often used for nasal dorsal and sidewall lesions that are not acceptable for primary closure. These flaps provide good color match and texture and are well suited for small defects less than 1.5 cm. A note flap is one

example of a transposition flap that is ideal for the sidewall and dorsum (Fig. 7). The laxity of the surrounding skin in these regions allows for flap transposition with minimal distortion of the surrounding tissues. The note flap is designed adjacent to the defect and incised and transposed as a single flap. As with other forms of closure, it is important to widely undermine the surrounding tissue in the sub-SMAS plane to minimize tension on the closure. The donor site is closed first, which allows for transposition of the flap and closure with minimal tension. The standing cone is removed after the flap is inset to prevent the removal of excess tissue.

Bilobed flap

The bilobed flap is a double-transposition flap commonly used for small defects less than 1.5 cm, as described by Zitelli.[4] The bilobed flap allows for

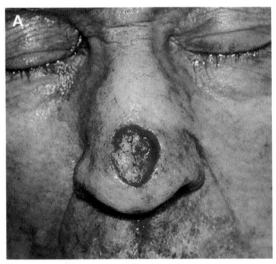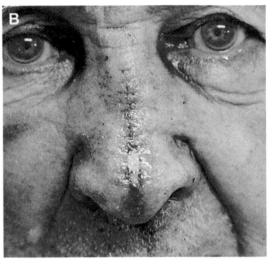

Fig. 4. (*A*) Midline defect of the dorsum and tip. (*B*) Partial primary closure of defect with placement of a full-thickness skin graft taken from the standing cone to complete the closure. Placement of the skin graft avoids excess tension at the midpoint of the defect.

the rotation of skin over a greater distance than is possible with a single transposition flap and is especially useful for defects where skin is less mobile, with good color and texture match. The blood supply for bilobed flaps is random and the flap can be medially or laterally based. The flap should be planned so that donor scars are in a vertical orientation if possible. The design of the flap requires meticulous measurements of the defect and selection of an appropriate pivot point. The pivot point is placed at a distance equal to the diameter of the defect. The first lobe is designed to equal the size of the defect and the second lobe is designed to be approximately half the size of the defect in an orientation 90° to 100° from the distal edge of the defect. Bilobe flaps are useful for repairing skin defects of the caudal sidewall using the lax skin along the nasal sidewall. The surgeon may estimate skin laxity by pinching the lateral nasal skin between the thumb and index finger.[5] Caution should be used in planning bilobe flaps in patients with thick sebaceous skin because there is a higher risk of flap necrosis, trap-door deformity, and depressed scars.

Dorsonasal (Reiger) flap
The dorsonasal, or nasal glabellar flap, was first described by Reiger[6] in 1967 and has been modified by several subsequent authors. The flap is a rotational flap with both random and axial blood flow. A large area of surrounding tissue is undermined to allow for a superolaterally based, rotation advancement flap of nasal and glabellar skin. The dorsonasal flap is used mostly used for middle or lower third defects. The flap is ideal for lax skin in the nasal dorsum, glabellar, and nasal bridge.

The releasing incision is placed in the subunit junction of the nasofacial sulcus, and can be extended into the cheek to increase advancement of donor skin.[7] Dissection is performed beneath the musculature of the nose to separate the flap from the periosteum and perichondrium for maximal rotation, and protect the blood supply to the flap. The donor defect in the glabella is closed primarily or in a V-Y fashion. Because the dorsonasal flap is a pivotal flap, a standing cone defect is created at the inferior aspect of the pedicle, which can be excised. Care must be taken to avoid excessive tension caudally, which may create distortion or rotation of the nasal tip or a prominent supratip depression (**Fig. 8**).

Interpolated Flaps

Paramedian forehead flap
The paramedian forehead flap is one of the most versatile and often-used nasal reconstructive option. The forehead flap is used almost exclusively for large surface area defects of the nasal dorsum and sidewall. Any nasal subunit can be reconstructed with this technique, including the internal vestibular lining. Full-thickness defects of the dorsum and sidewall generally require a separate reconstruction of the internal lining and structural support with subsequent external coverage using a forehead flap (**Fig. 9**).

The forehead flap is elevated preserving a narrow pedicle of 1.5 cm width, which captures the supratrochlear artery, and allows for a wide arch of rotation to reach proximal defects of the nasal dorsum, as well as distal defects of the nasal tip. This flap is usually performed in 2 stages, a flap

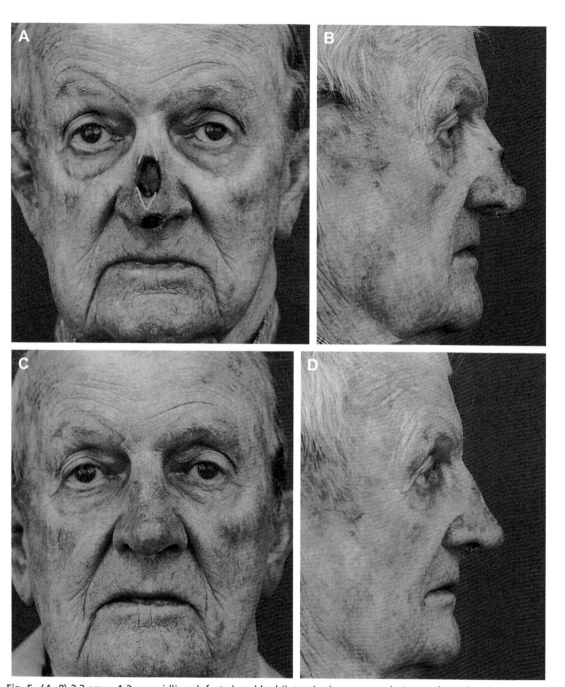

Fig. 5. (*A*, *B*) 2.3 cm × 1.3 cm midline defect closed by bilateral advancement (primary closure) with excision of the standing cutaneous deformity cephalad and caudal to the defect. (*C*, *D*) 1-month postoperative result. There is a subtle depression on the profile view. Caution should be taken with primary closure to avoid excess tension, which will result in a more obvious depression on lateral view.

inset stage and then subsequent pedicle division 3 to 4 weeks later. Additional procedures may be performed before pedicle division to thin and contour the flap while preserving the proximal blood supply. Further details of forehead flap reconstruction of nasal defects are described by Park elsewhere in this issue.

COMPLEX AND FULL-THICKNESS DEFECTS

Nasal defects involving the dorsum and sidewall of the nose may involve adjacent facial units including the forehead, medial canthus, eyelids, and cheek. It is beyond the scope of this review to include reconstructive options for each of these

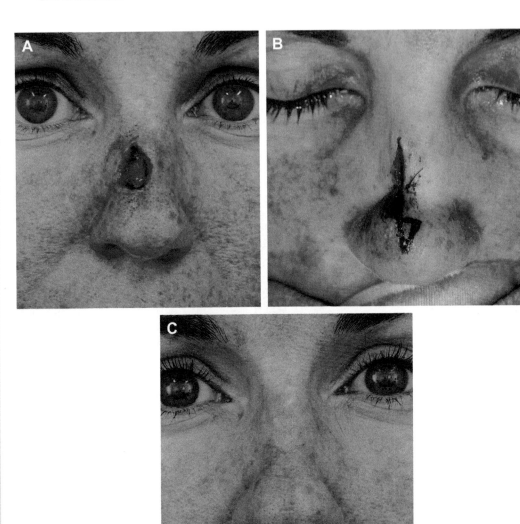

Fig. 6. (*A*) 1.4 cm × 1.1 cm paramedian defect closed by bilateral advancement. (*B*) Inferior standing cone is excised on the median side of the defect to reposition the inferior scar into a midline position. (*C*) 6-month postoperative result.

additional areas. However, these adjacent areas should be analyzed during reconstructive planning to ensure preservation of the distinction between the aesthetic borders of these facial units. For example, large nasal sidewall defects often extend into the cheek. It is best to perform reconstruction of the cheek component of the defect by performing a cheek advancement flap and then reconstruct the nasal component of the defect with a forehead flap. This allows for preservation of the nasal facial junction, which would not occur if the entire defect were to be closed with a forehead flap.

Full-thickness defects require reconstruction of all layers to adequately preserve the form and function of the nose. In addition to external lining, plans need to be formed for replacement of the internal lining and recreation of the structural support (bone/cartilage) of the nose.

Internal Lining

Pericranial flap

The pericranial flap receives its blood supply from the supratrochlear and supraorbital vessels. After making a coronal incision, the skin flap is elevated

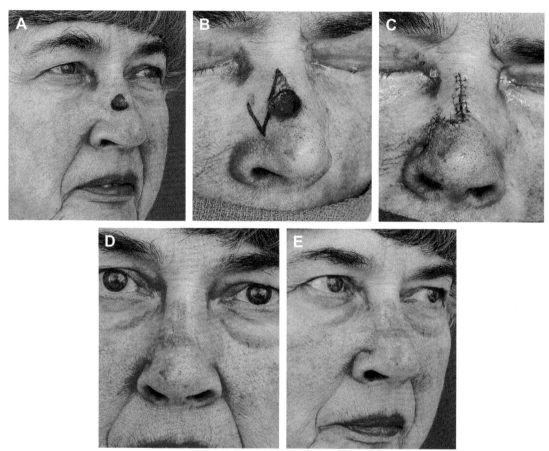

Fig. 7. (*A*) 1.2 cm × 1.0 cm defect of the right sidewall closed with a note transposition flap. (*B*) Flap is drawn with anticipated standing cone excision cephalad to the defect. (*C*) Intraoperative photograph of transposed flap. (*D*, *E*) 1-week postoperative result.

in a subgaleal plane toward the brow. Lateral elevation is performed just above the deep temporal fascia with blunt elevation to protect the frontal branch of the facial nerve, which lies in the temporal parietal fascia just superficial to the plane of dissection. The lateral elevation is connected to the central subgaleal elevation by dissecting through the conjoint tendon. Separate incisions are then created for the pericranial flap, which is elevated to the orbital rim in a subperiosteal plane. Additional length of elevation may be achieved by removing the inferior bridge of bone at the supraobital foramen.

The pericranial flap can be used for internal lining to fill in nasal defects, cover implants, and provide vascular flow to bone grafts.[8] Defects that require both internal and external lining may be closed using a pericranial flap for internal lining that is harvested from one side of the forehead and a forehead flap harvested from the opposite side for external covering. Bilateral forehead flaps are another option, where one forehead flap provides the internal lining and the other provides external coverage.[5]

Mucoperichondrial flaps

Mucoperichondrial flaps harvested from the nasal septum may be used to recreate the internal lining of nasal dorsal and sidewall defects. These flaps may be based off the posterior blood supply of the posterior septal branch of the sphenopalatine artery or from the caudal septum based off the septal branch of the labial artery. These flaps are limited by the arc of rotation required to reach the dorsal defects and care must be taken to preserve a broad base of the flap while making cuts to free up the flap. **Fig. 9** shows a posteriorly based mucoperichondrial septal flap that was freed by creating incisions along the dorsal septum, the caudal septum, and the maxillary crest. A broad posterior base was preserved and the anterior tip of the flap was reflected posteriorly and laterally to fill the defect of the internal lining. Note that the perichondrium is reflected laterally

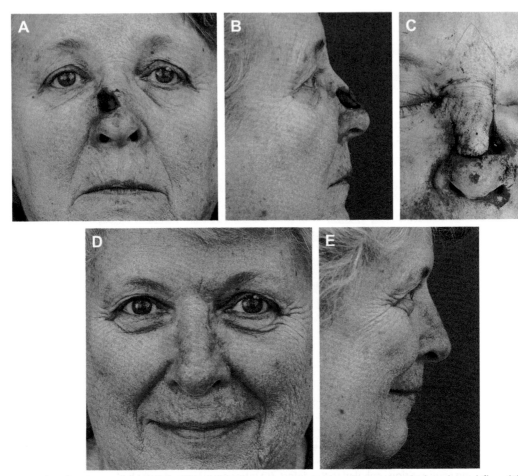

Fig. 8. (*A, B*) 2.0 cm × 1.5 cm defect involving the dorsum and sidewall closed with dorsal nasal flap. (*C*) Flap is elevated in sub-SMAS plane over the dorsum and advanced. There was excess tension across the dorsum, so the incision was extended into the glabella (*green*). The glabellar donor site was closed primarily. (*D, E*) 2-month postoperative result.

as the flap is turned over when it is reflected back into the defect. In this case the septal cartilage was harvested to provide structural support in the area of the resected nasal bones. The pedicle was divided as a staged procedure.

Structural Support

Reconstruction of full-thickness nasal defects requires the use of materials that are durable to provide structural support, resist forces of respiration, and scarring. Alloplastic materials may be used and can reduce surgical time, eliminate donor site morbidity, and be shaped into different forms. The use of alloplastic material is often avoided, however, because of the higher risk of infection, extrusion, and migration. Autogenous grafting is the preferred method for nasal reconstruction.

Split calvarial bone grafts

Split calvarial bone offers rigid reconstruction of the skeletal framework for large defects of the nasal dorsum and sidewall. Calvarial bone grafts are unique because they are from membranous bone that exists only in the bones of the cranial vault and skull base and last longer than endochondral bone.[9]

Split calvarial bone graft is versatile and has a large donor source that can provide up to 24 cm² of graft material with relatively straightforward harvest techniques. It is indicated for nasal dorsal reconstruction when defects involve large portions of the nasal bones, particularly at the bony-cartilaginous junction. For harvest, the donor site is marked out 4 to 5 cm lateral to the midline and a trough is drilled with a cutting burr around the bone graft. Curved osteotomes are then used to separate the outer table from the inner table, through the diploic layer. The

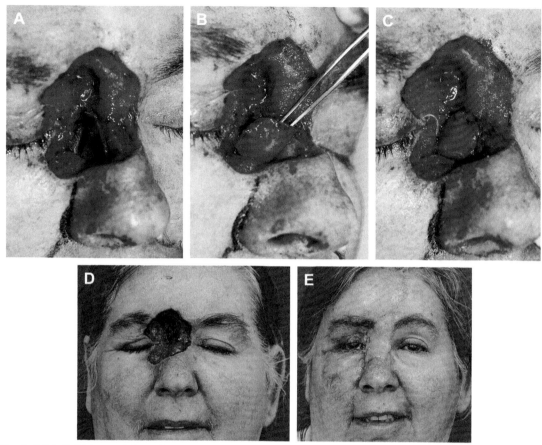

Fig. 9. (*A*) Full-thickness defect of nasal sidewall and dorsum extending into the right medial canthus, upper and lower eyelids, cheek, and forehead. (*B*) Septal flap elevated and rotated to create and internal lining for the nasal defect. (*C*) Septal flap sutured in place. Septal cartilage was used for structure before forehead flap coverage. (*D*) Preoperative photograph (*E*) 1-month postoperative result after septal flap, cartilage graft, forehead flap, cheek and lower lid advancement, brow and upper lid advancement, and skin graft at medial canthus.

split calvarial bone graft can then be shaped as needed to reconstruct the contours of the nasal dorsum and fixated to the radix with a titanium plating system.

Costal grafts, septal cartilage
Smaller defects may be reconstructed with osseous or cartilaginous costal grafts. Costal cartilage grafts are limited in size and may susceptible to warping, migration, and resorption. These undesirable outcomes are less likely with osseous costal grafts. In cases with small defects of the nasal bone and an intact osseocartilagenous junction, septal or rib cartilage may be used for reconstruction. Larger defects should be reconstructed with calvarial bone grafts.

Free Tissue Transfer

For various reasons, patients may delay excision of skin cancers resulting in large composite defects including total or near total rhinectomy defects. Reconstruction of these defects may be performed with free tissue transfer. Free tissue transfer requires microsurgical expertise and is more time consuming. However, with the rapid advancement of microsurgery techniques there is a promising outlook for these difficult defects, such as composite free flaps that can be used to repair full-thickness nasal defects in a single stage. Examples of complex defects requiring free tissue transfer are described elsewhere in this issue.

SUMMARY

As with all nasal reconstruction, nasal dorsal and sidewall defects require a thoughtful analysis of the characteristics of the defect and surrounding tissues. Simple techniques can often be used to reconstruct defects in this area and achieve excellent outcomes. Keys to successful reconstruction in this area, for both simple and complex defects, include protection or reestablishment of the support at the osseocartilagenous junction, maintenance of the transitioning thickness of the skin and soft tissues throughout this region, and preservation of the aesthetic borders with other facial units whenever possible. Consideration of these regional characteristics and the technical pearls described will help the surgeon achieve successful outcomes during reconstruction of the nasal dorsal and sidewall subunits.

REFERENCES

1. Burget GC, Menick FJ. Aesthetic reconstruction of the nose. St Louis (MO): Mosby-Year Book; 1994.
2. Wei FC, Mardini S. Flaps and reconstructive surgery. Philadelphia (PA): Saunders; 2009.
3. Park SS. Reconstruction of nasal defects larger than 1.5 centimeters in diameter. Laryngoscope 2000; 110(8):1241–50.
4. Zitelli JA. The bilobed flap for nasal reconstruction. Arch Dermatol 1989;125:957–9.
5. Baker SR. Reconstruction of the nose, . Local flaps in facial reconstruction. 2nd edition. St Louis (MO): Mosby-Year Book; 2007. p. 415–7.
6. Reiger RA. A local flap for repair of the nasal tip. Plast Reconstr Surg 1967;40:147–9.
7. Johnson TM, Swanson NA, Baker SR, et al. The Rieger flap for nasal reconstruction. Arch Otolaryngol Head Neck Surg 1995;121(6):634–7.
8. Argenta LC, Friedman RJ, Dingman RO, et al. The versatility of pericranial flaps. Plast Reconstr Surg 1985;76(5):695–702.
9. Emerick KS, Hadlock TA, Cheney ML. Nasofacial reconstruction with calvarial bone grafts in compromised defects. Laryngoscope 2008;118(9):1534–8.

Reconstruction of Nasal Tip and Columella

Callum Faris, MBBS, MRCS, DOHNS[a],*,
Hade D. Vuyk, MD, PhD[b]

KEYWORDS

- Nasal reconstruction • Skin cancer • Nasal tip • Columella
- Inner lining • Nasal defect

TIP RECONSTRUCTION

Tip defects are common, bearing a potential for considerable aesthetic and functional deformity. Of the 850 nasal defects treated in the authors' department, 325 involved the nasal tip, of which 70 were through-and-through defects. Because of its unique individual characteristics, reconstruction of the nasal tip is a challenging endeavor. The range of reconstructive options varies in complexity from simple grafting to 3- or 4-stage reconstruction with regional flaps. To sculpture a structure that simulates the nasal tip while allowing normal nasal function, the reconstructive surgeon is impelled to turn to current rhinoplasty knowledge and expertise. This expertise involves the application of both functional and aesthetic nasal analysis and modern rhinoplasty techniques to the reconstructive problem. Indeed, nowhere is the line between nasal reconstruction and rhinoplasty so blurred than in rehabilitation of defects of the nasal tip.

Tip Anatomy

The nasal tip is a biconvex structure. It is unique in that it is the only nasal subunit that shares a common border with all remaining subunits of the nose (columella, dorsum, ala, soft triangle, sidewall) (**Fig. 1**).

The shape and position of the nasal tip is determined both by the structure and position of the alar cartilages and by its skin, soft-tissue covering. Differences in skin characteristics, even within the nasal tip, can be appreciated. The majority of the nasal tip lies within a thicker skin zone, richly populated with sebaceous glands. The lower portion of the infratip lobule and soft triangle (separate subunit but juxtaposition to the tip subunit) lie within a zone with skin that is thinner, smooth, nonsebaceous, and adherent to the underlying cartilage.[1] Obviously, as the replaced alar cartilage must mimic normalcy, the choice of skin covering must fit the preexisting state.

In frontal view, the nasal tip unit consists of 2 halves or subunits. In profile, one may discern the supratip and infratip lobule. The lower lateral cartilage (LLC) largely determines these transitions from one area to another and thus contributes to the development of the double break, tip defining point, and supratip break point (**Fig. 2**). The transition of the medial crus to the intermediate crus forms an angle, which translates as a double break. This point is the most anterior point of the columella in profile and determines the transition from columella to infratip region. The highest point of the domal segment corresponds to the tip-defining point on each side. This pair of tip defining points is usually manifested externally by light reflexes. The supratip lobule ranges from the tip-defining point to the supratip break point. As the cephalic edge of the lateral crus slopes posterior it meets the dorsal septum producing the supratip breakpoint. This landmark defines the junction of the nasal dorsal and tip subunit. The transition from ala to nasal tip may best be assessed in basal view and is marked as the deepest point in this concave area (**Fig. 3**).

It may be clear that the shape of the cartilages translate as surface characteristics with, in

The authors have nothing to disclose.

[a] Department of Otolaryngology, Southampton University Hospitals, NHS Trust, Tremona Road, Southampton, Hampshire, UK SO16 6YD

[b] Department of Otolaryngology & Facial Plastic Reconstructive Surgery, Tergooi Hospitals, Rijksstraatweg 1, 1261 AN, Blaricum, The Netherlands

* Corresponding author. 11 Carbis Close, Port Solent, Portsmouth, Hampshire, PO6 4TW, UK.

E-mail address: callumfaris@gmail.com

Facial Plast Surg Clin N Am 19 (2011) 25–62

doi:10.1016/j.fsc.2010.10.012

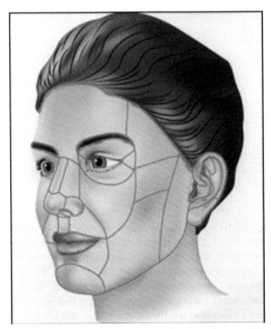

Fig. 1. Facial subunits. (*From* Vuyk HD, Lohuis, PJFM. Facial plastic and reconstructive surgery. 1st edition. Hodder Arnold; 2006. No. 1; with permission.)

general, gently flowing hills and valleys. The transition in shape from convex to concave does represent the borders of the nasal tip subunit. The delineation of the boundaries on the nose between concave and convex surfaces, which results in differences in light reflection and shadowing,

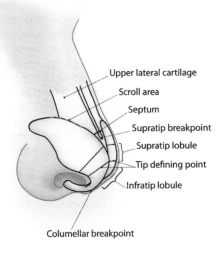

Fig. 2. Oblique view showing cartilaginous framework of nasal tip.

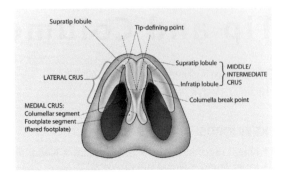

Fig. 3. Basal view showing relationship to underlying cartilaginous framework.

may be clear or sometimes less defined. However, they present opportunities to hide the reconstructive scars in areas where a transition is expected, making them less readily apparent to the eye.

Placing the scar in the previously mentioned areas might imply enlargement of the defect. Indeed, given the advantage of scar camouflaging one may go so far that if 25% to 50% or more of the nasal subunit is involved, the excision of the remaining subunit is considered.[2,3] For example, smaller defects limited to one-half of the nasal tip may be converted to a hemi-tip unit defect. The unaffected other half remains, and can be used as a template to mirror exactly the reconstruction. The vertical midline scar naturally divides the tip into an equal left and right half. For more extended tip defects, the whole nasal tip may be resurfaced. It must be stressed that if the transitions of the subunit are not clear, the aesthetic sense helps to delineate a further resection so that the size of the tip remains in harmony with the remaining nasal dimensions. Defects of the nasal (hemi or total) tip unit dictate more extensive reconstruction with the forehead flap. This point is subsequently discussed in more detail.

Tip Dynamics

In reconstruction of the nasal tip, a basic understanding of tip dynamics is helpful to appreciate the changes that occur by resections and of the steps one should follow in reconstructing the changes in nasal tip shape, position, and function. For example, skin-only resection may lead to loss of tip projection. Similar to external rhinoplasty, the skin has been lifted off the alar cartilages and thus one of the minor tip support mechanisms (skin-cartilage attachment) is damaged. Specifically in large resections, when part or all of the alar cartilage is missing, the reconstructed LLC must bear the weight of the whole reconstruction and withstand the retractile forces that will inevitably accompany healing and scar formation. It follows that, similar to reprojecting the nasal tip in rhinoplasty, the reconstructed cartilage tip complex must have a strong base and lateral components that ensure adequate nasal function. An overview of cartilage reconstruction follows.

Reconstructive Options

In reconstruction of the nasal tip, the authors aim for optimal aesthetic outcome (shape, position, scar, contour) with preservation of the nasal airway. The reconstructive plan will have to take

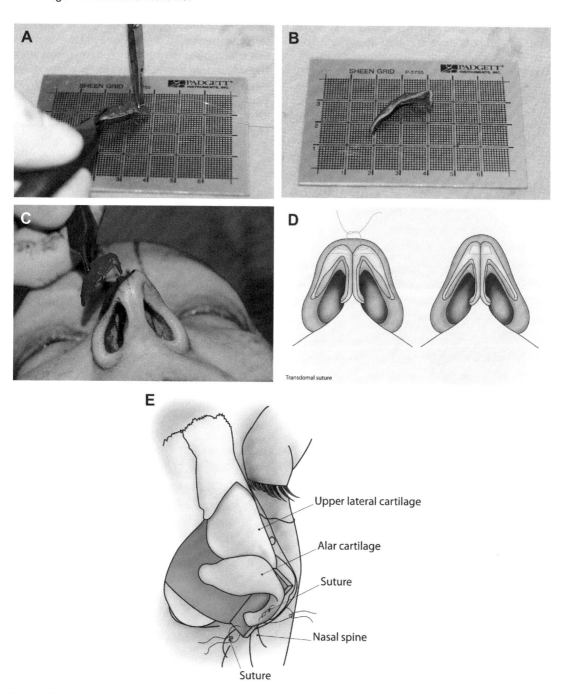

Fig. 4. (*A*) 5 or 6/0 PDS transdomal sutures help to recreate the curvature of the alar cartilage. (*B*) Graft aims to mirror the contralateral crus. (*C*) Shaped ear cartilage graft shown. (*D*) Transdomal sutures from rhinoplasty. (*E*) Example of added tip support with strut either free floating in between the remaining medial crura or fixed to septum or butt hole sutured to the spine.

into account tumor characteristics and patients' wishes.

Cartilaginous framework for tip reconstruction

The review of the anatomy and tip dynamics aims to help the reader appreciate the importance of the interaction between the reconstructed cartilaginous framework and external appearance of the nose. The authors have come to appreciate how even small changes in the reconstructed cartilaginous framework impact the tip shape and position.

The small loss of tip projection after skin-only excision, even with an intact underlying alar cartilage, can be compensated for by small tip grafting. As in rhinoplasty, grafts that contact the skin must be made to blend in to the remaining cartilage structure smoothly. Covering of tip grafts with perichondrium is considered. If the alar cartilage is damaged or missing it must be reconstituted. Ear cartilage harvested from the cymba concha is well suited because it has a preformed curvature. The Mustarde principle of suture shaping ear

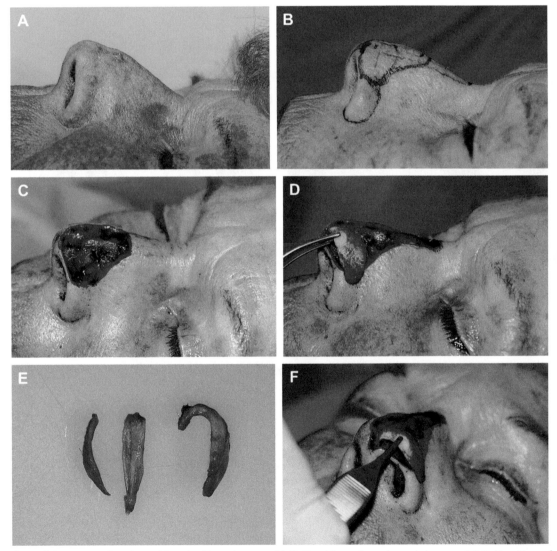

Fig. 5. (A) Preoperative view of basal cell carcinoma of left tip, side wall, and nasal dorsum. (B) Delineation of defect and nasal sub units. (C) Defect encompassing left hemi-tip and encroaching slightly on the right tip and left ala as well as lateral nasal wall and dorsum. (D) Excision of nasal dorsum continued to include the whole of the subunit and ear cymba cartilage before shaping. (E) On left and right side, cartilage grafts taken from the cymba concha. In the middle, the resected cartilaginous hump seen is from below. (F) The scored and sutured shaped curvature of the conchal cartilage mimics the contour required.

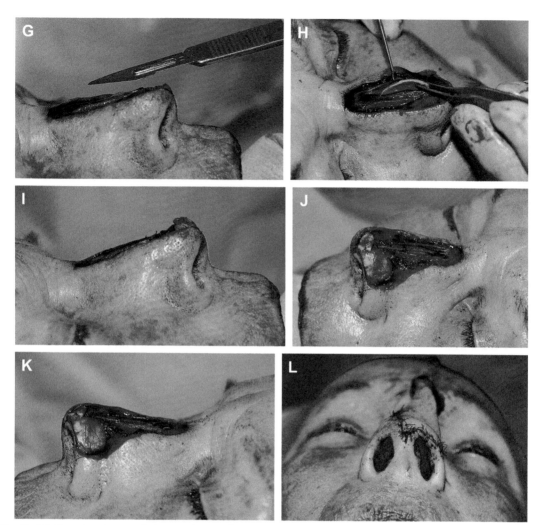

Fig. 5. (*G*) Dorsal reduction balances the profile. Further tip reprojection with tip grafts is anticipated. (*H*) Spreader grafts maintain middle nasal vault width and nasal function. (*I*) Onlay tip graft sutured as in rhinoplasty to enhance profile. (*J–L*) The reconstructed nasal skeleton in place. Skin coverage with forehead flap.

cartilage in combination with scoring is applicable to bend or straighten the neo-alar cartilage (**Fig. 4**A–C). This principle uses suture techniques from rhinoplasty, such as transdomal suturing, to mold the cartilaginous free grafts (see **Fig. 4**D). Septal cartilage is ideal to extend the length of these ear cartilages more laterally, which gives support even onto the piriform aperture to preserve nasal valve function. Septal cartilage can be used to support the nasal tip in the columella region as a strut (see **Fig. 4**E) or even septal extension graft, the latter offering maximum support.

To reposition and gain further support, the neo-alar is also fixed to the contralateral alar cartilage with interdomal sutures, which controls the width of the nasal tip. Essentially any of the tools used in rhinoplasty[3,4] may be used depending on the experience of the surgeon.

At this stage it is important to make an assessment of the contractile forces on the lower two-thirds that will be exerted during the healing phase. To further support the free alar rim, alar rim grafts may come into play. Similarly, the soft triangle may need cartilaginous support. Spreader grafts or butterfly grafts are added so as to maintain nasal airway. For example, a butterfly graft beautifully repositions the recreated alar cartilages more laterally and opens up the external nasal valve.[5]

Grafts in the alar-sill region that extend laterally from the neo-alar to the septal spine may be the final link in recreating a cartilage ringlike structure from the columella, tip, lateral wall, and sill, which may offer maximum control over position, shape, and function. One may also appreciate that apparent tip position is also related to the height and shape of the nasal dorsum.

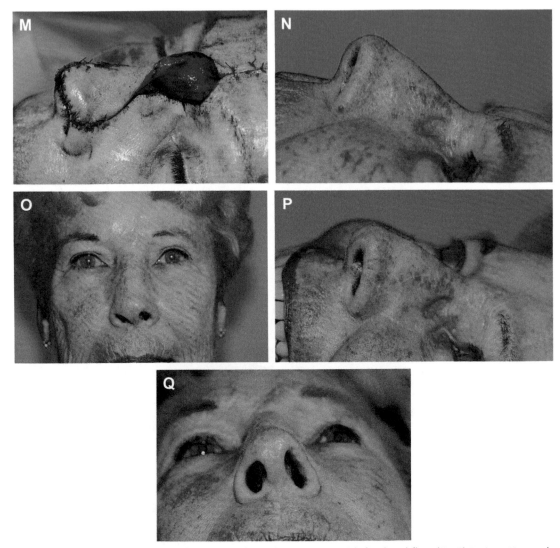

Fig. 5. (*M*) The reconstructed nasal skeleton in place. Skin coverage with forehead flap. (*N–Q*) Patient 13 months following surgery. Patient happy with result, function is impeccable. Profile improved, not perfect but harmonious. Maybe a slight tilt of the nasal tip has occurred because of the strong reconstruction on the left side.

To get an aesthetically balanced outcome, an overprotected nasal dorsum may be lowered to compensate for loss of tip projection while harmonizing with the recreated nasal tip. When the cartilaginous dorsum is lowered and the upper laterals become detached from the dorsal septal edge, spreader grafts may be needed.

Apart from aesthetic goals, the authors work hard to maintain function or even correct it at the time of reconstruction. Any septal deviation or preexistent valve abnormality may become a potential problem, even after a well-executed reconstruction, if not corrected or compensated for. Moreover, the authors have come to realize that functional problems after nasal reconstruction are not easy to deal with. Because of the different anatomy and scarring, the rhinoplasty techniques applied are less effective.

The application of the reconstruction options presented here must be based on a clear appreciation of the preoperative situation. This appreciation includes evaluation of the patients' airway and possibly pre-excision, 4-view photograph documentation. Preoperative aesthetic analysis may suggest the reconstructive possibilities and needs. For example, nasal-tip rotation or nasal-dorsal reduction create a relative excess of the skin soft-tissue envelope and help to diminish the size of the defect, which may then allow for a simpler reconstruction. The precise reconstitution of the cartilaginous framework cannot be overstated because this directly relates to the final results.

An example is given of a reconstructed alar cartilage, including tip grafting and dorsal reduction, with the application of spreader grafts (**Fig. 5**), and another case with cartilage butterfly-type reconstruction (**Fig. 6**).

Nasal lining reconstruction

In through-and-through defects, 3 different layers are missing. The 3 components include lining, cartilage framework, and skin covering. If the different layers are reconstructed separately, each can be manipulated, shaped, and placed to contribute to the best possible outcome. Nasal-tip defects with inner lining defects often result from inferior and lateral extensions of the tumor onto the infratip lobule and the adjacent soft triangle, thereby reaching and growing over the nostril margin into the nose. Alternatively, lateral impingent of the tumor deep into the alar subunit may also result in nasal cavity involvement. Direct

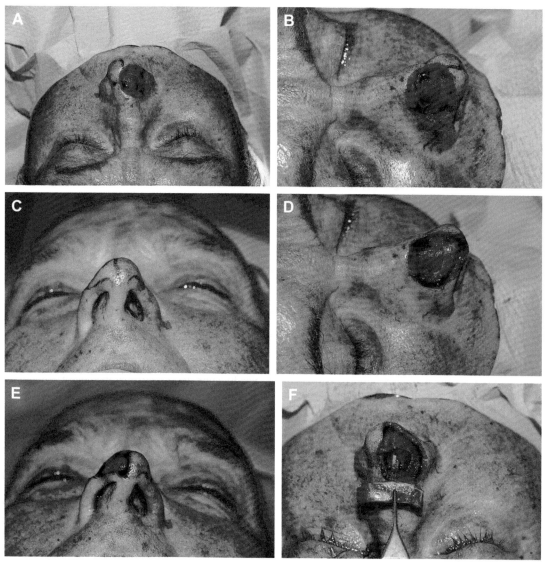

Fig. 6. (*A, B*) Defect involving tip, nasal dorsal subunit, and side-wall subunit. Inner lining intact but there is partial deficiency in upper lateral and lower lateral cartilages. (*C*) Alar margin, soft triangle not involved. Note the deviation of the anterior septum putting the nasal valve at risk after reconstruction. (*D, E*) Remainder of right hemi-tip excised. (*F*) Butterfly graft fashioned from concha cartilage to reconstruct the cephalic portion of the alar cartilage in proper position. This maneuver aims to maintain nasal valve function.

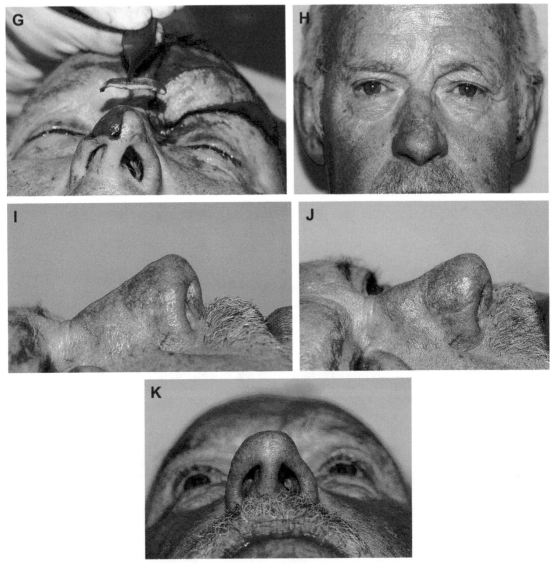

Fig. 6. (*G*) Butterfly graft fashioned from concha cartilage to reconstruct the cephalic portion of the alar cartilage in proper position. This maneuver aims to maintain nasal valve function. (*H–K*) Postoperative result. Good nasal function. Slight widening of the external nasal valve can be discerned. No middle nasal vault collapse. Contour of tip and function excellent. Scars well hidden in aesthetic subunit borders.

deep extension into the vestibule of isolated nasal-tip lesions is unusual because of the barrier afforded by the lower lateral cartilages and their perichondrium.

The considered lining options follow a logical reconstructive ladder from simple to more intricate. Small defects can be left to heal by secondary intention. Primary closure may, although infrequently, be an option. Caution must be exercised not to significantly diminish the internal diameter of the nasal airway.

Skin grafts can be applied onto the defect wound edges, which in a subsequent stage will serve as lining. After 2 or 3 months, when the wound edges have been skin covered and healed, the previous graft can be developed from superior to inferior and hinged into the lining deficit. Skin grafts can also be applied to the undersurface of skin flaps used for skin covering in the first stage of the reconstruction. There is a slight risk of graft failure. A second, intermediate stage is used for placement of cartilage grafts.[6] The simplicity of this is alluring, but one has to be exact with the cartilage shape and position because at the third stage pedicle division is performed precluding further cartilage reshaping.

Skin-cartilage composite grafts offer 2 layers for reconstruction, but they are difficult to shape while placing the skin part of the graft exactly in the lining defect. However, in defects of less then 1 cm that involve the free border of the columella, soft triangle, and tip, they have an outstanding record. Ideally, some remaining lining will enhance vascular growth and increase the chance of survival.

Flaps have the advantage of carrying blood supply to support primary cartilage grafting. However, these flaps must be thin and supple to follow the desired contour and not impinge on the nasal airway. For clarity, the authors conceptualize flaps for lining by categorizing them according to donor site rather than flap type or tissue movement. Thus the possible *donor sites* include

Septum (ipsilateral or contralateral)
Lateral nasal wall (inside or outside)
Adjacent facial units (melolabial fold, forehead)

Of the septal flaps, only the ipsilateral anterior-based septal flap offers enough tissue and reach to be of value for tip reconstruction (**Fig. 7**). The inside of the lateral nasal wall may yield tissue

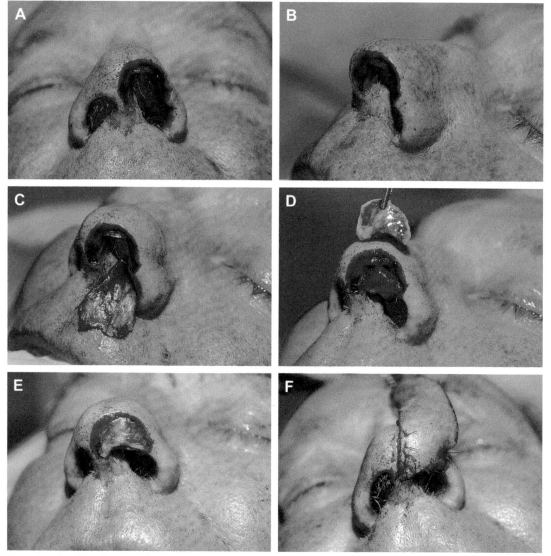

Fig. 7. (*A, B*) Full thickness defect of alar columella and nasal tip defect. (*C*) Anteriorly based septal flap based on the branches of the superior labial artery. (*D*) Septal flap used to reconstruct the inner lining sutured in place. Ear cartilage sculpted to reconstruct the missing part of the alar cartilage and soft triangle. Note part of the cartilage placed in the soft triangle is nonanatomic. (*E*) Cartilage in situ. (*F*) Forehead flap inset into defect.

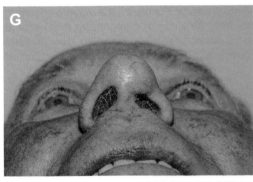

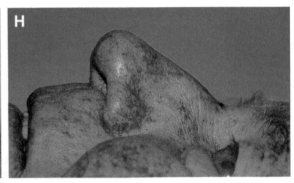

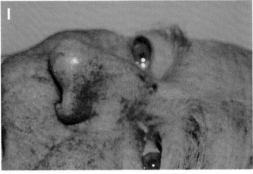

Fig. 7. (G–I) 1-year postoperative result.

often moved caudally as bipedicled mucosal flaps or more rarely as an anteriorly pedicled inferior turbinate flap. The outside of the lateral nasal wall offers ample tissue to be developed from superior to inferior and hinged into the lining defect. A major advantage is that the inside of the nose is not taken apart. These thicker flaps are sturdy and thin spontaneously over time.[7]

For tip defects, the forehead flap may be folded inward as lining. In an intermediate stage, the bulky flap is incised caudally, divided, and thinned aggressively.[8] Cartilage can be added at that stage. The pedicle is divided at the final stage (Fig. 8).

The authors suggest that tip-cartilage reconstitution is so demanding that a 3-layer, 3-stage reconstruction yields the best possibilities for an aesthetic shape. The precise cartilage grafting done at the first stage can be improved upon at 3 weeks during the intermediate stage. The forehead flap left pedicled superiorly can be lifted completely out of the wound bed and thinned as necessary. Cartilage can be shaped, refined, and added if needed.

Of course, the exact choice of reconstruction of the defect depends upon patient and defect factors. Patient factors, such as diabetes or smoking, make the fragile vestibular and septal flaps more prone to fail. Sometimes multiple lining options are used to compliment each other.

Skin resurfacing Nasal-tip defects may be classified according to the location, size, and depth of the defect. As cartilage framework and lining reconstruction have already been discussed, the focus turns specifically to skin covering. Again, adherence to a general reconstructive ladder listing the multiple options available from simple to more intricate is suggested (second intention healing, primary closure, skin grafts and local/regional flaps).

The choice and application of these techniques logically parallels the defect size. Thus, defects are subdivided into small (1 cm or less), moderate (1.0 to 1.5 cm), and large defects (greater than 1.5 cm). Again, there are no distinct cutoffs between the 3 categories, but these distinctions are not arbitrary.

The authors' preferred options in reconstruction of the nasal tip are free skin/composite grafting and regional flaps (the forehead flap). For smaller defects (<1 cm), skin grafting (including composite skin-fat and skin-cartilage grafts) as well as local flaps are commonly used. Full-thickness skin grafts are taken from the melolabial fold or forehead region. These areas provide the best match in color, texture, thickness, and sebaceous glands. Local flaps are developed in the middle and upper nasal vault, if the defect is slightly larger (1.0 to 1.5 cm) or when patients present with recipient sites that are not ideal (patients with diabetes or who smoke), indeed

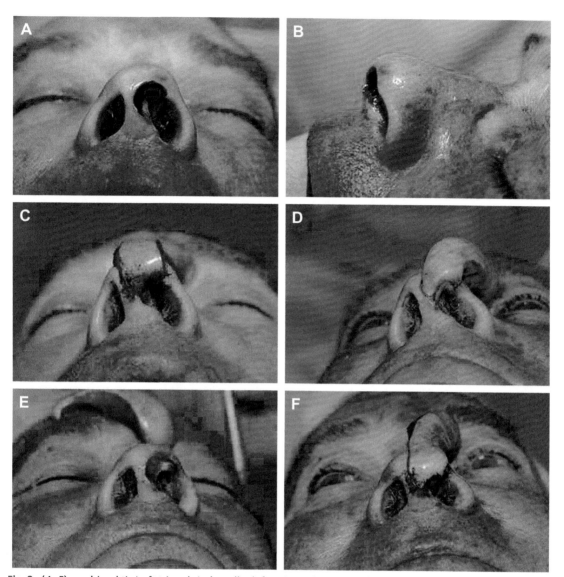

Fig. 8. (A, B) combined tip/soft triangle/columella defect, inner lining is deficient. (C) Following first stage. Folded forehead flap has been used to reproduce inner lining. No cartilage is placed in the defect yet. (D) At second stage, the idea site for the alar margin is marked and then incised elevating the remaining forehead flap. (E) After elevation of the proximal forehead flap one can appreciate the reconstructed inner lining. This neo-lining is then thinned and sculptured with a cartilage graft to prevent retraction. (F) The distal portions of the residual forehead flap is then thinned to improve the contour match and replaced over the cartilage graft. The pedicle will then be divided at the third stage (not shown).

local or regional flaps are good alternatives to skin grafts. In larger defects (>1.5 cm), the subunit principle is often applied and a forehead-flap reconstruction is executed.

Small skin defects (≤1 cm)

Secondary intention healing Because of its simplicity and the possible excellent results, secondary intention healing has to be considered

in any defect. Secondary intention wounds heal by the process of filling in the defect with granulation tissue, re-epithelialization, and scar maturation. The best possible results are related to shape, depth, and size of the defect. Small superficial wounds in concave areas in fair patients with thin skin can do extremely well.[9] The nasal tip, however, is mostly convex, largely covered with a thicker often sebaceous quality of the skin, which

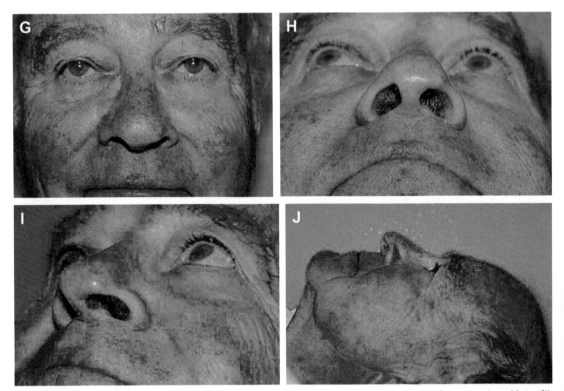

Fig. 8. (*G*) 1-year postoperative appearance. (*H*) No asymmetry of alar margins. (*I*) No alar retraction. (*J*) Profile demonstrates good columella-alar relationship.

does not favor secondary intention healing. However, to demonstrate the possibilities of second intention healing, a rare case is presented (**Fig. 9**).

Primary closure Primary linear closure is a rare possibility only in lax abundant skin. If the skin covering is thick and sebaceous it is also immobile and unaesthetic scars must be anticipated. In the supratip-dorsum junction a horizontal closure may be acceptable. Lateral dog-ear excision and tip rotation are logical sequelae. This scar will come to lie in relaxed skin tension lines (RSTLs) and in the aesthetic subunit boundaries. A vertical midline with dog-ears projected superior and inferior is a variation. On any other part of the tip a linear closure, even if following the RSTL, must be discouraged. Closure tension will flatten and even indent the natural convex surface of the nasal tip. The scar will be perceived readily as an interruption of the smooth, convex contour of the nasal tip. If simplicity is sought rather then aesthetics, the defect may be partly closed by superior and inferior dog-ear excision and horizontal skin advancement. A skin graft may cover the remainder of the defect. Alternatively, the excised dog-ears can be applied.[10]

Skin grafts When secondary intention healing or primary closure is not suitable, skin/composite grafts are the next option, having distinct advantages over local flaps in most cases.

Skin/composite grafts are quick to perform and multiple donor sites are available. The aim is to reproduce the color/texture match with maximal contour. Full-thickness skin grafts (FTSGs) have been used but may unfortunately lack volume, which can produce quite obvious contour defects on the convex nasal tip. Alternatives include skin/perichondrial, skin/fat, and skin/cartilage composite grafts. The ideal donor site will depend on what portion of the nasal tip is deficient.

Full-thickness skin grafts: The use of FTSGs in nasal-tip reconstruction is well established.[11,12] This option continues to be an excellent choice for several reasons. It is a simple single-stage technique. Survival rates range from 70% to 90%[13,14] and depend on recipient site factors, patient factors, and technique. The recipient site should ideally be well vascularized (subcutaneous tissue, fascia) with a lack of infection. Patient health factors that adversely affect graft survival include diabetes mellitus, smoking, and malnutrition. Technique factors, such as antibiotic

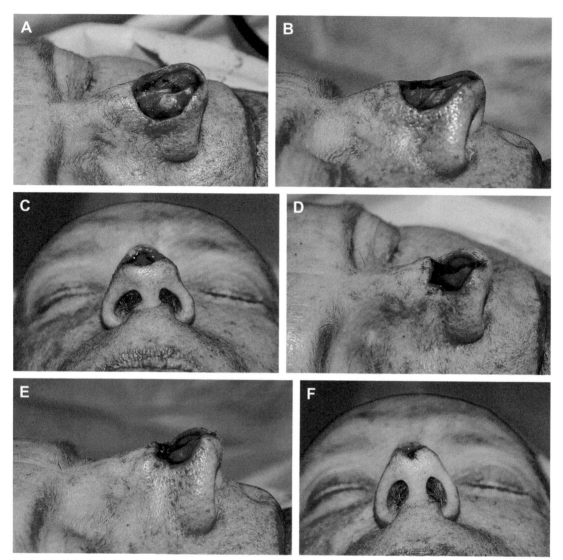

Fig. 9. (*A–C*) Defect after basal cell carcinoma excision. The patient was awaiting a second renal transplantation. Because of the possible delay, he did not want a multiple-stage forehead flap reconstruction. (*D–F*) Approximation of wound edges with some tip rotation sets the stage for second intention healing over a period of 4 weeks. Note that cartilages were exposed. Moist environment is essential to prevent desiccation and filling in with granulation tissue.

prophylaxis; careful handling of the graft; strict hemostasis while avoiding too much cautery; antibiotic/saline irrigation of graft and recipient site before placement; sutures that eliminate shear between the graft and recipient site (but risk bleeding); and a soft, not overly pressured bolster (often with Steri-Strips only [3M, St Paul, Minnesota]), help reduce graft failure.

FTSGs involve a specific set of challenges. Typically, the skin of the convex nasal tip is thick and sebaceous. What then is the ideal donor site and graft type to reduce the often patchwork postoperative appearance caused by color mismatch and contour defects?

Various donor sites for FTSGs are available, such as the preauricular and postauricular regions, conchal bowl, melolabial, forehead, and supraclavicular region. The forehead and melolabial fold possibly represent the most closely matched site for nasal-tip reconstruction in terms of surface characteristics and sebaceous glad population.[12,15,16] The donor-site scar can be well hidden in the melolabial crease or forehead rhytids with minimal aesthetic compromise.

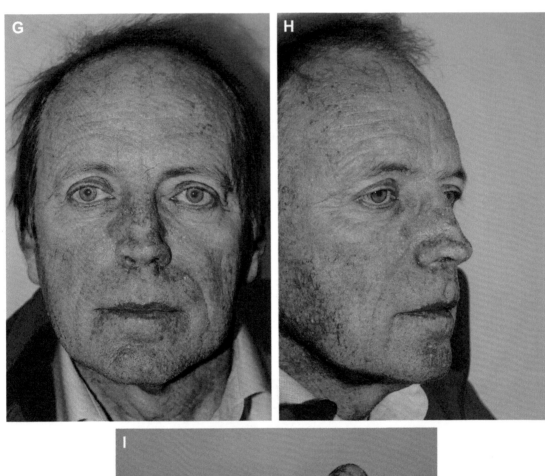

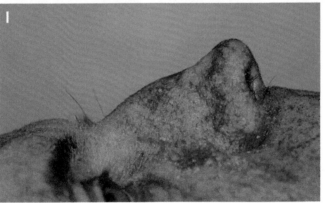

Fig. 9. (*G–I*) Patient received a new kidney. This 3-month postoperative view testifies to natures healing capacity.

Composite skin grafts are of the follwing 3 types:

Skin-fat composites grafts: Classical teaching suggests that skin grafts must be defatted to enhance blood vessel growth and survival. But thinner skin grafts are associated with contour deficits. The question arises whether it is possible to retain subcutaneous fat while aiming for an enhanced contoured reconstruction.[17,18] In **Fig. 10**, the authors present a case of tip reconstruction using a composite skin-fat graft to effect optimal tip contour.

The complete survival rate of these skin/fat composite grafts are in the range of approximately 80%.[17] But even if the superficial parts do not seem to survive completely, the overall postoperative result show good contour. A degree of hypopigmentation and some loss of sebaceous glands may accompany these grafts. Dermabrasion may reduce some of the color mismatch or contour discrepancy.[15] Given the possibilities

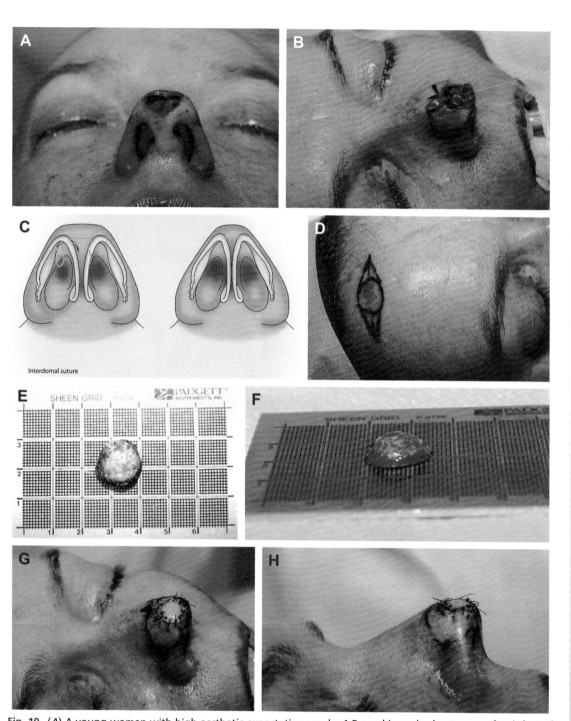

Fig. 10. (*A*) A young woman with high aesthetic expectations and a 1.5-cm skin and subcutaneous fat defect of the nasal tip. Alar cartilages are intact. (*B*) Interdomal suturing is performed to diminish the size of the defect to 1 cm. (*C*) Interdomal sutures used to narrow width of alar domes. (*D*) Donor site marked, centered over forehead rhytid, lateral burrows triangle excision marked. (*E*) Composite skin-fat graft. (*F*) Subcutaneous fat retained on the undersurface of the graft to improve contour. (*G*) The skin graft carefully manipulated and sutured in with 6-0 fat-absorbing sutures. Skin/fat composite graft is defatted incrementally until the contour exactly matches surrounding skin. (*H*) Tip projection and contour maintained. A small bolster is lightly applied with sterile strips for 4 days.

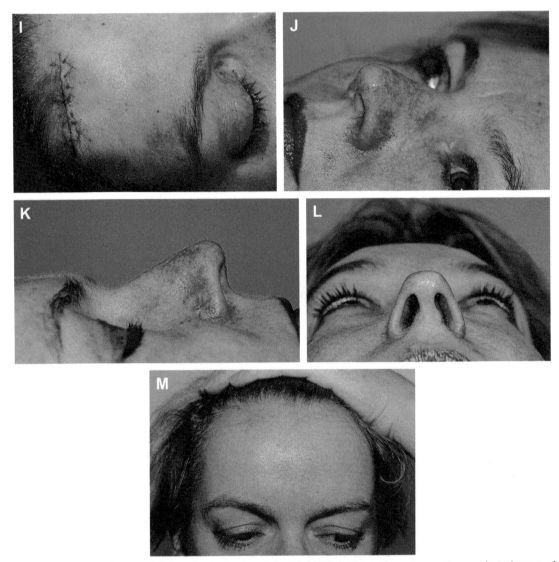

Fig. 10. (*I*) Primary closure of donor site in forehead rhytid. (*J*) The 10-month postoperative result A degree of hypopigmentation but excellent contour. (*K*) Tip projection is maintained. (*L*) Smooth contour and maintenance of tip convexity. (*M*) Minimal donor-site morbidity.

and minimal risks involved, skin-fat composite grafts are an excellent option for deep nasal-tip defects less than 1 cm in diameter.

Perichondrial cutaneous composite grafts: Perichondrial cutaneous composite grafts (PCCGs) are composite grafts (usually harvested from the conchal bowl) consisting of skin and a thin perichondrial layer. Its use is based on the theory that if one maintains the perichondrial plexus in a skin perichondrial composite it may allow for quicker revascularization of the graft, lower graft failure rates, and less retraction. Indeed, clinical studies suggest tendency of improved graft

take.[12] The conchal bowl donor site is easily managed by second intention healing.

Skin/Cartilage composite grafts: Composite chondrocutaneous grafts are an excellent alternative to other grafts in specific circumstances.

They contain skin and cartilage usually harvested from the helical root. The benefit of including cartilage is the inherent shape and support. These characteristics can be used in reconstructing rims that otherwise are complex to reproduce. Skin/cartilage composite grafts do, however, have an increased metabolic demand and most authors agree that they have a somewhat higher failure rate than

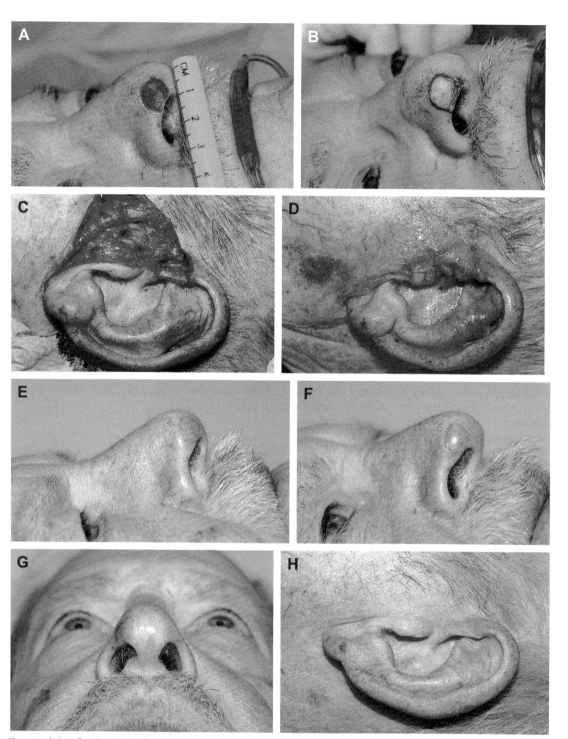

Fig. 11. (*A*) Soft-triangle defect abutting the free soft-triangle margin. (*B*) Auricular composite chondrocutaneous graft taken from root of helix. The cartilage dimensions extend laterally just beyond the skin to be inserted in the lateral wound edges. These extensions will provide support against scar contraction forces. (*C*) Donor site reconstructed with a small cartilage strip harvested from the scapha region and a cheek advancement flap. (*D*) Flap is seen in place in early 5-day postoperative picture. (*E*) Aesthetic outcome at 5 months. (*F*) No alar notching. (*G*) Symmetry of nares, no distortion of nasal tip. (*H*) Donor-site morbidity is minimal.

FTSG or PCCGs. However, much depends on patient selection. Skin/cartilage composite grafts are not used in patients who smoke or have diabetes, and the authors limit their size to a maximum of 1 cm. Ideally, some inner lining remains to increase the graft's vascular support. Thus, for nasal reconstruction the indication for skin cartilage grafts are partial defects of the columella, soft triangle, and alar rim where one requires not only replacement of skin but also a definite shape. In **Fig. 11**, the authors present a case where a soft-triangle defect is reconstructed with a chondrocutaneous graft.

Moderate-size defects (1.0–1.5 cm)

Local flaps Local flaps attempt to transfer tissue from tissue reservoirs in the upper nasal vault or medial cheek where skin laxity exists to the lower third where the thick sebaceous skin of the nasal tip offers minimal mobility. Most local flaps for nasal reconstruction do not conform to the aesthetic unit borders or the RSTLs. As most flaps do pincushion to a degree, this will unmask the complex unaesthetic incisions. Most importantly, the nasal skin envelope may not tolerate reduction in the upper two-thirds to reconstruct the lower third. Indeed, local flaps may cause unaesthetic pushes and pulls, which can lead to alar retraction and tip deformity/asymmetry.

Bilobed flaps: Compared with uni-lobed transposition flaps, a double-lobed or even sometimes triple-lobed flap does extend the distance of tissue transfer. However, it must be recognized that although flaps are denominated as to their primary type of movement, these double-transposition flaps do move largely by a rotational component. In that sense, a double-transposition and a rotation flap are, apart from the garlanded type of incision of the former, quite similar. The geometric basis of the modern bilobed flap does demonstrate that clearly (**Fig. 12**).[19] The rotational angles are limited to 50° for each flap (100° in total), which decreases the buckling around the pivotal point and the greater pull that occurs with the previous bilobed designs. Adherence to a precise geometric plan helps execution and sets the stage for optimal healing. The primary defect needs to be accurately measured in diameter and arcs of rotation for the transposition calculated and drawn. The plan further includes a total rotation between 90–110 degrees, and wide undermining into the surrounding tissues to prevent pin cushioning. The dog-ear is removed last. For laterally placed defects, the flap's secondary defect should come to lie perpendicular to the alar margin. Careful planning and execution is asked for. Small

inaccuracies in vector alignment and length of the primary and secondary flap can have dramatic effects and produce asymmetric retraction.[20,21] Defects of 1.5 cm are the utmost limit for this flap or too much distortion and scarring is to be anticipated. Cases are presented in **Figs. 13** and **14**.

Regional flap

Nasal-dorsal (glabellar) flap: The nasal-dorsal (glabellar) flap is a rotation flap, which at least encompasses the nasal dorsum up to the nasofrontal angle. More extended rotation may yield tissue from the glabella to be moved into the nasal unit.[22] The vascular pedicle is centered on the angular artery located at the upper part of the lateral nasal wall. It is typically based ipsilateral to the lesion to improve flap rotation. The flap and surrounding tissue of the nasal vault are undermined widely in the sub-superficial musculoaponeurotic system (sub-SMAS) plane, similar to rhinoplasty. In the glabella region a transition in dissection plane is made to a more superficial subcutaneous plane. The thicker glabellar skin does come to lie opposite the thin skin of the medial canthal area. Generally, differences in

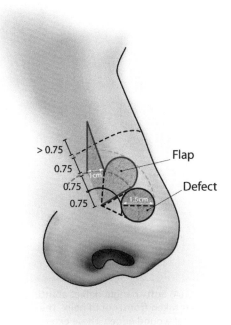

Fig. 12. Bilobed orientation on nasal vault for reconstruction of nasal supratip defect. Note the relationship of the radius of defect (0.75 mm) to the arcs of rotation.

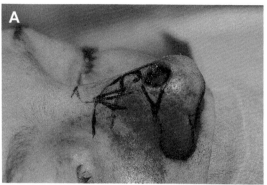
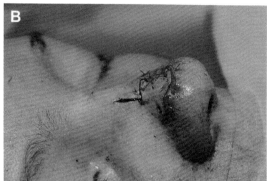
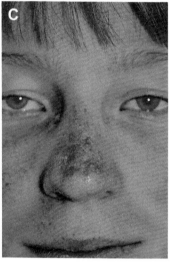

Fig. 13. (A) Bilobed planned according to geometric design. Given the youth of the patient and the tight skin, the primary lobe of the flap in retrospect may need to be slightly oversized, rather then the exact dimensions of the defect. (B) Questionable skin laxity and possible undersizing of flap lead to suboptimal tension on closure. (C) 15-month postoperative result. Acceptable outcome, complex incisions slightly visible.

skin thickness must be accounted for or corrected by thinning of the flap and additional soft-tissue grafts.[23] Judicious excision of a standing cutaneous deformity is one of the last maneuvers to prevent alar retraction. The secondary defect in both lateral nasal wall regions is closed by cheek advancement. The nasal-dorsal rotation flap is only indicated in patients with lax skin over the dorsum and cheek regions. It is suggested that this flap should be limited to defects less than 1.5 cm in diameter located in the distal half of the nasal dorsum and nasal tip. The preferably centrally located defects, may extend to (but not beyond) the supratip lobule. Defects less than 1 cm from the alar rim do risk free alar border displacement.[24] The wide dissection gives an unparalleled exposure to perform any rhinoplasty maneuver. More specifically, a large nasal skeleton with an under-rotated tip and an overprojected dorsum may be reduced. Secondary

movement of the tip upwards, by means of a rotation control suture, facilitates defect closure and takes some tension off the closure. Similarly, dorsal reduction does reduce the size of the nasal skeleton relative to the skin soft-tissue envelope and also aids closure.

Because it is a dependent flap it may fill with lymphoid fluid, which takes a year to resolve. The scars are not in the RSTL, but the versatile blood supply and one stage of the procedure are a definite vote for this flap.[22] **Fig. 15** presents a typical case of the use of the nasal-dorsal (glabellar) flap (see **Fig. 15**).

Large skin defects (≥1.5 cm) A defect that is greater than 1.5 cm signifies the movement above a threshold to a bigger reconstructive issue.

It is suggested that reconstruction is more reliably achieved in these instances with excision of

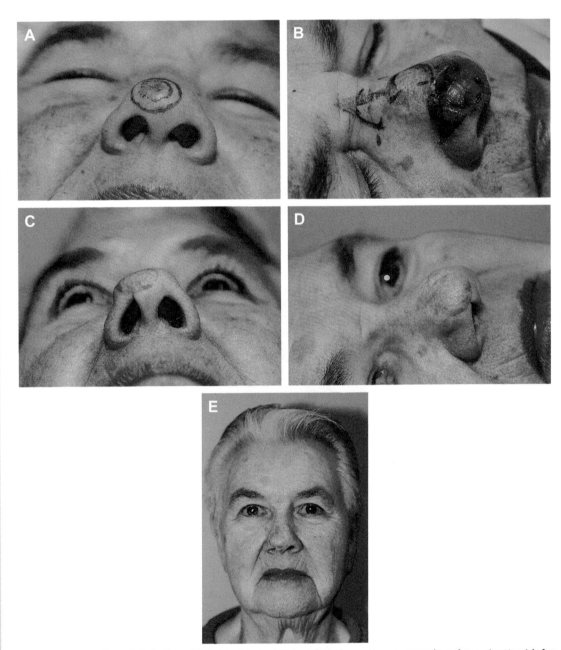

Fig. 14. (*A*) Central nasal tip lesion of 1.4 mm. A large bilobed flap chosen to accommodate the patient's wish for a 1-stage closure. (*B*) Bilobed flap planned using geometric design, including dog-ear excision deferred to end of procedure. How much tissue can you move? (*C–E*) A 2-year postoperative result. Some distortion of the soft triangle. Unaesthetic complex incisions are made more obvious by some pin cushioning despite undermining around the defect.

the hemi-tip on one or both sides and resurfacing with a forehead.[25] The forehead flap offers ample tissue for reconstruction facilitating the application of the subunit principle where smaller defects are enlarged, aiming to place the final scars in the favorable boundaries of the tip subunit. This, however, may convert a possible 1-stage reconstruction to a more complex 2- or 3-stage reconstruction. As all flaps contract to a degree, it elevates the skin in a convex shape, which ideally

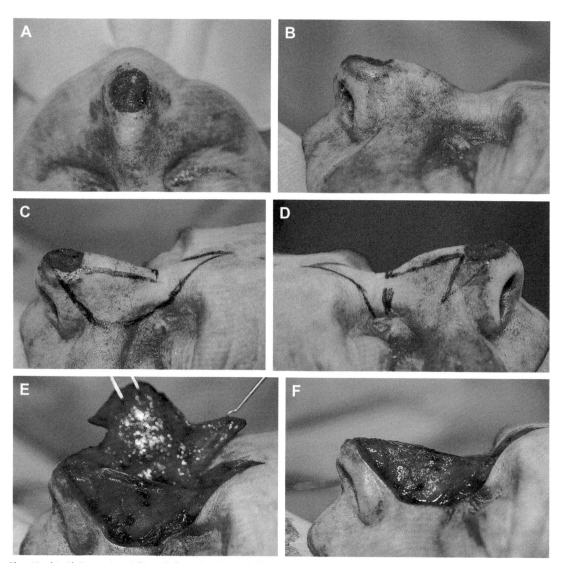

Fig. 15. (*A, B*) Supratip midline defect, the ideal defect for dorsal glabella flap. (*C, D*) Flap planned with back cut in glabella region, preplanned dog ear. Nasal dorsal artery and dorsal lowering is also outlined. (*E*) Flap elevation in sub-superficial musculoaponeurotic system plane. Cartilaginous and bony overprojection are reduced to facilitate closure. (*F*) Profile view demonstrates improved dorsal contour.

mimics the natural contour of the subunit (tip and alar). Appropriate thinning, contouring of the flap with cartilage framework, matching flap edges to the recipient site, and bracing the flap's marginal scars with thin platforms of cartilage are important techniques to master if any reconstruction is to succeed.[26] When considering the subunit principle, multiple factors come into play. Skin with actinic damage may well camouflage skin grafts for similarly damaged skin or incisions associated with local flaps not adhering to the subunit borders[27] and in these instances a more simple reconstruction may be a valid alternative. It is of

note that, because of its insufficient reach and limited size, the melolabial flap is reserved for alar defects that encompass only some lateral part of the nasal tip.

Forehead flap For large defects of the nasal tip, the authors almost exclusively use the forehead flap for skin coverage. This flap is unrivaled in its robustness, skin color, and texture match for reconstruction of the nasal tip. As suggested, this provides the confidence to apply the subunit principle if indicated. The authors may indeed extend the defect to include the adjacent subunits

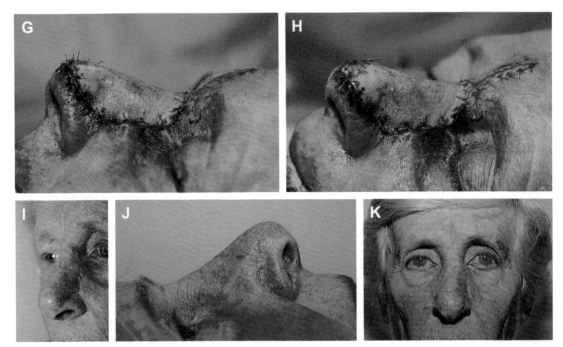

Fig. 15. (*G*) Dorsal profile following flap inset. (*H*) Glabella incision closed in straight line. The non-RSTL closure line clearly visible. (*I–K*) The 8-month postoperative showing near optimal aesthetic result for this reconstructive method. The incisions are only visible to a slight degree. Dorsal profile is, however, greatly improved. A small tendency of the alar free margin to come up together with the rotated tip can be noted.

(soft triangle, alar) even if minimally (only 25%) involved. Large skin tip defects frequently coexist with cartilaginous defects of the alar cartilages and occasional inner-lining defects. Synchronous repair of these accompanying defects is mandatory and will not be repeated.

In the authors' practice, the current design of a forehead flap consists of a superior medial donor site and a vertically drawn pedicle, which at the level of the brow is less then 1.5 cm and as small as 1.2 cm in width and is placed just above the midline subsequently bending toward the lateral nasal sidewall half way between the medial canthus and the nasal dorsum. The flap pedicle is not extended more than 0.5 cm below the brow level. The pedicle is placed contralateral to the defect so that the flap does not impede vision. Anatomic studies have shown the rich dense vascular supply in the medial forehead from the supratrochlear and dorsal nasal arteries and angular artery.[28–30] Of interest is the description of the central and para-central artery and vein, which may be key to the current design.[31] The resulting vertical midline scar in the forehead is camouflaged by its position delineating a natural border between the 2 halves of the forehead. A small offset pedicle facilitates rotation while

maintaining proper length. The purpose of extending the pedicle just below the brow level is to gain further length. Admittedly, the flap then has similarities to the older midforehead flap design (which also did not contain a supratrochlear artery) and still shares its unparallel survival rate. The authors have not seen vascular problems in any of their primary forehead flaps.

The forehead flap is raised in the suprapericranial plane. Incisions are beveled outward to increase the subcut vascular support and to facilitate closure. Sufficient length to reconstruct the nasal tip is achieved often without extending into the hair-bearing scalp. The distal part of the flap is thinned at the first stage. A total of 2 to 3 mm of subcutaneous fat, however, may enhance a more normal aspect of the reconstructed surface. When tip defects coexist with columella defects, the requirement of extension of the forehead flap into the hair-bearing scalp is to be expected.

Enough skin is available to reconstruct the entire nasal envelope based on 1 pedicle. When the width of the forehead flap is greater than 4.5 cm, primary closure of the forehead donor site is not possible. Intraoperative tissue expansion of the remaining lateral forehead regions and dissection into the temporal pockets help facilitate closure. At the second or third stage of the procedure, the forehead can be further closed and the forehead scar revised. Although the authors aim for complete closure of the donor site, a superior midline forehead defect left to heal by secondary intention, despite its convexity, may usually yield acceptable aesthetic results to the patients.[32]

Whether the flap is divided in the second or at a third stage is optional. It depends on the degree of thinning of the flap and sculpting cartilage framework that is required. In the authors' practice, most nasal tip reconstruction requires a 3-stage approach for optimal aesthetic results. The intermediate stage may involve partial or total lifting of the flap off of the reconstructed nasal framework, which gives ample room for additional thinning and contouring of the flap, afforded by the enhanced blood supply resulting from the delay phenomenon. As suggested, the cartilage tip

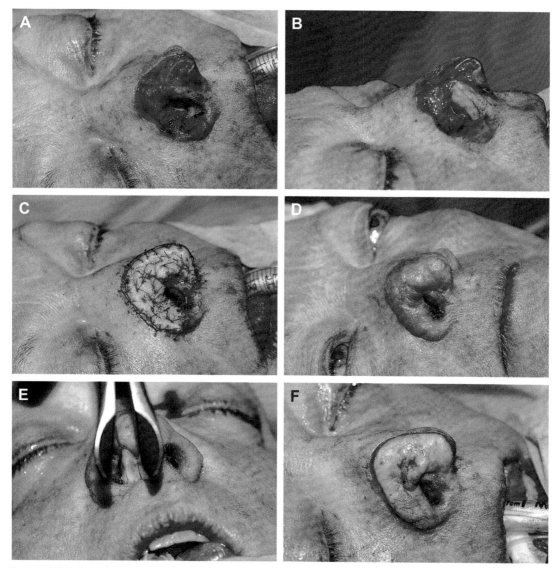

Fig. 16. (A) Full-thickness defect of the nasal tip, alar, and soft triangle. This defect is approaching a hemi-nasal defect and requires a demanding reconstruction. (B) Profile view demonstrates degree of inner lining missing. (C) To bring in more tissue for lining reconstruction in a preliminary stage a FTSG is placed over the defect. (D) Following healing of FTSG. Note that some retraction of the remaining ala/sill has occurred. (E) Septal deviation, clinically significant, to be corrected in the same stage. (F) FTSG incised, elevated, and folded in to reconstruct inner lining defect.

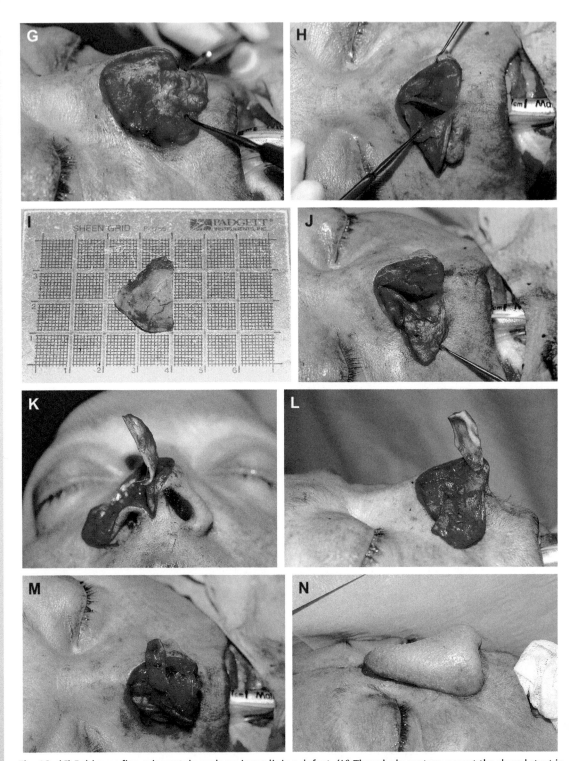

Fig. 16. (*G*) Fold over flap adequately replaces inner lining defect. (*H*) The whole septum except the dorsal strut is taken out to be placed more caudally in the midline. (*I*) Cartilage septal graft to recreate the caudal strut. (*J*) Neo-septum in midline caudal position will provide additional support for the alar and sidewall reconstruction. (*K, L*) Neo-alar cartilage harvested from the cymba of the ear, reattached to neo-septum. (*M*) Butterfly graft added for lateralization of the reconstructed cartilaginous side wall. (*N*) Initial forehead flap is oversized so as not to deform the initially fragile cartilaginous reconstruction.

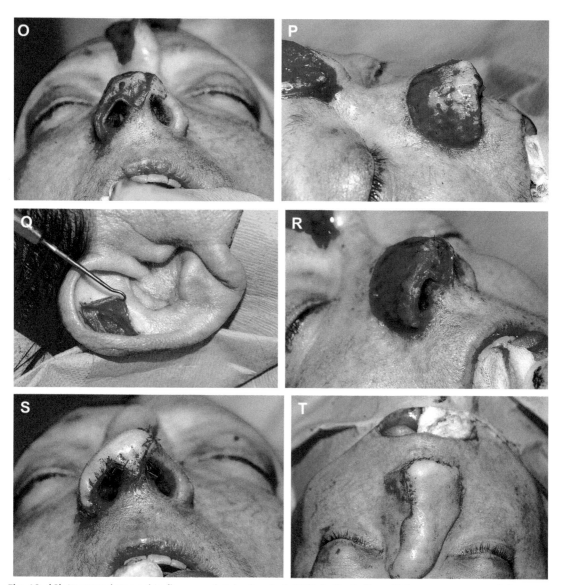

Fig. 16. (O) At second stage skin flap completely elevated. (P) Note the bulky soft-tissue component of the reconstruction after flap elevation. This component will need to be progressively thinned and further sculpted with cartilage to create ideal framework for the forehead flap, which will be replaced again. (Q) Further cartilage grafts taken from scapha for tip grafting. (R) Molding of the lateral cartilage grafts, tip graft added. (S) Basal view following decrease of lateral cartilage ring dimension to harmonize both sides, flap thinning, and inset. (T) Frontal view following flap thinning and inset.

framework may also need more sculpturing or adding of cartilage. The timing of the second and third stage is 3 to 4 weeks and 6 to 8 weeks, respectively, after the initial operation. At the final stage the flap pedicle is divided and only a small portion of the pedicle base is worked into the inter-brow/nasal area. The following two case studies (**Figs. 16** and **17**) sum up the extensive possibilities of current day nasal reconstruction

a posttraumatic defect from the war zone in Iraq (**Fig. 16**) and a previous forehead flap reconstruction performed elsewhere (**Fig. 17**).

COLUMELLA RECONSTRUCTION

Columella defects may be congenital, infectious, traumatic, or surgical. The obvious aesthetic deformity may be compounded by loss of tip

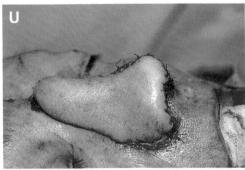
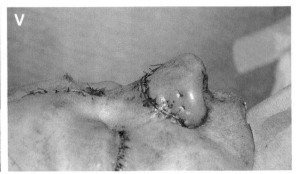
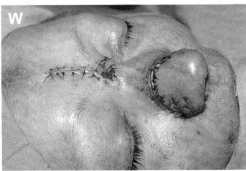

Fig. 16. (*U*) Profile view showing supratip break and good contour match. (*V*) At last stage the pedicle is severed and set in. (*W*) Some light mattress sutures to eliminate dead space. Good contour and function to be anticipated.

support. Again, the whole range of reconstructive options may apply: primary closure, second intention healing, skin/composite grafts, skin flaps, and even microvascular techniques.[33–35]

Columella Anatomy

The columella extends from the infratip lobule to the nostril sill. The cartilaginous portion of the columella is composed of the medial crus demonstrating some flaring caudally to form the medial crural footplates (see **Figs. 2** and **3**). The width of the columella is largely determined by the distance between the medial crura and the flare of the crural footplates (see **Fig. 3**). The columella is crucial in tip support. Indeed, the medial crura do figure prominently in both the tripod and M-Arch concept.[36,37]

The skin of the columella is thin and adherent to the underlying cartilage. The columella skin is continuous with the membranous septum. The position and shape of the septum obviously has impact on the columella. The blood supply is derived from the superior labial arteries giving off the paired columella and anterior septal branches. In the lateral view a 2-mm columella show is ideal. From the anterior view a gull wing appearance is suggested by both ala and the columella.

Skin Resurfacing

When considering the various reconstructive options, including the application of the subunit principle, several variables can be taken into account. The skin of the columella, infratip lobule, the soft triangle and alar margin is thin. These areas are also non-sebaceous, giving the skin a more smooth quality.[1] This skin lends itself well to reconstruction with full-thickness skin and composite grafts. Grafting of defects larger than 1 cm with composite grafts leads to suboptimal survival.[38] Experience with open rhinoplasty has shown that scars in the columella region can be well hidden even when not conforming to subunit transition zones.[39–41]

Cartilaginous Framework and Tip Support

Defects of the columella often involve deficiencies of one or both medial crura, which are often essential in tip support. To avoid loss of tip position, reconstruction of the cartilaginous support is required. The actual amount of cartilage needed to reconstruct the support mechanism is minimal in small defects. A free cartilaginous strut from the septum or pinna (see **Fig. 4E**) and coverage with full-thickness skin grafts or skin flaps[1] may be all that is needed. For small columella, vestibular, and soft-triangle defects, an auricular composite graft is ideally suited. As the defect increases in size, the resultant demand on the cartilaginous framework increases. A more elaborate and stronger cartilaginous support must be strived for. Rhinoplasty techniques may be useful in these situations. Septal extension grafts,[42] subtotal septal repositioning,[43] or a rib cartilage neo-septal/spreader graft structure[44] may be indicated. These grafts do find suture-fixated caudal support on the nasal spine.

Common Types of Defects Classified by Reconstructive Need

In attempt to rationalize reconstructive options to a manageable framework the authors categorize the defect depending on deficient structures that

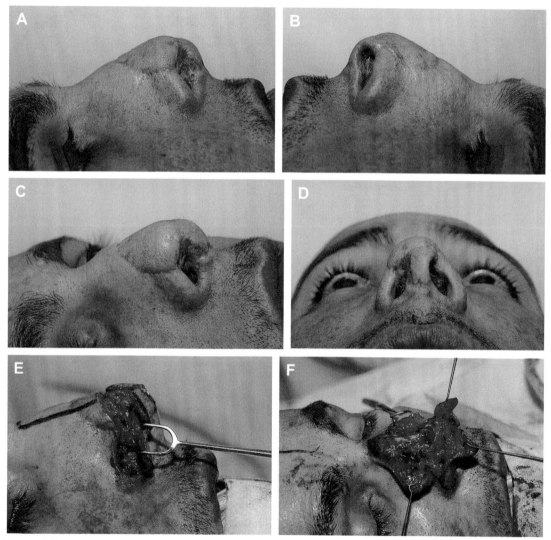

Fig. 17. (A) Post-traumatic defect from war zone in Iraq. Previous forehead flap reconstruction carried out elsewhere. There is scarring retraction and notching of alar margins presents a through and through defect on both sides. (B) Loss of tip projection, tip defining point, supratip break point, columella break point. (C) Unaesthetic appearance with significant scarring and asymmetry of alar margins and alar retraction. (D) Scarring has produced buckling of the alar cartilages. (E) Subunit excision of alar, soft triangle, tip is planned, which will be developed into hinge flaps that will be the inner lining on both sides. (F) Because of retraction, the nasal length is not adequate. The excess skin is folded over for inner lining.

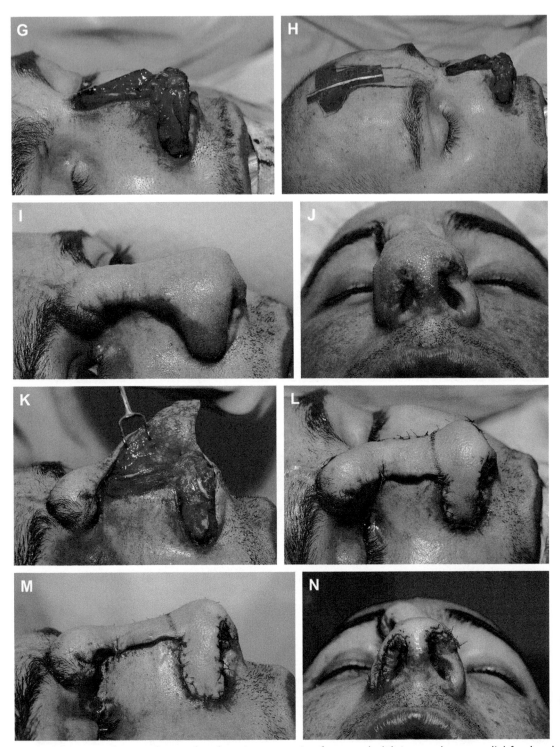

Fig. 17. (*G*) Free cartilage grafts are placed to give supporting framework. (*H*) A second para medial forehead flap is planned. In those cases, Doppler studies are available to know if supratrochlear artery is viable. (*I*) Flap initially bulky following first stage. (*J*) Basal view following first stage. (*K*) At second stage, flap elevated, thinned, framework also sculpted. Flap is left attached distally at columella only. (*L*) End of second stage showing significant reduction in the thickness of the flap and improved contour. (*M*) Reduction in flap thickness shows acceptable profile view, however further thinning will be required for optimal aesthetic result. (*N*) Basal view at the end of second stage showing significant reduction in the thickness of the flap and improved contour that is required.

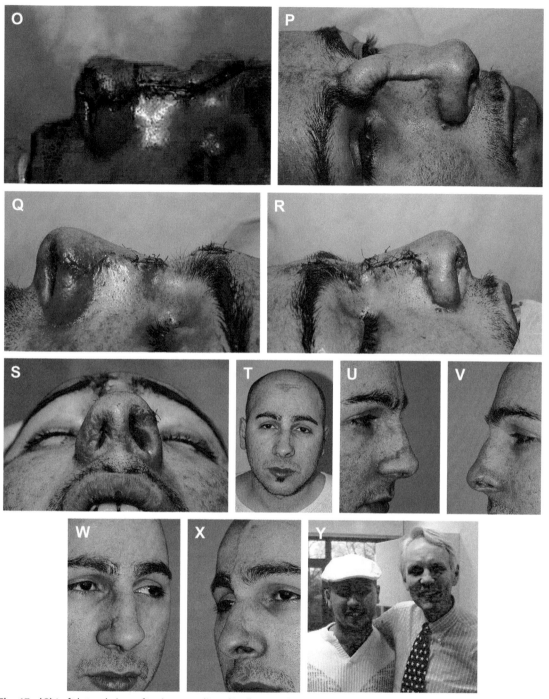

Fig. 17. (*O*) Left lateral view after intermediate (2nd) stage thinning, further thinning will be required at the final (3rd) stage (see fig. 17Q) for comparison. (*P*) Beginning of third stage again demonstrates the importance of thinning the flap at the second stage. Edema and flap retraction has again increased the bulkiness of the flap, which will now require further careful thinning. (*Q*) Third stage, the pedicle is divided and flap is thinned and set in to dorsal contour. The left alar flap is partly lifted again, thinned, soft tissues sculpted, and flap trimmed. (*R, S*) Note the distal attachment of the flap has not been elevated to allow thinning of the cephalic portion of the flap. (*T*) 17-month postoperative good alar symmetry without alar retraction or notching. Donor-site morbidity of second forehead flap minimal. (*U, V*) Aesthetic male profile view with maintenance of the supratip break point of tip defining point (transition from supratip to infratip lobule) and columella break point. (*W, X*) Oblique views showing good outcome of the reconstructed alar and soft triangle, using the subunit principle. (*Y*) Delighted patient in after operation with senior author.

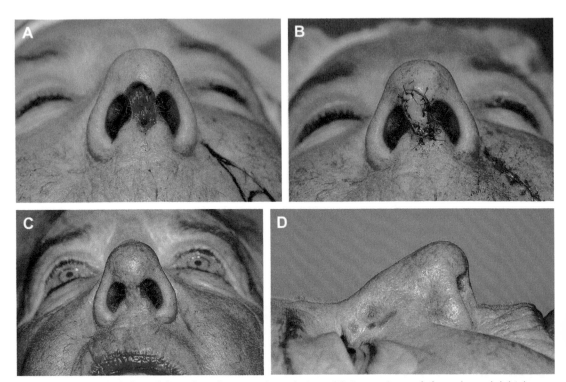

Fig. 18. (*A*) Skin-only defect of the columella approximately 1 cm. (*B*) Composite graft from the melolabial crease to maximize contour and color match. (*C*) Excellent 12-month postoperative result. (*D*) Good contour match.

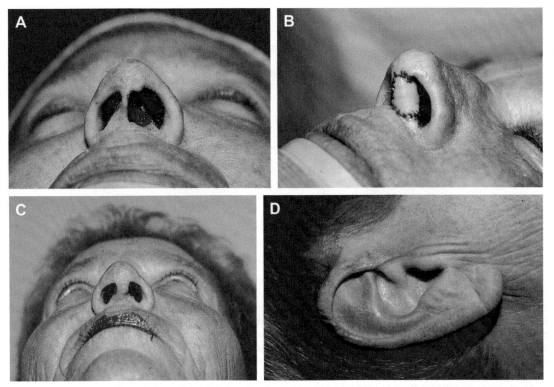

Fig. 19. (*A, B*) Skin cartilage defect of the left hemi-columella repaired with composite skin cartilage graft taken from the helical root. (*C, D*) 12-month postoperative result showing excellent outcome with minimal scaring.

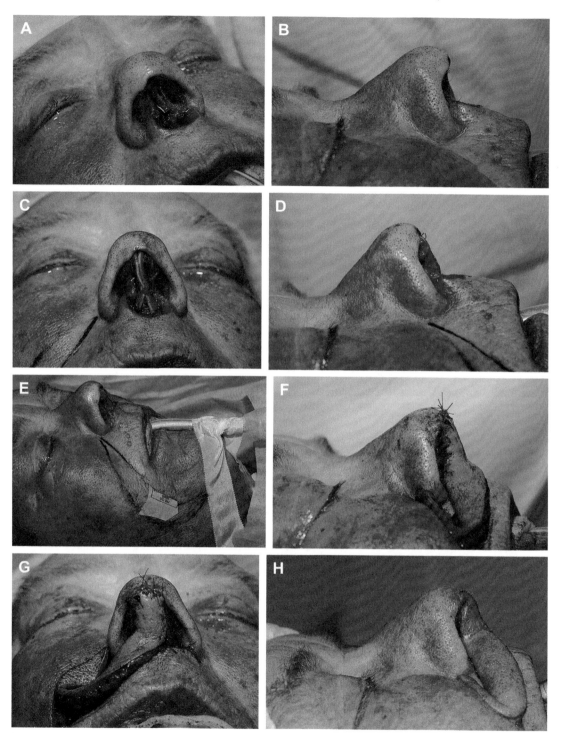

Fig. 20. (*A*) Complete loss of columella subunit with limited extension onto philtrum and infratip lobule. Medial crus of alar cartilages have been resected. (*B*) Profile view shows the loss of tip support and degree of tissue loss from the columella. (*C*) Bilateral medial crus are reconstructed with conchal cartilage, note normal flaring of footplates is reproduced to achieve an anatomic reconstruction. (*D*) Correct alar/columella relationship. (*E*) Subcutaneous melolabial flap planned with aid of template of the columella defect. (*F, G*) Interpolated flap is inset. (*H*) At second (intermediate) stage excess soft tissue requires thinning.

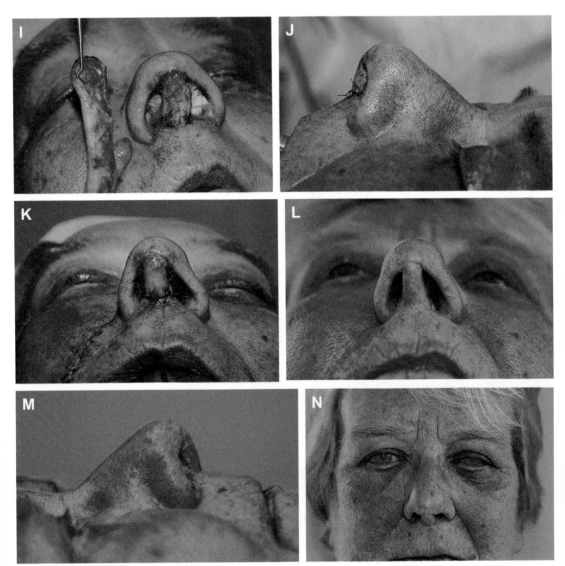

Fig. 20. (*I*) Intermediate second stage, the interpolated subcutaneous-based melolabial flap is raised and cartilage strut is inset and the flap is thinned. (*J*) Third stage pedicle is divided and discarded. (*K*) Donor site closed primarily. (*L*) The 13-month postoperative result, complete reconstruction of columella subunit. (*M*) No columella retraction, ideal columella show (columella/alar relationship). (*N*) Good contour, minimal donor-site morbidity.

will dictate optimal reconstructive choice. Of course some reconstructions will be suitable in more than 1 category.

Skin defects
Given a matching donor site, skin grafts are excellent substitutes for effectively replacing the thin,

smooth skin of the columella. However, skin-graft contracture may produce a skeletonized, unnatural appearance to the reconstructed columella. A composite skin and subcutaneous fat graft may indeed provide a more natural outcome. Although a slightly higher population of sebaceous glands is found in the melolabial donor site, it does match

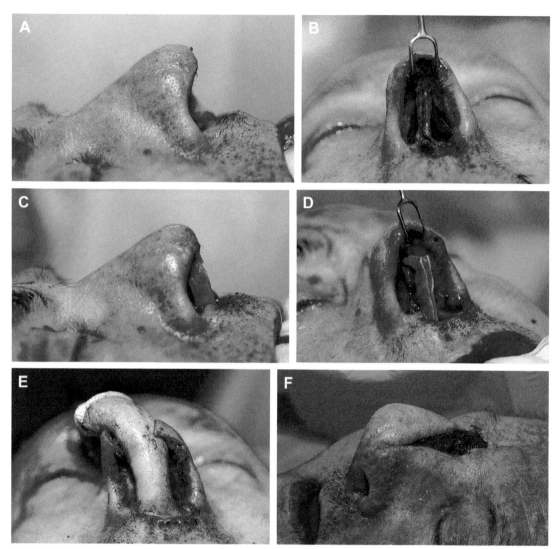

Fig. 21. (*A*) Combined tip columella defect. (*B*) Complete loss of columella (skin and medial crura) and a proportion of alar sill. (*C*) Columella strut fashioned and fixed to residual septum from spreaders from auricular cartilage and alar cartilages (rib grafts not used because of patient's age). (*D*) Cartilage frame work/neo-septum in situ. (*E*) Forehead flap used for skin coverage, note that the tip skin was split to inset in flap. (*F*) At second stage patient declined intermediate stage.

fairly well with the original columellar skin. **Fig. 18** presents a composite skin-fat graft to the columella.

When the skin defect is larger than 1 cm, alternatives to skin grafts must be sought. Various local flaps, such as the subnasale,[45–47] alar rim, and nostril sill flaps,[48] transpose tissue from the columella base and peri-columella areas. They, however, provide limited amounts of skin, both in terms of width and lengths. Regional flaps (nasolabial, naso-facial, and forehead) offer abundant tissue to resurface the columella. A unilateral

melolabial flap is sufficient to resurface the entire subunit, providing both contour and color match.

Skin-cartilaginous defects

For minor skin-cartilaginous columella defects, free auricular composite grafts are beneficial in view of their good color and skin-type match (**Fig. 19**). With the inclusion of the cartilage, the tip support is enhanced.

For larger skin-cartilaginous defects, the entire subunit skin/medial crus may require

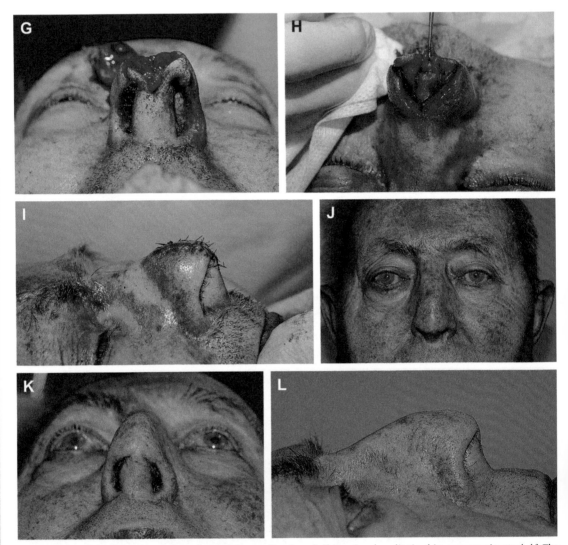

Fig. 21. (*G*) Pedicle divided and discarded. (*H*) Tip grafts placed. (*I*) Previously split tip skin reapproximated. (*J*) The 17-month postoperative result. (*K*) Slightly bulky reconstruction caused by the fact that the patient also declined further thinning. (*L*) Some loss of tip projection, a hanging columella result from the inability to thin the columella in an intermediate procedure.

reconstruction. Much attention must be given to robustly reconstructing the cartilage framework for support and contour purposes (**Fig. 20**).

Alternatively to the nasolabial flap, a naso-facial flap may be considered. This flap is harvested from the naso-facial sulcus with a subcutaneous inferior pedicle centered on the angular artery. The facial artery, vein, and investing muscular tissues are isolated as far inferiorly as the alar crease. The flap is then tunneled subcutaneously under the alar crease into the columella defect.[49]

For skin coverage of larger defects, either bilateral nasolabial flaps[50,51] or a forehead flap may be applied. If this coverage is not sufficient, it can be combined with bilateral septal mucoperichondrial flaps. A forehead flap, which is folded into the vestibular defect, will initially be too thick and may need thinning over time. A forehead flap does provide enough tissue to reconstruct a concomitant tip defect while reaching as far as the columellar base (**Fig. 21**).

When the columella defect is associated with significant upper-lip tissue loss, an Abbe flap

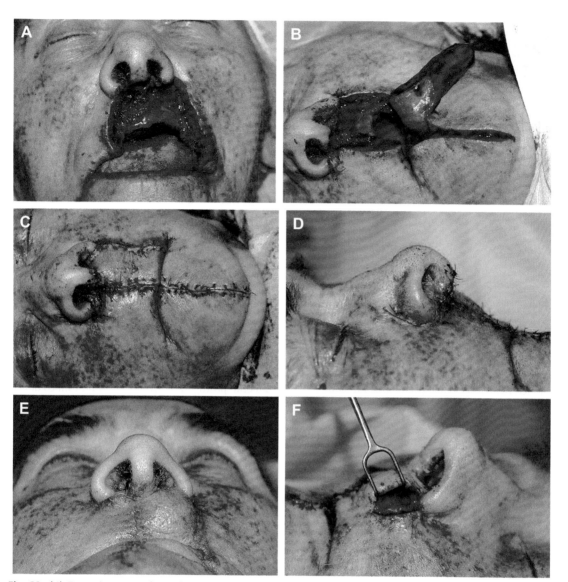

Fig. 22. (A) Extensive upper-lip, columella, and left-vestibular defect. The columella was skin defect only and therefore cartilaginous framework reconstruction not deemed necessary. Extended Abbe flap applied. If required, the Abbe flap may provide for a complete columella reconstruction. (B) Large full-thickness upper-lip columella defect repaired with Abbe flap. (C) Flap set in at first stage, reconstructing inferior aspect of columella. (D) Loss of support of basal columella causes inferior displacement and bowing. (E) At second stage, significant pincushion deformity can be seen. (F) Lip pedicle severed and set in. Excess subcutaneous tissue of the flap excised and columella repositioned with oval membranous septal excisions.

extended onto the chin region does provide enough tissue to reconstruct part of the columella with the same technique (**Fig. 22**).[52] The vascular supply of the extended Abbe flap is based on a circumoral labial arcade made up of bilateral inferior and superior labial arteries. The vascular supply of the inferior cutaneous territory encompasses the skin of the entire lower lip, chin, and extending to the submental skin, which indeed can be pedicled on this flap.[53]

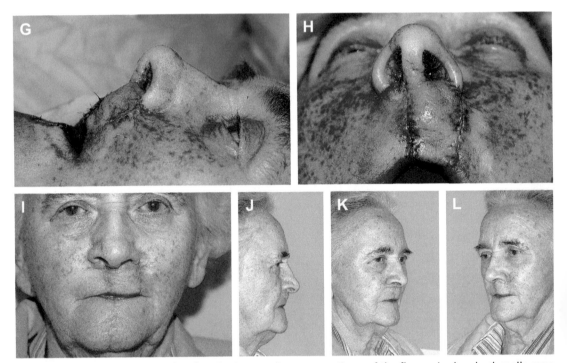

Fig. 22. (*G–H*) Lip pedicle severed and set in. Excess subcutaneous tissue of the flap excised and columella repositioned with oval membranous septal excisions. (*I–L*) The 3-month postoperative result, no significant columella retraction.

SUMMARY

Reconstruction of the nasal tip and columella is a complex task. Patients have 2 aims: a tumor-free nasal tip and a reconstruction that does not draw attention away from the eyes. To attain this goal the surgeon must adapt what remains after complete tumor removal, replacing the skin, cartilaginous framework and inner lining. A purely anatomic reconstruction is often insufficient because healing forces must be accounted for. To avoid late contraction extra anatomical cartilage grafts to buttress the reconstruction are often required. Using rhinoplasty skills (cartilage grafting and suture techniques), the ability to replace kind with kind, understanding the contraction of the soft-tissue envelope with scarring, and placing scars in favorable locations are tools to create the best possible result.

REFERENCES

1. Burget GC. Aesthetic reconstruction of the tip of the nose. Dermatol Surg 1995;21(5):419–29.
2. Burget GC, Menick FJ. The subunit principle in nasal reconstruction. Plast Reconstr Surg 1985;76(2): 239–47.
3. Vuyk HD, Lohuis PJFM. 1st edition. Facial plastic and reconstructive surgery, vol. 1. London: Hodder Arnold; 2006.
4. Toriumi DM, Checcone MA. New concepts in nasal tip contouring. Facial Plast Surg Clin North Am 2009;17(1):55–90, vi.
5. Andre RF, Vuyk HD. The "butterfly graft" as a treatment for internal nasal valve incompetence. Plast Reconstr Surg 2008;122(2):73e–4e.
6. Menick FJ. Lining options in nasal reconstruction. Operat Tech Plast Reconstr Surg 1998;5(1): 65–75.
7. Cannady SB, Cook TA, Wax MK. The total nasal defect and reconstruction. Facial Plast Surg Clin North Am 2009;17(2):189–201.
8. Menick FJ. The evolution of lining in nasal reconstruction. Clin Plast Surg 2009;36(3):421–41.
9. van der Eerden PA, Lohuis PJ, Hart AA, et al. Secondary intention healing after excision of nonmelanoma skin cancer of the head and neck: statistical evaluation of prognostic values of wound characteristics and final cosmetic results. Plast Reconstr Surg 2008;122(6):1747–55.
10. Lee KK, Mehrany K, Swanson NA. Fusiform elliptical Burow's graft: a simple and practical esthetic approach for nasal tip reconstruction. Dermatol Surg 2006;32(1):91–5.

11. Gloster HM Jr. The use of full-thickness skin grafts to repair nonperforating nasal defects. J Am Acad Dermatol 2000;42(6):1041–50.

12. van der Eerden P, Simmons M, Zuur K, et al. Full-thickness skin grafts and perichondrial cutaneous grafts following surgical removal of cutaneous neoplasms of the head and neck. Eur Arch Otorhinolaryngol 2010;267(8):1277–83.

13. Rustemeyer J, Gunther L, Bremerich A. Complications after nasal skin repair with local flaps and full-thickness skin grafts and implications of patients' contentment. Oral Maxillofac Surg 2009; 13(1):15–9.

14. Robinson JK, Dillig G. The advantages of delayed nasal full-thickness skin grafting after Mohs micrographic surgery. Dermatol Surg 2002;28(9):845–51.

15. McCluskey PD, Constantine FC, Thornton JF. Lower third nasal reconstruction: when is skin grafting an appropriate option? Plast Reconstr Surg 2009; 124(3):826–35.

16. Dimitropoulos V, Bichakjian CK, Johnson TM. Forehead donor site full-thickness skin graft. Dermatol Surg 2005;31(3):324–6.

17. Hubbard TJ. Leave the fat, skip the bolster: thinking outside the box in lower third nasal reconstruction. Plast Reconstr Surg 2004;114(6):1427–35.

18. Menick FJ. 1st edition. Nasal reconstruction art and practice, vol. 1. St Louis: Mosby Elsevier; 2008.

19. Zitelli JA. The bilobed flap for nasal reconstruction. Arch Dermatol 1989;125(7):957–9.

20. Cho M, Kim DW. Modification of the Zitelli bilobed flap: a comparison of flap dynamics in human cadavers. Arch Facial Plast Surg 2006;8(6):404–9 [discussion: 410].

21. Zoumalan RA, Hazan C, Levine VJ, et al. Analysis of vector alignment with the Zitelli bilobed flap for nasal defect repair: a comparison of flap dynamics in human cadavers. Arch Facial Plast Surg 2008; 10(3):181–5.

22. Bitgood MJ, Hybarger CP. Expanded applications of the dorsal nasal flap. Arch Facial Plast Surg 2007; 9(5):344–51.

23. Zimbler MS, Thomas JR. The dorsal nasal flap revisited: aesthetic refinements in nasal reconstruction. Arch Facial Plast Surg 2000;2(4):285–6.

24. Rohrich RJ, Muzaffar AR, Adams WP Jr, et al. The aesthetic unit dorsal nasal flap: rationale for avoiding a glabellar incision. Plast Reconstr Surg 1999; 104(5):1289–94.

25. Menick FJ. A 10-year experience in nasal reconstruction with the three-stage forehead flap. Plast Reconstr Surg 2002;109(6):1839–55 [discussion: 1856–61].

26. Burget GC. Modification of the subunit principle. Arch Facial Plast Surg 1999;1(1):16–8.

27. Singh DJ, Bartlett SP. Aesthetic considerations in nasal reconstruction and the role of modified nasal subunits. Plast Reconstr Surg 2003;111(2):639–48 [discussion: 649–51].

28. Shumrick KA, Smith TL. The anatomic basis for the design of forehead flaps in nasal reconstruction. Arch Otolaryngol Head Neck Surg 1992;118(4): 373–9.

29. Kelly CP, Yavuzer R, Keskin M, et al. Functional anastomotic relationship between the supratrochlear and facial arteries: an anatomical study. Plast Reconstr Surg 2008;121(2):458–65.

30. Reece EM, Schaverien M, Rohrich RJ. The paramedian forehead flap: a dynamic anatomical vascular study verifying safety and clinical implications. Plast Reconstr Surg 2008;121(6):1956–63.

31. Kleintjes WG. Forehead anatomy: arterial variations and venous link of the midline forehead flap. J Plast Reconstr Aesthet Surg 2007;60(6):593–606.

32. Burget GC, Menick FJ, editors. Aesthetic reconstruction of the nose. 2nd edition. St Louis (MO): Mosby; 1994. p. 57–92.

33. Ozek C, Gundogan H, Bilkay U, et al. Nasal columella reconstruction with a composite free flap from the root of auricular helix. Microsurgery 2002; 22(2):53–6.

34. Livaoglu M, Karacal N, Bektas D, et al. Reconstruction of full-thickness nasal defect by free anterolateral thigh flap. Acta Otolaryngol 2009; 129(5):541–4.

35. Walton RL, Burget GC, Beahm EK. Microsurgical reconstruction of the nasal lining. Plast Reconstr Surg 2005;115(7):1813–29.

36. Anderson JR. A reasoned approach to nasal base surgery. Arch Otolaryngol 1984;110(6):349–58.

37. Adamson PA, Litner JA, Dahiya R. The M-Arch model: a new concept of nasal tip dynamics. Arch Facial Plast Surg 2006;8(1):16–25.

38. Lin SD, Lin GT, Lai CS, et al. Nasal alar reconstruction with free "accessory auricle". Plast Reconstr Surg 1984;73(5):827–9.

39. Adamson PA, Smith O, Tropper GJ. Incision and scar analysis in open (external) rhinoplasty. Arch Otolaryngol Head Neck Surg 1990;116(6):671–5.

40. Adamson PA. Open rhinoplasty. Otolaryngol Clin North Am 1987;20(4):837–52.

41. Friedman GD, Gruber RP. A fresh look at the open rhinoplasty technique. Plast Reconstr Surg 1988; 82(6):973–82.

42. Toriumi DM. New concepts in nasal tip contouring. Arch Facial Plast Surg 2006;8(3):156–85.

43. Andre RF, Vuyk HD. Reconstruction of dorsal and/or caudal nasal septum deformities with septal battens or by septal replacement: an overview and comparison of techniques. Laryngoscope 2006;116(9): 1668–73.

44. Ahmed A, Imani P, Vuyk HD. Reconstruction of significant saddle nose deformity using autogenous costal cartilage graft with incorporated mirror

image spreader grafts. Laryngoscope 2010;120(3): 491–4.

45. Jung DH, Chang GU, Baek SH, et al. Subnasal flap for correction of columella base deviation in secondary unilateral cleft lip nasal deformity. J Craniofac Surg 2010;21(1):146–50.

46. MacFarlane DF, Goldberg LH. The nasal floor transposition flap for repairing distal nose/columella defects. Dermatol Surg 1998;24(10):1085–6.

47. Mavili ME, Akyurek M. Congenital isolated absence of the nasal columella: reconstruction with an internal nasal vestibular skin flap and bilateral labial mucosa flaps. Plast Reconstr Surg 2000;106(2):393–9.

48. Gillies H. The columella. Br J Plast Surg 1949;2(3): 192–201, illust.

49. Sherris DA, Fuerstenberg J, Danahey D, et al. Reconstruction of the nasal columella. Arch Facial Plast Surg 2002;4(1):42–6.

50. Yanai A, Nagata S, Tanaka H. Reconstruction of the columella with bilateral nasolabial flaps. Plast Reconstr Surg 1986;77(1):129–32.

51. Nicolai JP. Reconstruction of the columella with nasolabial flaps. Head Neck Surg 1982;4(5): 374–9.

52. Naficy S, Baker SR. The extended Abbe flap in the reconstruction of complex midfacial defects. Arch Facial Plast Surg 2000;2(2):141–4.

53. Kriet JD, Cupp CL, Sherris DA, et al. The extended Abbe flap. Laryngoscope 1995;105(9 Pt 1): 988–92.

Reconstruction of Alar Defects

Jason D. Bloom, MD[a],*, Evan R. Ransom, MD[b],
Christopher J. Miller, MD[c]

KEYWORDS

- Nasal reconstruction • Nasal ala • Flap reconstruction

ANATOMY

Successful reconstruction of the nose depends on a thorough understanding of the anatomic and functional components of the ala. The crescentic alar groove serves as a topographic landmark that frames the ala and separates this convex structure from the surrounding cosmetic subunits. The ala abuts the nasal tip anteriorly and the nasal sidewall superiorly. The alar groove deepens as it extends posteriorly. This posterior portion of the alar groove is often called the alar-facial sulcus and separates the ala from the cheek and hairless apical triangle of the lip.

The ala is a critical cosmetic and functional landmark. The distal free margin of the alar lobule and the transition from the shadows of the alar groove to the reflection of the convex surface of the ala are important visual landmarks. The ala also frames the lateral aspect of the external nasal valve, a critical path for airflow during inspiration. Altered position of the ala during reconstructive surgery can compromise function of the external nasal valve. Relative to the nasal tip and sidewall, the alar tissue is more compliant, because it does not contain cartilage.[1] The alar lobule consists of skeletal muscle and fat enveloped by dermis and epithelium on both the vestibular and external aspects.[2] The lower lateral cartilage does not cross the alar groove and it is not part of the alar lobule.[2] The lack of an intrinsic osseous-cartilaginous skeleton and the complete absence

of support at its distal free margin make this delicate structure particularly susceptible to distortion during reconstructive surgery.

Although the alar lobule does not contain cartilage, the ala gains dynamic and static support from the close relationship of its muscles with the osseous-cartilaginous framework of the nose.[1] A brief description of the osseous-cartilaginous framework is helpful. The nasal bone and maxilla frame the pyriform aperture. The paired upper lateral cartilages are firmly stabilized as they flare laterally from cartilaginous septum and fix to the deep aspect of the nasal bone. The intercartilaginous ligament stabilizes the cephalic margin of the lateral crura of the lower lateral cartilages to the caudal aspect of the upper lateral cartilages.[3] The lower lateral cartilages gain additional stability from loose connective tissue that links the domes of the lower lateral cartilages and possibly from direct connection of the medial crura with the caudal septum.[3] A fascial system, called the pyriform ligament, stabilizes the entire cartilaginous framework by connecting the lateral cartilages with the pyriform rim.[4]

The alar lobule essentially suspends from this osseous-cartilaginous framework as a network of skin and skeletal muscles. The actions of skeletal muscles on the position of the nasal ala remain poorly understood.[1,4,5] The dilatator naris muscle is the main muscular component of the alar lobule. The dilatator naris muscle originates from the lateral crus of the lower lateral cartilage and inserts

[a] Division of Facial Plastic and Reconstructive Surgery, Department of Otolaryngology, New York University Medical Center, 550 First Avenue, NBV Suite 5E5, New York, NY 10016, USA
[b] Department of Otorhinolaryngology: Head & Neck Surgery, University of Pennsylvania Health System, 3400 Spruce Street, 5 Silverstein, Philadelphia, PA 19104, USA
[c] Division of Dermatologic Surgery, Department of Dermatology, Perelman Center for Advanced Medicine, University of Pennsylvania Health System, 3400 Civic Center Boulevard, Suite 1-330S, Philadelphia, PA 19104, USA
* Corresponding author.
E-mail address: bloomj@gmail.com

Facial Plast Surg Clin N Am 19 (2011) 63–83
doi:10.1016/j.fsc.2010.10.009

directly onto the alar skin.[1] Contraction of this dilatator naris muscle opens the nostril and may indirectly, via the intercartilaginous ligament, affect the caudal margin of the upper lateral cartilage and internal nasal valve.[1] The alar portion of the nasalis muscle originates from the fossa incisiva of the maxilla and inserts on the alar skin and accessory cartilages near the pyriform aperture. Contraction of this muscle may dilate the nasal valve area by drawing the accessory cartilages, and by extension, the lateral crura, laterally.[1] By contrast, the transverse portion of the nasalis muscle does not insert on the nasal cartilages and it mainly stabilizes the valve area by moving nasal skin. Additional dynamic support to the ala may come from the levator labii superioris alaeque nasi, which pulls the ala superiomedially,[5] and from the levator labii superioris muscle, which partially inserts on the vestibular skin of the nasal vestibule and widens the nostril by pulling it superolaterally.[4]

In addition to the structural and supporting tissue of the ala, the sensory and motor innervation, vascular supply, and lining all play intricate parts in the nasal alar anatomy. The dilator naris anterior, levator labii superioris alaeque nasi, and alar nasalis muscles are innervated by the buccal branch of the facial nerve (CN VII). The sensory innervation to the caudal and lateral portions of the nose are supplied by the external branch of the anterior ethmoidal nerve (branch of V1) and branches of the infraorbital nerve (V2).[6] The vascular supply to the nasal ala is derived from multiple branches of both the external and internal carotid artery systems. The facial artery gives off the superior labial and angular arteries, both of which contribute blood supply to the ala. Branches of the infraorbital artery, lateral nasal artery, and the external nasal branch of the anterior ethmoid artery also supply blood to the ala.[6,7]

In addition, because the nasal ala borders a free margin, the undersurface of the ala incorporates a combination of nasal vestibular skin and mucosal lining, going further into the nose. The importance of an intact nasal lining should not be underestimated, because if it is not replaced during a nasal reconstructive procedure, the nasal ala can become distorted from the contraction of this intranasal tissue void.

The structure and support of the nasal valves are linked to the anatomy and function of this area of the nose. The external nasal valve has been described as the area bounded by the caudal edge of the upper lateral cartilage superolaterally, the nasal ala and attachment of the lateral crus laterally, the caudal septum and columella medially, and the nasal sill inferiorly.[8] This area is variable and dependent on the shape, size, and strength of the lower lateral cartilage. Located just superior to the external nasal valve is the site of greatest resistance in the entire human airway, the internal nasal valve. Anatomically, the internal nasal valve is the cross-sectional area bounded superiorly by the upper lateral cartilage, cartilaginous nasal septum medially, anterior head of the inferior turbinate laterally, and nasal floor inferiorly. This valve angle is normally between 10 and 15 degrees in whites, but tends to be more obtuse in ethnic African Americans and Asians. The cross-sectional area of the internal nasal valve is about 0.73 cm.[2,9]

ANALYSIS OF THE ALAR DEFECT

The reconstructive surgeon must carefully analyze the defect to determine precisely what is missing. Originally described by Manson and colleagues,[10] nasal reconstruction should be viewed as a 3-part approach. The overlying skin, structural framework, and internal lining should be evaluated individually before developing an operative plan. Furthermore, the nostril free margin, contour, and relationship of the external nasal valve are vital to both a functional and aesthetic alar reconstruction. Preoperative recognition of whether reconstruction of the defect needs skin coverage, nonanatomic cartilage support, internal lining, or a combination of these allows for optimum results.

The skin of the nasal ala is thick and sebaceous. The skin in the region of the ala is also tightly adherent to the underlying muscles of facial expression. Consequently, the skin of the ala affords considerably less mobility or laxity compared with the skin of the nasal sidewalls and dorsum. To achieve aesthetic reconstructions of alar tissue, the surgeon strives to recruit skin with a similar thick texture and sebaceous character, such as the skin immediately adjacent to the defect or from the more distant melolabial fold and forehead.

Other factors that may influence reconstructive options of soft tissue defects include the quality of the wound bed and patient history. Patients who have prior nasal scars in the vicinity, current smokers, or those with a history of radiation to the area of the defect require an especially judicious choice of reconstruction. In such patients, the surgeon may limit the risk of necrosis by avoiding skin grafts, by delaying a flap before transfer, or by lengthening the amount of time between the flap transfer and pedicle division and insetting.[11]

In addition to the soft tissue defect, the surgeon must assess the status of theosseous-cartilagenous skeleton, which provides critical support to the ala. If portions of the lower lateral cartilage are missing or if the defect is sufficiently close to the alar margin, there is an increased risk of distortion and alar retraction or notching. Loss of structural support at the alar rim can lead to distortion of the position of the free alar margin and functional problems, such as external nasal valve collapse. To prevent these issues, the use of cartilaginous grafting to repair a deficient lateral crus or nonanatomic alar batten grafts placed at the time of primary reconstruction help to prevent external valve collapse and alar retraction.[12,13] Nonanatomic free cartilage grafts both add structural support and provide a scaffold over which the skin can mold for an aesthetic contour.

The third and final aspect of alar defect analysis pertains to the nasal lining. If the nasal mucosal lining is missing and not replaced, contraction and distortion of the alar reconstruction is likely. Besides the obvious scar contracture that can occur, lining tissue is vital to providing a vascular supply to free cartilage grafts that are used in the reconstruction of full-thickness alar defects. If the cartilage does not have an adequate blood supply on either side of the graft, the cartilage has a high risk for necrosis.[13] Small holes in the mucosal lining can sometimes be closed primarily, if the lining is able to be freed up and advanced. However, larger defects often require other tissue and various flaps for repair. Multiple techniques can fill lining defects with intranasal mucosa, such as bipedicled, septal mucoperichondrial, and turbinate flaps.[13,14] In addition, skin grafts, turn-in flaps, and local tissue flaps can replace missing lining, but often require delayed cartilage grafting or subsequent contouring procedures.[14]

The size of the defect relative to the remaining portions of the subunit may also influence reconstruction options. Burget and Menick[15] introduced multiple principles for reconstruction of the cosmetic subunits of the nose, including the idea that if a defect involved more than 50% of the surface area of any subunit, the entire subunit should be resected. These investigators and others have demonstrated that strict adherence to this principle of complete cosmetic subunit repair is not always necessary.[11,16] The reconstruction must preserve and restore normal contour. In some instances, the surgeon can best preserve the subtle shadows and reflections of the ala by leaving intact skin. For example, it is often better to leave a millimeter or 2 of the alar-facial groove than to resect it and try to recreate it during the reconstruction.

RECONSTRUCTIVE OPTIONS

After methodically evaluating the characteristics of the patient and defect, the surgeon must then choose the most aesthetic reconstruction. For the sake of simplicity, we use a reconstructive ladder to organize reconstruction options from the most basic to the most complex.

Healing by Secondary Intension

Even small defects of the ala often demand considerable time and attention to achieve an excellent cosmetic result. When a simpler option is desirable, the surgeon may consider second intention healing (**Fig. 1**). Studies have shown that, in certain circumstances, healing by secondary intension can produce functional and even cosmetic results equal to or better than those achieved with a flap or graft repair.[17,18] Healing by secondary intention can result in acceptable scars for defects in concavities and subtle indentions of the face and nose.[19] Accordingly, Zitelli[17,18] has described the regions of the alar crease as a suitable location for healing by secondary intention. Other investigators have used second intention healing for small defects (<5 mm) in the area of the nasofacial sulcus or in the alar-facial crease.[18,20,21]

Because all scars contract, the surgeon must always account for the possibility that second intention healing will result in alar retraction or obstruction and compromise of the internal or external nasal valves.[22] Larger and deeper defects and a location near the alar rim portend a higher risk for such complications. Second intention healing should be avoided in these instances. As a crude physical test, the surgeon should push the alar rim superiorly. If the rim contracts easily, second intention healing will likely lead to a poor outcome. In most cases, the free margin of the ala will resist the force of scar contraction only for wounds that are shallow (ie, defect involved only epidermis and dermis) and at least 3 mm superior to the alar margin.

Concave surfaces do not always lend themselves to second intention healing. The surgeon must take caution when allowing wounds to heal in the concavities that frame the ala. Webbing that can result from scar contraction can ablate concavities and distort contour. Deep defects at the alar-facial crease are especially susceptible to this type of webbing.

The scars that result from second intention healing are predictably smooth and shiny. The light that reflects from these scars is predictably more harsh, compared with the more subtle reflections as light scatters from the normally

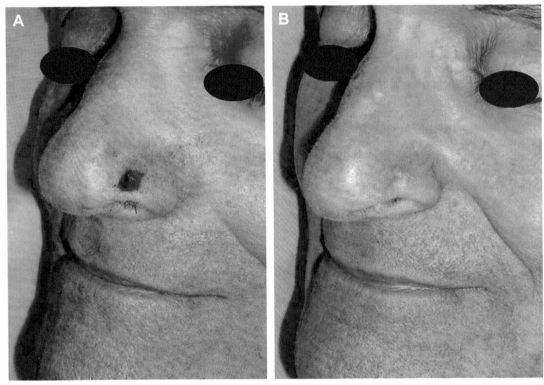

Fig. 1. (*A*) Small shallow defect involving the anterior aspect of the alar groove. (*B*) 4-month postoperative result after secondary intention healing.

textured and sebaceous skin of the ala. Larger, pale, and shiny scars from second intention healing can attract undue attention. The surgeon must prepare the patient for these predictable qualities of the scar.

Full-thickness Skin Graft

Another conservative reconstructive option would be to consider a full-thickness skin graft (FTSG) for an alar defect (**Fig. 2**). Although FTSGs may provide adequate coverage for an alar defect,

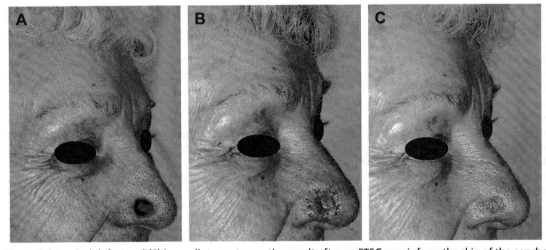

Fig. 2. (*A*) Surgical defect and (*B*) immediate postoperative result after an FTSG repair from the skin of the concha cavum. (*C*) 2-month postoperative result showing the graft with reasonable texture and contour, but a color discrepancy that is typical of skin graft reconstructions.

especially in a patient who may not be medically suitable for a long procedure, it is often difficult to match the texture, color, and thickness of the alar skin. With these difficulties of FTSGs noted, there have been data to support the use of these grafts for shallow nasal tip and alar defects.[23]

With time, FTSGs may frequently develop a depressed, shiny, or patchlike appearance. With this in mind, the surgeon must go back to the functional and cosmetic goals of the patient to produce the optimal result. FTSGs do work well, however, for small, partial-thickness defects of the alar rim with the underlying skeletal muscles still intact.[24] Possible FTSG donor sites include, pre- and postauricular skin, the supraclavicular area and even the melolabial fold. Other excellent donor sites for an FTSG to the nasal ala are the conchal bowl of the ear or the skin of the forehead, given their thicker skin texture, high density of sebaceous glands, and actinic damage similar to the nasal ala, in the case of the forehead skin.[24,25] For an FTSG to have the best aesthetic outcome, it is suggested that a template of the defect be created with the foil from suture packaging or a nonadherent dressing (Telfa). This template allows for the graft to be fashioned exactly according to size, so that it is not too large, causing a pincushion effect or too small, leading to necrosis from tension in securing it to the defect edges. FTSGs are harvested and raised in the subdermal plane and contain the epidermis, dermis, and a very minimal amount of subcutaneous fat, which can be trimmed extensively to reduce the flap bulk. Sufficient contact between the dermis of the FTSG and the recipient defect bed is critical to the processes of imbibition, inosculation, and neovascularization. Therefore, careful defatting of the FTSG helps to improve its survival.

Once transferred into the defect, these grafts are secured to the wound bed with absorbable suture. The donor sites are then closed primarily without tension after minimal undermining. After the graft has been secured in place, it is usually bolstered in place with Xeroform gauze for 5 to 7 days to prevent any shearing forces that may dislodge the graft from the underlying bed and to apply gentle compression to the graft site. This technique assists in optimizing graft adherence and eliminates any dead space under the graft.

Primary Closure

Although primary closure may be a viable option for defects of the loose skin over the nasal dorsum and supratip, few defects of the nasal ala allow this option. Three factors usually preclude this option.

First, because the dermis intermingles with the underlying skeletal muscle of the ala, the skin is relatively stiff and immobile. Second, primary closure almost always threatens the position of the free margin. Primary closures oriented parallel to the alar margin elevate the rim. When primary closures are oriented perpendicular to the rim, the free margin exposes the standing cone and causes a slight downward push at the free margin. Third, primary closures, especially when oriented perpendicular to the free margin, can cause buckling of the soft tissue toward the vestibule, effectively decreasing the size of the external nasal valve. For primary closure in the alar subunit, these problems can cause both cosmetic distortion of the alar free margin and even compromise of the nasal valve from distortion of the nasal cartilages.[21] The lower lateral cartilages usually have enough intrinsic support to overcome wound contracture, but the distortion created from a primary closure could have ill effects on the alar-columellar relationship and nasal tip rotation.[26]

One-stage Flap Reconstructions

Alar advancement-rotation flap

There are few flaps derived entirely from within the alar subunit, and these must be reserved for small defects (eg, approximately 3–4 mm in width). An advancement-rotation flap with the arc based along the alar groove is one such flap. The ideal defect for this flap is located in the anterior half of the ala and is no wider than 3 to 4 mm (**Figs. 3 and 4**). To decide whether this flap will provide a good result, first draw a standing cone from the inferior aspect of the defect extending perpendicularly to the alar rim. If the angle of the standing cone at the alar rim exceeds 20 to 30°, then the flap is likely to distort the contour at the alar margin, and the advancement-rotation flap is a poor reconstructive option.

Next, extend the defect in a narrow column superiorly until it meets the alar groove. From the point where this extension of the defect intersects with the alar groove, the arc of the rotation flap can be cut laterally toward the alar-facial sulcus. The flap should then be undermined immediately superficial to the vestibular mucosa, so that the flap contains epidermis, dermis, and the muscles of facial expression. The flap is then rotated to close the defect. A secondary defect will form in the alar groove. The larger the arc of rotation, the larger the secondary defect will become. To close the secondary defect, the cheek is advanced medially. Care should be taken to keep the tension vectors of these sutures parallel to the alar rim.

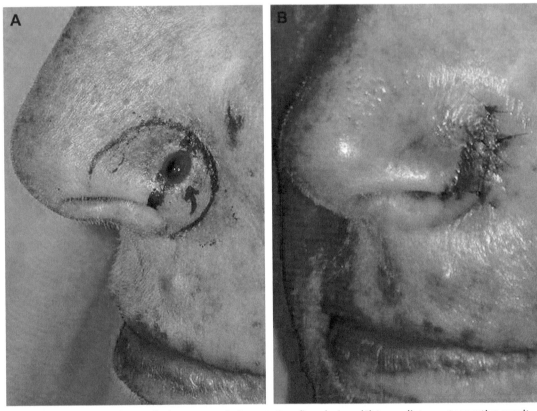

Fig. 3. (*A*) Small alar defect with the proposed alar rotation flap design. (*B*) Immediate postoperative result.

The main advantages of using this local flap are that it is a 1-stage flap with excellent color, thickness, and texture skin match.[27] Also, the arc of the rotation flap is nicely disguised by the natural concavity of the alar groove. However, the flap has some distinct disadvantages. The vertically oriented arm to close the defect and the standing cone can cause a slight downward push at the free margin. If the defect is too large (>1 cm) or the nasal tip cartilages are flimsy, this may lead to buckling of the alar rim and subsequent distortion of that lower lateral cartilage and nasal tip, when the local tissue is advanced for reconstruction.[27] Buckling of the soft tissue or lower lateral

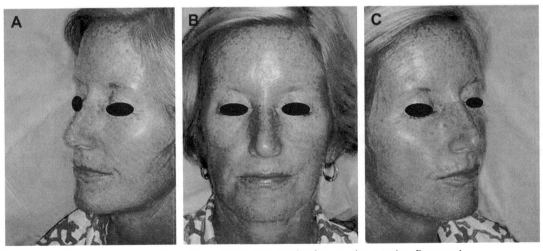

Fig. 4. (*A–C*) Three views of the 3-month postoperative result after an alar rotation flap repair.

cartilage toward the vestibule effectively decreases the size of the external nasal valve. The flap predictably causes a postoperative flattening of the alar rim, which may improve by 2 weeks after surgery and completely resolve by 6 months.[27]

V to Y island pedicle advancement flap

The V to Y island pedicle advancement flap is another option for 1-stage reconstruction of small (<0.5 cm) alar defects that are confined entirely to the alar cosmetic subunit. The ideal defect for this flap is located in the anterior half of the ala and is no wider than 0.5 cm. The greatest advantages of this flap are the superb color and textural skin match from the adjacent skin within the same subunit.[28] Anatomically, this myocutaneous flap maintains the transverse portion of the nasalis muscle pedicle that is supplied by the rich vasculature from the lateral nasal artery, fed by branches of both the angular and infraorbital arteries.

The basic design of this flap involves sliding a muscle-based skin paddle from laterally on the nasal ala to reconstruct a small defect that is more medially located. The secondary defect that is then created by transferring this tissue is closed in a linear fashion. The reconstructive surgeon must remember that the movement of this flap is in a direction that parallels the free nostril margin so that the nostril is not pulled up or retracted when attempting to close the defect. In addition, if there is an insufficient amount of tissue that is able to be recruited laterally, a second medially based flap can also be used to create a bipedicled modification of this technique. When performing this flap reconstruction, the triangular flap is tapered to a 30° point and it is sharply dissected with a knife, down to the muscle layer, providing significant flap mobility. Once the underlying nasalis muscle has been identified, the flap is lifted in a submuscular plane, maintaining the skin-muscle attachment to the triangular flap and its blood supply.[28] The surrounding alar subunit may be undermined to allow for adequate tissue movement and closure.

Using this flap to repair certain alar defects needs to be chosen wisely. It is best used for medial alar defects not involving the free alar margin. This is because as the flap gets closer to the nostril margin, the circulation is increasingly compromised and there is a dense adherence of the tissues, limiting the flap movement. Some investigators recommend designing these flaps at least 3 to 5 mm away from the alar margin to prevent retraction of the alar rim.[28] This flap prevents many of the functional problems that can exist with other flaps involving the compromise of the nasal valves and especially in dilating the nostril. It seems that even though the nasalis muscle is involved in nostril dilation, the redundancy of the muscle fibers that contribute to this act help to maintain this function.[28]

Rhombic flap

By transposing skin from the surrounding cosmetic subunits, the surgeon can avoid distortion of the alar rim and preserve the volume of the ala. The rhombic flap is a single-lobed transposition flap that can rarely be used for alar reconstruction. Although this flap can present the advantage of transposing like tissue to the area for reconstruction, it has multiple disadvantages for defects of the ala. First, the donor site for the rhombic flap usually needs to be the skin of the nasal sidewall, immediately superior to the alar groove. The tension to close the secondary defect at the donor site can compromise the nasal valve by causing medial deviation of the lower lateral cartilage on that side.[21] Second, it is difficult to avoid blunting of the alar groove when using the rhombic flap.

Bilobe flap

In contrast to the rhombic flap, the second lobe of the bilobe flap places the tertiary defect further from the alar groove and rim, thereby allowing closure with less risk of nasal valve compromise. Tension to close the tertiary defect on the loose skin of the proximal nose carries less risk of nasal valve collapse, because the underlying nasal bone affords more stability compared with the lower lateral cartilage on the distal nose. Rather than transposing the flap along a 180° axis of rotation, as originally described, the bilobe flap should be designed to rotate along a 90° or 100° axis (**Figs. 5** and **6**).[15,29] With this design improvement, each of the lobes of the bilobe flap transposes approximately 45°. In addition to decreasing the size of the standing cone, the decreased arc of transposition results in less secondary motion at the primary defect and less risk of elevating the alar rim.

The bilobe flap for alar reconstruction is best suited for defects of the anterior and middle aspects of the ala. Defects that are too far lateral on the ala often demand that the bilobe flap cross directly over the alar crease, a penalty that is best avoided. The bilobe flap can be based off either a medial or lateral blood supply, depending on the needs of the defect site. For most alar defects, a medially based pedicle is preferable (**Figs. 7** and **8**). The medially based pedicle allows a flap design that does not cross over the alar crease and helps avoid nasal valve

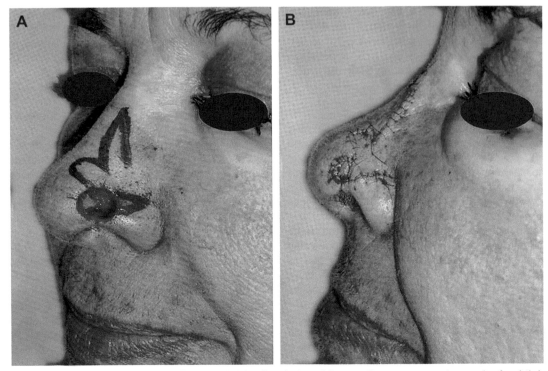

Fig. 5. (*A*) Surgical defect and laterally based bilobe flap design. (*B*) Immediate postoperative result after bilobe flap repair.

problems. Robinson and Burget[30] have written that in reconstruction of the lower third of the nose or the nasal sidewall, any flaps that cross or come within 1 mm of the alar crease are at risk for postoperative nasal valve obstruction. After transposition of the flap, the alar crease should be located right between the first and second lobe of the bilobe flap, diminishing the possibility of blunting the contour of the alar groove. With even with the most careful flap design, the surgeon must take pains to avoid distortion and elevation of the free margin of the ala.

Nasolabial groove transposition flap (single-stage melolabial fold flap)

The melolabial fold flap can be used as a single-stage flap to reconstruct alar defects as large as

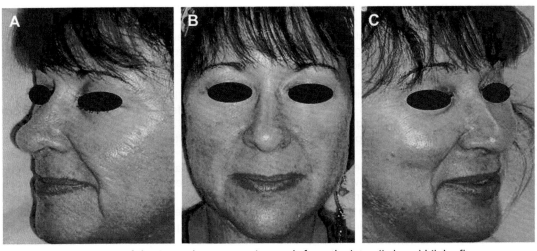

Fig. 6. (*A–C*) Three views of the 6-month postoperative result from the laterally based bilobe flap.

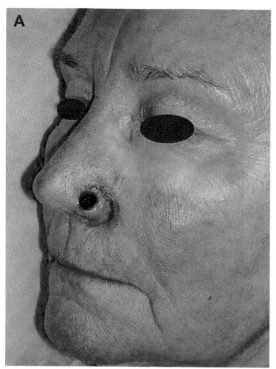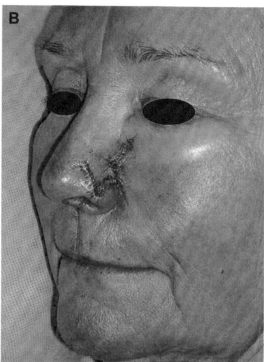

Fig. 7. (*A*) Surgical defect before a medially based bilobe flap. (*B*) Immediate postoperative result after bilobe flap repair.

2.5 cm.[31] This 1-stage, superiorly based, transposition-advancement flap receives its random pattern, but robust blood supply from the distal branches of the angular and facial arteries, as they perforate through the levator labii superioris alaeque nasi muscle.[32] The skin of the melolabial fold serves as an ample donor site flap that has a great tissue match for skin of the nasal ala.[32,33]

The ideal defect for the single-stage melobial transposition flap involves the alar groove. A small island of lateral ala must be present to anchor the advancing cheek skin and close the donor site, so defects that extend all the way to the lateral aspect of the ala and alar groove may best be reconstructed with another flap option. The medial aspect of the flap is designed to correspond to the melolabial crease, and the flap should taper down to a 30° point inferiorly. The horizontal width of the flap on the cheek should exactly match the width of the alar defect and should be extended no further than where the defect and the nasojugal fold intersect. The nasal sidewall skin is also excised up to the nasojugal sulcus, at a 30° angle maximum, to facilitate the medial transfer of the flap into the defect site.[32] Once these cuts have been made, the flap is elevated in the standard subcutaneous plane and advanced medially over a small island of native ala (**Figs. 9** and **10**).

To ensure this flap is well contoured, some basic techniques must be used. To ensure a tension-free closure, a tacking suture should be placed from the dermis of the underside of the advancing flap to the thick fascia and muscle along the rim of the pyriform aperture. As the suture is gently tightened, this will take the tension off of the flap and also recreate the contour and concavity of the nasofacial sulcus. Even a mild over-correction in this area can be tolerated, as the tissues tend to relax with time. Next, the donor site defect is closed and the distal flap is thinned aggressively to allow tissue match of that aspect of the flap into the alar defect. In addition, the skin of the nasal tip, ala, and sidewall is undermined and the flap is trimmed to fit the defect exactly, although it can be important to leave this area of the flap slightly redundant to push back the ala and accentuate the alar crease.[32]

Compared with other flap choices, this is a great reconstructive option, given the excellent tissue match, ability to hide the donor scar in the melolabial fold, and because it is a 1-stage procedure. Disadvantages include the possibility of blunting the alar groove and a high risk for pincushioning if the flap is not sized appropriately. Moreover, without meticulous suturing technique, the rounded scar where the flap insets at the ala tends to invert.

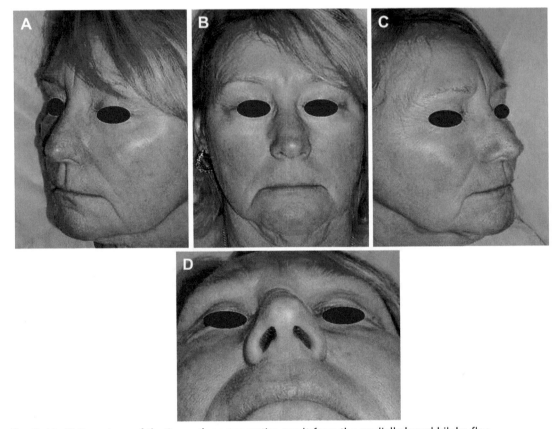

Fig. 8. (A–D) Four views of the 3-month postoperative result from the medially based bilobe flap.

Two-stage Flap Reconstructions

Interpolated paranasal flap

When the surface area and depth of the alar defect are great or when the preservation of the contour is not possible with a single-stage flap, a 2-stage interpolation flap may be necessary. The interpolated paranasal flap is a random pattern skin flap with an inferior pedicle based on the rich blood supply of the angular artery. The donor skin for this flap is located in the nasofacial sulcus, where the nasal sidewall and cheek facial subunits meet.

When deciding whether to reconstruct the alar defect with the interpolated paranasal flap through a spot-filling approach or by resurfacing the entire subunit, Cook[34] has described his extensive experience with the favorable cosmetic results achieved solely by replacing the tissue to fill the defect. It has also been suggested that this flap be mapped exactly according to the template or even slightly smaller. This technique of under sizing the flap has reduced the instances of pincushioning that have been seen.[35] If the defect involves more than 50% of the surface area of the ala, the surgeon may consider removing the remaining portions of the alar subunit. A template of

the contralateral nasal ala may be used to design a flap that is symmetric in size. Whether reconstructing the entire alar subunit or spot-filling the defect, always ensure that the template is sized appropriately by placing it over the alar defect.

With the template resting over the alar defect, it should then be rotated approximately 90° superiorly and laterally and transferred to the nasofacial sulcus on the affected side. After doing so, the portion of the template corresponding to the alar rim faces medially and the portion of the template corresponding the anterior portion of the alar defect is closer to the medial canthal angle. The horizontal width of the flap design should equal the vertical height of the defect on the ala. A surgical marking pen can be used to trace the outside edge of the template onto the skin of the nasofacial sulcus. The template must be placed superiorly enough to ensure that the distal portion of the flap reaches the most anterior aspect of the alar defect when it is rotated counterclockwise into the defect.

The medial incision for the flap begins just lateral to the alar groove and is carried superiorly in the nasofacial sulcus toward the medial canthus. The

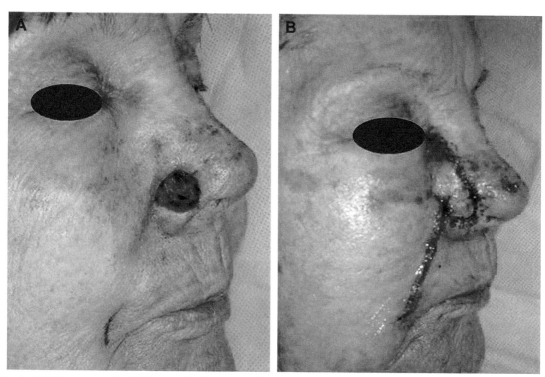

Fig. 9. (*A*) Right alar defect following Mohs surgery. (*B*) Immediate postoperative result after a 1-stage nasolabial transposition flap reconstruction.

standing cone superior to the template should have a maximum angle of 30° at its apex. To preserve the blood supply to this flap, it is elevated in the deep subcutaneous plane, immediately over the levator labii superioris alaeque nasi and the nasalis muscles. The flap should be thinned judiciously, but the distal aspect of the flap may be thinned down to the dermis. Once the medial cheek and nasofacial sulcus have been undermined so that the donor site may be closed, a tacking stitch may be placed on the underside of the advancing cheek flap to secure it medially. The flap is then swung inferiorly and medially into the alar defect, trimmed as necessary, and then secured with a layered suture closure.

The pedicle is usually left intact for about 3 weeks and the patient then returns for division and insetting. For the second stage of the reconstruction, the proximal flap is divided, thinned, and inset to cover the lateral aspect of the defect. As a general rule, it is best to deepen the defect site if possible, rather than thinning the flap pedicle too aggressively and compromising its blood supply. The flap is next inset in a layered fashion from laterally to medially. The pedicle is then removed with a fusiform excision and closed with the incision in the melolabial fold.

There are multiple advantages to using this flap versus other reconstructive options. Because the blood supply to this flap comes from an inferiorly based pedicle, and not from above, like the interpolated melolabial flap, non–hair-bearing tissue can be swung into the defect from the nasofacial sulcus and lateral nasal sidewall. Additional benefits of this flap are that it has a rich vascular supply from branches of the facial and angular artery and that the axis of rotation is less than 90°, allowing for less torsion and constriction of the pedicle.[35] The medial cheek pad is also spared with this approach, decreasing some of the asymmetry of the melobial fold, which is common after a melolabial interpolation flap.[35]

Interpolated melolabial flap (superiorly based nasolabial flap)

Although the paranasal interpolated flap uses the skin from the nasofacial sulcus as its donor site, the melolabial interpolation flap uses the skin from the melolabial fold as its donor site. In contrast to the paranasal interpolated flap, which has an inferiorly based pedicle, the melolabial interpolation flap has a superiorly based pedicle. The skin of the melolabial fold is an excellent color and texture match for the ala, and the flap preserves the alar-facial

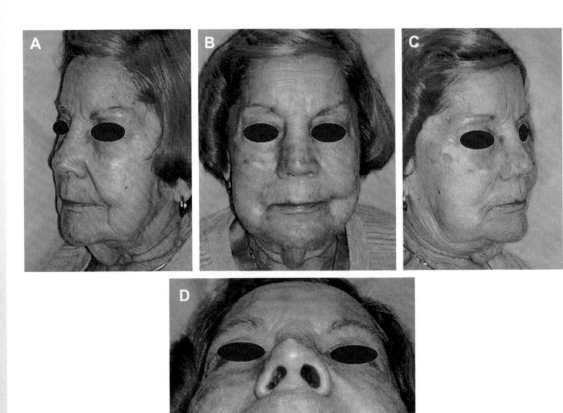

Fig. 10. (*A–D*) Four views of the 6-month postoperative result from the 1-stage nasolabial transposition flap.

sulcus.[20] The interpolated melolabial flap remains the workhorse flap for replacement of the alar subunit.[35] This flap has often been referred to as the first choice option when reconstructing cutaneous defects of the entire nasal ala, largely because of its generous donor site tissue availability.[35] The flap is a random pattern flap that has its vascular source based on the abundant blood supply coming from the perforating branches of the facial and angular arteries, as they come through the levator labii muscle.

This is a 2-stage procedure. The first stage involves transferring the flap into the defect site, usually along with the placement of a cartilage batten graft for support. When considering the flap design, the base is created with an incision that extends superiorly to just above the nasolabial crease on the side of the defect and about 5 mm lateral to the alar-facial sulcus, with the medial border of the donor flap lying in the melolabial fold.[36] It is recommended that a template is created from the contralateral ala and that this template is centered directly over the midportion of the nasolabial fold at approximately the level of the oral commissure (**Figs. 11** and **12**). The flap width should be equal to the vertical height of the nasal alar defect to ensure a good size match, and the lateral incision should parallel the nasolabial fold. This melolabial flap has been described both as a peninsula of skin or as a true island, based solely on the subcutaneous pedicle.[37] Alternatively, epidermis and dermis can be left on the superiorly based pedicle at the time of initial transfer.[20,38] This pedicle can be interpolated, as is the case of the flap described, or it can even be tunneled subcutaneously in some cases. In addition, in cases of full-thickness alar defects, this flap may also be used for both internal lining and external skin cover by turning over the most distal aspect of the flap for the internal lining and then using the mid or more proximal portion of the flap to cover the external defect.[39]

When replacing the entire alar subunit, a nonanatomic cartilage batten graft is usually necessary to brace the alar rim against the forces of flap contraction. Excellent donor sites include the conchal bowl or the antihelix. Cartilage from these

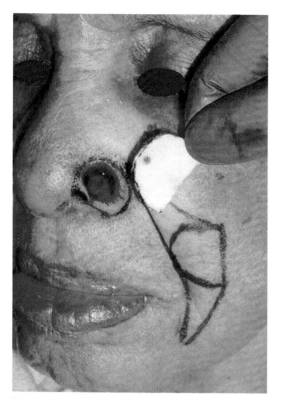

Fig. 11. Views of a partial surgical defect, delineation of the nasal alar subunit, and template for the entire alar subunit. A 2-stage nasolabial interpolation flap reconstruction planned and design transposed on the patient's cheek.

sites can be trimmed and shaped to preserve and restore the contour of the alar rim, then secured to the vestibular mucosa with interrupted sutures. Cartilage batten grafts may not be necessary if a substantial portion of the ala remains intact and a spot-filling flap is used.

The flap is elevated in a subcutaneous plane and thinned distally to a millimeter or two of subcutaneous fat to create the appropriate thickness match for the defect site. Next, the flap is rotated superiorly and medially to cover the alar defect. This flap has a wide angle of rotation, and it can be rotated about 150°.[20] A standing cone is removed inferiorly at the donor site, and the secondary defect is then undermined to allow closure in a layered fashion at the melolabial fold.[40]

The pedicle of the flap usually remains in place for 3 weeks. The second stage involves the division of the pedicle, thinning of the proximal flap, and insetting to the alar-facial sulcus. The base of the flap is divided and the skin of the flap base can be used to reconstruct the curvature of the lateral ala and alar base, if that was part of the

original defect. Excess skin at the base of the flap must be trimmed to fit exactly in the defect. The more proximal aspect of the flap can be thinned at this second stage. The base of the pedicle is excised and closed primarily along the melolabial fold or nasofacial sulcus.

Advantages of this flap include the excellent color and skin match of the local tissue, as well as the rich vascular supply that traverses this area. However, there are reasons why some reconstructive surgeons may tend to use other flaps for alar reconstruction. One disadvantage to using this flap is that in men, the flap may transfer hair-bearing skin from the donor site to the ala. Although laser hair removal is possible after the reconstruction, light or gray hair is difficult to remove with the laser. Another possible downside to using this flap is the postoperative facial asymmetry that results in the nasolabial folds.[41]

Paramedian forehead flap

The paramedian forehead flap can give excellent results for alar reconstruction.

Compared with the paranasal and melolabial interpolation flaps, which both have a random blood supply in their pedicles, the paramedian forehead flap is an axially based flap. The flap pedicle contains the supratrochlear artery and has a robust and reliable blood supply. If Doppler sonography is not available, the artery reliably originates at the medial brow, in the transverse crease formed with contraction of the corrugator muscle.[36] The pedicle is then constructed with a 1.1- to 1.5-cm base that is centered on the artery.

After making a template of the alar defect, the template design is transferred just below the hairline and centered on the pedicle of the supratrochlear artery. A nonanatomic, free, cartilage batten graft should be sutured to the alar margin, as necessary. The conchal bowl and antihelix are convenient donor sites. Incisions are then made around the flap pedicle and its distal margin before the flap is lifted. The most distal aspect of the flap is dissected in the subdermal or subcutaneous plane. Variable amounts of subcutaneous fat are left, according to the desired thickness. The dissection then deepens to a subgaleal or subfrontalis plane to avoid transection of the supratrochlear artery and its branches, which lie superficial to the frontalis muscle and galea at the level of the mid and superior forehead. As the dissection continues toward the orbital rim, blunt dissection lifts the corrugator off the frontal bone and leaves the artery intact. The flap is then rotated medially and inferiorly almost 180° and inset onto the nasal defect. The donor site on the

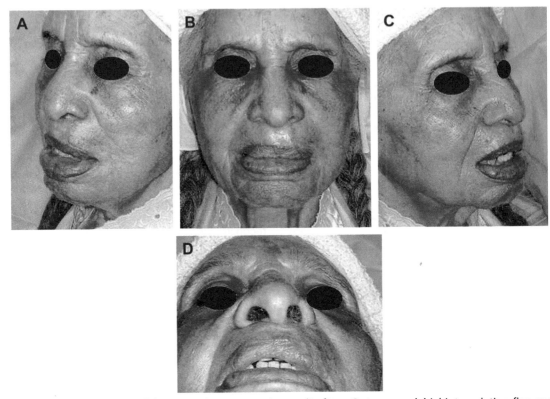

Fig. 12. (*A–D*) Four views of the 6-month postoperative result after a 2-stage nasolabial interpolation flap and free conchal cartilage graft reconstruction.

forehead is closed primarily, as tension allows. A standing cutaneous deformity can be excised superiorly to close the forehead donor site. If the surgeon is unable to close the forehead donor site, this may be left open to granulate by secondary intention with good results.[14]

This pedicle is left connected for about 3 to 4 weeks before division and inset. At that point, the pedicle is divided, and the flap is trimmed and inset at both the proximal aspect of the nasal defect and at the donor site at the medial brow.

The paramedian forehead flap is a dependable and robust flap to resurface large alar defects and those encompassing multiple distal nasal subunits. Compared with the interpolated flaps discussed earlier, there are some benefits and disadvantages. The axial blood supply of the paramedian forehead flap has been suggested for situations where a reliable blood supply is necessary, such as defect sites that have been irradiated or in patients who are diabetics or smokers.[42] One disadvantage with this flap, however, is the long forehead scar that may leave some patients unhappy. Many prefer the donor site incision to be hidden in the melolabial fold. In a series reported by Arden and colleagues,[42] they compared the paramedian

forehead flap with the melolabial interpolation flap. They found the melolabial donor site scar to be objectively superior to the paramedian forehead flap donor site, in terms of scar length and width. Also, 1 out of 3 patients in this study was dissatisfied with the result of the forehead scar.

SPECIAL RECONSTRUCTIVE CONSIDERATIONS AND COMPLICATIONS
Composite Grafts

Reconstruction of full-thickness defects demands replacement of the external skin envelope, the internal mucosal lining, and structural support.[7] Auricular composite grafts provide a 1-stage option to reconstruct small, full-thickness alar defects. Composite grafts are commonly taken from the helical crus, conchal bowl, or antitragus, and include the skin and underlying cartilage.[19] The donor site is chosen based on the geometry of the nasal defect and whether the cutaneous portion of the composite graft is used to reconstruct the external nasal skin or the internal lining. Composite grafts have a high metabolic demand and a high risk for necrosis. Therefore, it is generally recommended that auricular composite grafts do not exceed 1 cm in size to minimize the risk of necrosis.[7,43]

Obtaining the composite graft requires careful measurements and planning, with selection of the appropriate donor site based on contour match and tissue availability. It is generally appropriate to take a graft that is slightly larger than the defect (approximately 2 mm in all dimensions), to account for the expected wound contracture and to decrease the likelihood of notching during the healing process.[6] After transferring a template of the alar defect to the desired donor site on the ear, the skin and/or cartilage is excised. It is frequently desirable to harvest a cartilage graft that is larger than the overlying skin paddle. The excess cartilage on either side of the skin can be inserted into pockets on either side of the defect in the fashion of a tongue-and-groove joint. These pockets help to stabilize the graft and also increase the surface area of contact with vascularized tissue. Inset of the graft requires meticulous closure in layers, including the internal lining and external skin. For very small cartilage grafts, sutures through the cartilage itself are usually unnecessary, although larger grafts may benefit from fixation to the native nasal framework (eg, lower lateral cartilage).

Reconstruction of the donor site defect depends on its size. Smaller defects may be closed primarily, whereas larger defects may require skin grafts (eg, thin full-thickness graft) or a postauricular advancement flap.[19] Auricular composite grafts larger than 1 cm are infrequently needed, but may be taken from the conchal bowl. In such cases, the donor site requires a more advanced repair; for posterior defects, a local advancement flap of postauricular skin, and for anterior defects, a thin FTSG. To limit donor site deformity, however, larger cartilage grafts are generally harvested as free cartilage alone.

Composite grafts have also been used with great success for repair of nostril or nasal vestibule stenosis.[44,45] This procedure is rarely required in primary repair, but is an extremely useful technique for secondary reconstruction in patients with unacceptable cosmesis as a result of scar contracture or previously operated congenital defects. Graft harvest is performed as described earlier, although the graft size and donor site may differ somewhat. Placement of composite auricular grafts for nostril stenosis involves dissection and elevation of the alar-facial groove and alar base. The cutaneous component of the composite graft is used to augment the nasal vestibule. In combination with local flaps and V to Y advancements, satisfactory results have been shown for a wide range of deformities.[46]

Stabilization of free composite grafts is required to avoid shearing forces and to ensure survival. Methods to stabilize the graft include intranasal and external bolsters and even intranasal packing with a standard dental roll or a piece of emollient-impregnated gauze that is rolled to an appropriate size.[6] External bolsters are also useful, in particular for the recreation of the alar-facial sulcus and the depression that separates the superior ala from the nasal sidewall.[47] These may be secured with a fine-gauge, unbraided, synthetic suture, and should be left in place for approximately 1 week.

For reconstruction of large defects that include the nasal ala and portions of neighboring subunits, such as the columella, tip, or sidewall, composite auricular cartilage grafts may also be used in combination with local or regional flaps. In cases where a combination of reconstruction techniques are used, the composite graft is typically used for alar replacement, with the cutaneous portion of the graft used as an internal lining and the local/regional flap tissue used for external lining (eg, paramedian forehead flap for resurfacing of the tip and alar rim, with a composite graft for alar replacement and lining). In such cases, general adherence to the subunit principle ensures adequate cosmesis.[12,19] As these composite grafts are at increased risk for failure, meticulous technique is necessary.[11,16] Necrosis of a composite graft used for internal lining can sabotage the reconstructive efforts.

Free Cartilage Grafts

Free cartilage grafts are used much more frequently than composite grafts. When external skin is provided by a local flap and adequate mucosa exists for internal lining, nonanatomic free cartilage grafts are frequently necessary to preserve the position of the alar margin and to brace it against contraction. Free grafts for alar reconstruction are most commonly taken from the contralateral ear, either from the antihelix or the conchal bowl (**Fig. 13**). These grafts may be harvested using either an anterior or posterior incision through the skin of the ear. Hydrodissection of both the anterior and posterior auricular skin with local anesthetic facilitates harvest of the cartilage. Once the skin is carefully elevated, sharp dissection is used to excise the free cartilage graft. The free cartilage can then be sutured to the vascularized lining of the nose and covered with a vascularized flap for external cover. To ensure survival, vascularized tissue should nourish both sides of the cartilage.

Attention can then be turned to the donor site on the ear. After obtaining careful hemostasis, the

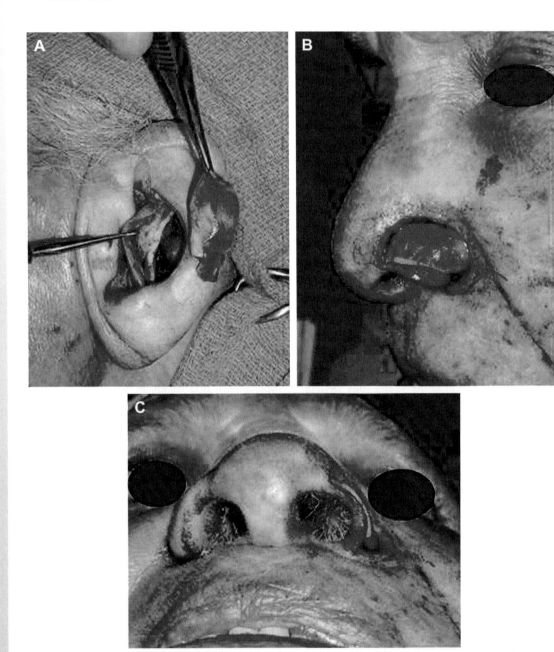

Fig. 13. (*A*) Conchal cartilage graft is harvested from the left ear donor site. (*B*) Free cartilage graft inset and sutured to the nasal lining mucosa. (*C*) Swimmer's view of cartilage graft displaying the appropriate thickness for restoration of the alar rim contour.

incision in the auricular skin can be closed with a simple layer of cutaneous sutures. Quilting sutures and a bolster dressing may be prudent to avoid hematoma, depending on the size of the cartilage graft.

Internal Lining Reconstruction

The nasal mucosa is essential for maintaining adequate nasal function and provides crucial blood supply to all types grafts and flaps. The function of the nasal airway is to warm and humidify inspired air, a mechanism that depends on adequate airflow and a healthy, large mucosal surface area.[7,9] Failure to adequately repair or reconstruct the internal nasal lining may lead to chronic crusting, infection, and poor healing.[13] These complications may eventually lead to graft necrosis. Because a significant contribution of the vascular supply to cartilage grafts is derived from the nasal mucosa, formally reconstructing this layer is essential. There is a high risk for contraction of the reconstruction used for external cover if there is a defect of the underlying mucosa.

A variety of donor sites and techniques exist for reconstruction of the internal nasal lining. The simplest option is a free septal mucosal graft, although these grafts must be small to ensure quick healing and survival. Free grafts are less desirable in situations where any doubt exists about the vascular supply of the remaining layers. Vestibular skin may be rotated as a bipedicled advancement flap for smaller alar reconstructions.[36] This flap is elevated roughly in an oval shape, beginning with an intercartilaginous incision (proximal to the alar defect) with the medial end roughly at the nasal septum and the lateral end at the floor of the vestibule. The wider middle portion of the mucosal flap is then rotated inferiorly into the reconstructed alar subunit, and the donor site is repaired with a thin FTSG.

When alar or distal nasal reconstruction demands a larger internal lining flap, as in the case of full-thickness defects, an excellent option is a hinge flap based on the ipsilateral septal mucosa.[7,36] This flap is based on a single wide pedicle at the anterior septal angle, and is raised by standard hydrodissection followed by submucoperichondrial dissection and mucosal cuts. The posterior cut defines the length of the flap, then the superior and inferior cuts determine its distal width. Once the flap is raised, it is folded (like a hinge) and sutured into the internal aspect of the defect. Ideally, this procedure is performed before reconstruction of the cartilaginous framework and external skin envelope, as the exposure and dissection is significantly easier at this point. A second step is generally required to divide and inset the flap, because the hinged portion can cause substantial nasal airway obstruction. This can be undertaken at the same time as pedicle division in cases where 2-stage local flaps (eg, paramedian forehead or melolabial) have been used.

The inferior turbinate is an alternative intranasal donor site for internal lining reconstruction.[43] The mucoperiosteum of the bony inferior turbinate is abundant, well vascularized, and may be harvested as a pedicled flap based at its head. This procedure begins with generous infiltration of local anesthetic followed by medialization (in-fracture) of the turbinate with a blunt elevator or knife handle. Incision is made along the superior aspect of the turbinate and the mucoperiosteum is elevated along the free edge. Subsequently, the bony turbinate is disarticulated from the lateral nasal wall using sharp osteotome dissection or

cutting sinus instruments, taking care to avoid transecting the flap and leaving a small amount of bone and soft tissue at the head of the turbinate. Once the bone is removed posteriorly, the remaining mucoperiosteum is mobilized and the flap is turned toward the alar defect. This is sutured in place and allowed to heal, although a second stage with pedicle division is necessary for large flaps causing significant nasal airflow obstruction.

When there is insufficient or inadequate intranasal graft materials, local flaps have also been used for internal lining reconstruction. In such cases, the donor tissue is not of the typical mucosal type. Two common examples are so-called turnover flaps, where a portion of a local skin flap is rotated into the defect and flipped 180° so that the skin surface faces the nasal passage. Although this can be an excellent option in cases where much internal lining is missing, the surgeon must ensure that the skin used for nasal lining is free of cutaneous neoplasms. It is unwise to place skin with similar actinic damage inside the nose where surveillance is difficult.[48] In addition, Menick[49] has written extensively about the 3-stage, turnover forehead flap as a source of both external cover and internal lining. In this situation, the distal end of the flap is folded over to form the ala, free margin, and the lining inside of the nostrils. Another option when a paramedian forehead flap is planned for the external layer reconstruction is to extend the local flap dissection to include the galea aponeurotica.[50] This layer can be raised with the overlying cutaneous tissue and then separated as its own pedicled layer when the skin flap is thinned. The galea is then used as an internal lining flap, with cartilage grafts placed in between this layer and the forehead skin. This reconstruction eventually becomes mucosalized, as the native nasal mucosa grows across the galea graft.[50] The galea-including paramedian forehead flap is most useful for larger distal reconstructions including portions of the ala and tip subunits, as the geometry of rotation and inset can be difficult in other areas, and ensuring the stability of cartilage grafts may be difficult. Other local pedicled flaps and even a second paramedian forehead flap from the other side of the forehead have been used alone or in combination to reconstruct large defects of the nasal lining.

Free microvascular reconstruction

In large, distal nasal reconstructions, some investigators have used radial forearm free flaps for internal nasal lining.[51] This flap is a free fasciocutaneous graft based on the radial artery and venae commitantes, and has been combined with local flaps and cartilage grafts to reconstruct complete defects of the distal third of the nose.[51] In addition, some interesting work has been done using free microvascular transfer of composite grafts from the helical root and preauricular skin.[52] This flap is based on the superficial temporal artery and vein, and may be harvested in a variety of configurations, including variable quantities of cartilage, skin, and even bone. Although beyond the scope of this article, these options at the top of the reconstructive ladder are mentioned as a last resort for massive defects or in cases where local graft tissues are not available or such reconstructions are contraindicated.

Structural Cartilage Grafts for Alar Reconstruction

Full-thickness alar reconstructions are exposed to significant contractile forces during the healing process. Without proper consideration and structural support, this may lead to significant alar retraction, alar notching, columellar show, and a poor cosmetic result. As with any surgery, the best treatment of a complication is prevention. This philosophy dictates that cartilage grafting be performed at the primary reconstruction to support the nose as it heals. In the case of alar retraction, prevention is best performed by placement of an alar rim graft (unless an auricular composite graft has already been used at the alar rim). These grafts are nonanatomic in the sense that they do not replace or reconstruct a specific piece of native cartilage.[53] Alar rim grafts are generally carved from free conchal cartilage, and when shaped to the appropriate size and contour, add significantly to the final cosmetic result.[43] These grafts should be thin (1–2 mm), and shaped using the contralateral ala as a template to determine length and curvature. Grafts should be placed at the reconstructed alar margin and secured with suture to the surrounding tissues to prevent migration during healing.

External nasal valve collapse may also accompany reconstruction of the nasal ala, especially when soft tissue flaps are large or poorly supported.[22] Reconstructions that involve the entire alar subunit or a portion of the lateral nasal wall are predisposed to this complication, and preventative techniques resemble those used for functional rhinoplasty. Alar batten grafts are linear, free cartilage grafts that may be carved from septal cartilage, or less commonly, conchal cartilage. The graft should be made long enough to span the distance between the lateral crus of the lower lateral cartilage and the bony edge of the pyriform aperture.[8] Depending on the size of the defect and the extent of the nasal

dissection, batten grafts may be placed via a precise pocket (closed technique) or directly onto the exposed framework (open technique).

The internal nasal valve (INV) is the narrowest portion of the airway and contributes about half of all airway resistance. Thus, any compromise of this area during the reconstructive process (including soft tissue bulk or internal lining flaps) results in significant functional loss.[22] The INV is actually a three-dimensional space bounded by the head of the middle turbinate, the floor of the nose, the cartilaginous septum, and the articulation of the upper lateral cartilage (ULC) with the septum. The angle formed by the ULC and the septum is typically 9° to 15°.[8] Narrowing of this angle results in significant increases in nasal airway resistance, corresponding to Poiseuille's law, which states that resistance to flow is proportional to the radius to the fourth power. Maintenance or augmentation of the INV is key to a satisfactory functional result of any nasal surgery. Thus, larger distal nasal reconstructions involving replacement or manipulation of the ULC must consider spreader graft placement as an adjuvant treatment. Again, depending on the size of the defect and the extent of the nasal dissection, spreader grafts may be placed endonasally (closed technique) or directly between the exposed quadrangular cartilage and ULC (open technique).

With larger defects that involve the nasal tip or columella, in addition to the ala, consideration must be given to the structural support of the distal third of the nose. This is particularly true when the resection margins have included a significant portion of the lower lateral cartilages, violating important tip support mechanisms (eg, the scroll region or the medial crural footplates). To avoid tip ptosis, the reconstructive surgeon must consider the tip support mechanisms disrupted by the surgical defect and the relative weight of the grafted tissues. In these cases, a columellar strut graft may be useful in providing strength to the reconstructed tip.[54] This simple cartilage graft may be carved from septal, conchal, or costal cartilage. The graft should be 2 to 3 mm wide, with the length determined by the preoperative or desired postoperative projection. The graft is placed in a precise pocket that is dissected between the medial crura of the lower lateral cartilage and rests on the maxillary crest. It should be secured with fine-gauge, synthetic, nonabsorbing suture.

Timing of Flap Takedown and Insetting

For any interpolated or 2-stage flap that is performed, the surgeon must decide the optimal time to perform the pedicle take down and flap inset. Most of the literature suggests that the 3 weeks after surgery is a safe time to take down the flap, but specific patient comorbidities, such as smoking, prior radiation, or diabetes, may warrant leaving an intact pedicle for a longer period of time. Also, less aggressive thinning of the flap during the initial procedure may be judicious in patients with a history of some of the comorbid issues. Despite variability in the time of take down and inset among surgeons, most of the vascular in-growth from the wound bed is adequate to divide the flap pedicle between 2 and 4 weeks after the initial procedure.[43] A quick test can be performed in the clinic to determine if the flap has engrafted itself to the defect wound bed. The surgeon can assess the color of the flap by constricting the pedicle at its base with a hemostat. If the color of the flap does not change, the flap has taken to the defect site and it is safe to severe the pedicle at that time. In addition, during the procedure of pedicle division, most surgeons lift up the proximal flap, thin it out aggressively, add contour and shape to the alar reconstruction with tacking and fixation sutures, and then inset the remainder of the flap. The flap should be adequately debulked at this point, using a scalpel blade to remove any excess fat and subcutaneous tissue, as well as granulation tissue, from the wound bed.[26] The flap can then be precisely trimmed to exactly fit the defect size, after the wound edges are freshened, and inset with interrupted cutaneous sutures.

Complications

In performing nasal reconstructive surgery, there are many issues that can lead to poor functional and cosmetic results. Although some complications such as infection, flap necrosis, and unsatisfactory cosmetic appearance can occur with many different flaps, this section address some of the complications or problems that can occur more specifically with alar reconstruction. Thorough preoperative assessment of the defect and reconstruction options, as well as proper surgical technique can limit the risk for most of these complications.

Decreased nostril or alar size

This problem can become an issue especially in cases where the surgeon is set to repair small defects that are confined to the alar subunit itself. As discussed earlier, primary closures, rotation-advancement flaps, and V to Y nasalis muscle island pedicle flaps all predictably shorten the size of the ala. Consequently, the alae can be asymmetric and the aperture of the external nasal

valve is decreased. When considering defect reconstruction with tissue that is entirely within and limited to the ala, these flaps, as well as those using just alar tissue, should be reserved for reconstructing defects with a horizontal dimension less than or equal to 0.5 cm.

Impairment of alar contour

The contour of the nasal ala is particularly difficult to replicate. The delicate convex ala is framed by the concave alar groove. The inferior free margin is particularly susceptible to distortion. If care is not taken, flaps for which donor tissue is taken from the nasal sidewall or cheek can blunt or ablate the alar groove superiorly or the nasofacial sulcus laterally. The surgeon must exercise caution when using 1-stage flaps with donor sites located outside the alar skin, such as a medially based bilobe flap or nasolabial transposition flap. If the chosen flap is likely going to blunt the alar contour, another flap that incorporates multiple stages or one that reconstructs the entire alar subunit should be considered.

Buckling of the lateral crus of the lower lateral cartilage into the nasal vestibule

Reconstruction options that decrease the volume of the ala in the anterior-posterior dimension often cause buckling of the lateral crus of the lower lateral cartilage into the nasal vestibule because of the strain put on the underlying cartilage with this type of closure. The problems associated with this can range from being asymptomatic to causing significant nasal obstruction. The reconstructive surgeon must be aware of this possibility and take steps to try and prevent or repair this issue. Free cartilage grafts can help to stabilize the position of the lateral crus. In many cases, either an alar strut graft can be placed between the vestibular mucosa and the undersurface of the lateral crus or an alar batten graft can be placed in a precise pocket, over top of the lower lateral cartilage, in the region of the INV. Horizontal mattress sutures securing the cartilage graft to the intrinsic lower lateral cartilage will help to bring the tail of the lateral crus out of the nasal cavity and relieve that aspect of the patient's nasal obstruction. In general, the surgeon can prevent buckling of the lateral crus by reconstructing with flaps that have volume equal to the size of the defect.

Distortion or retraction of the free alar margin

The complication of alar retraction usually occurs from either a weakened lateral crura of the lower lateral cartilage, from undersized flaps, from flap designs with secondary motion that pulls the alar rim superiorly, or from postoperative scar contracture.[54] Alar retraction can usually be prevented though careful planning during the reconstructive procedure. A cartilage graft, most often auricular concha, is usually placed along the alar rim or slightly superior to this, to brace the free alar margin and prevent a retraction of the ala, which can lead to a poor cosmetic outcome.

REFERENCES

1. Bruintjes TD, van Olphen AF, Hillen B, et al. A functional anatomic study of the relationship of the nasal cartilages and muscles to the nasal valve area. Laryngoscope 1998;108:1025–32.
2. Ali-Salaam P, Kashgarian M, Davila J, et al. Anatomy of the Caucasian alar groove. Plast Reconstr Surg 2002;110:261–6.
3. Han SK, Lee DG, Kim JB, et al. An anatomic study of nasal tip supporting structures. Ann Plast Surg 2004;52(2):134–9.
4. Rohrich RJ, Hoxworth RE, Thornton JF, et al. The pyriform ligament. Plast Reconstr Surg 2008;121: 277–81.
5. Hur MS, Youn KH, Hu KS, et al. New anatomic considerations on the levator labii superioris related with the nasal ala. J Craniofac Surg 2010;21(1): 258–60.
6. Jewett BS. Repair of small nasal defects. Facial Plast Surg Clin North Am 2005;13:283–99.
7. Baker SR, Naficy S. Principles of nasal reconstruction. St. Louis (MO): Mosby; 2002.
8. Lee J, White WM, Constantinides M. Surgical and nonsurgical treatments of the nasal valves. Otolaryngol Clin North Am 2009;42:495–511.
9. Walsh WE, Kern RC. Sinonasal anatomy, function, and evaluation. In: Bailey BJ, Johnson JT, Newlands SD, editors. Head & neck surgery – otolaryngology. Philadelphia: Lippincott Williams & Wilkins; 2006. p. 307–18.
10. Manson PN, Hoopes JE, Chambers RG, et al. Algorithm for nasal reconstruction. Am J Surg 1967;138:528.
11. Rohrich RJ, Griffin JR, Ansari M, et al. Nasal reconstruction – beyond aesthetic subunits: a 15-year review of 1334 cases. Plast Reconstr Surg 2004;114:1405–16.
12. Burget GC. Aesthetic restoration of the nose. Clin Plast Surg 1985;12:463–80.
13. Burget GC, Menick FJ. Nasal support and lining: the marriage of beauty and blood supply. Plast Reconstr Surg 1989;84:189–202.
14. Singh DJ, Bartlett SP. Nasal reconstruction: aesthetic and functional considerations for alar defects. Facial Plast Surg 2003;19(1):19–27.
15. Burget GC, Menick FJ. Aesthetic reconstruction of the nose. St. Louis (MO): Mosby; 1994.
16. Singh DJ, Bartlett SP. Aesthetic considerations in nasal reconstruction and the role of modified nasal subunits. Plast Reconstr Surg 2003;111:639–48.
17. Zitelli JA. Secondary intension healing: an alternative to surgical repair. Clin Dermatol 1984;2(3):92–106.
18. Zitelli JA. Wound healing by secondary intension: a cosmetic appraisal. J Am Acad Dermatol 1983; 9(3):407–15.
19. Sherris DA, Larrabee WF. Principles of facial reconstruction. A subunit approach to cutaneous repair. New York: Thieme; 2010.
20. Barlow RJ, Swanson NA. The nasofacial interpolated flap in reconstruction of the nasal ala. J Am Acad Dermatol 1997;36:965–9.
21. Kaufman AJ. Reconstruction of a defect of the nasal ala and alar crease. Dermatol Surg 2003;29:963–4.
22. Reynolds MB, Gourdin FW. Nasal valve dysfunction after Mohs surgery for skin cancer of the nose. Dermatol Surg 1998;24:1011–7.
23. Gloster HM Jr. The use of full-thickness skin grafts to repair nonperforating nasal defects. J Am Acad Dermatol 2000;42:1041–50.
24. Hendi A. Reconstruction of an alar rim defect. Dermatol Surg 2006;32:1179–80.
25. McCluskey PD, Constantine FC, Thornton JF. Lower third nasal reconstruction: when is skin grafting an appropriate option? Plast Reconstr Surg 2009;124: 826–35.
26. Weber SM, Baker SR. Management of cutaneous nasal defects. Facial Plast Surg Clin North Am 2009;17:395–417.
27. Zeikus PS, Maloney ME, Jellinek NJ. Advancement flap for the reconstruction of nasal ala and lateral nasal tip defects. J Am Acad Dermatol 2006;55: 1032–55.
28. Asgari M, Odland P. Nasalis island pedicle flap in nasal ala reconstruction. Dermatol Surg 2005;31: 448–52.
29. Zimany A. The bilobed flap. Plast Reconstr Surg 1953;11:424–34.
30. Robinson JK, Burget GC. Nasal valve malfunction resulting from resection of cancer. Arch Otolaryngol Head Neck Surg 1990;116:1419–24.
31. Zitelli JA. The nasolabial flap as a single-stage procedure. Arch Dermatol 1990;126:1445–8.
32. Lindsey WH. Reliability of the melolabial flap for alar reconstruction. Arch Facial Plast Surg 2001;3:33–7.
33. Younger RAL. The versatile melolabial flap. Otolaryngol Head Neck Surg 1992;107:721–6.
34. Cook J. Repair of an alar defect. Dermatol Surg 2003;29:1089–91.
35. Fisher GH, Cook JW. The interpolated paranasal flap: a novel and advantageous option for nasal-alar reconstruction. Dermatol Surg 2009;35:656–61.
36. Driscoll BP, Baker SR. Reconstruction of nasal alar defects. Arch Facial Plast Surg 2001;3:91–9.
37. Carucci JA. Melolabial flap repair in nasal reconstruction. Dermatol Clin 2005;23:65–71.
38. Baker SR, Swanson NA. Local flaps in facial reconstruction. St. Louis (MO): Mosby; 1995.

39. Iwao F. Alar reconstruction with subcutaneous pedicled nasolabial flap: difficulties, considerations, and conclusions for this procedure. Dermatol Surg 2005; 31:1351–4.
40. Kaporis HG, Carucci JA. Repair of a defect on the ala. Dermatol Surg 2008;34:931–4.
41. Cook JL. The undesirable influence of reconstructive procedures on the symmetry of the nasolabial folds. Dermatol Surg 2005;31(11 pt 1):1409–16.
42. Arden RL, Nawroz-Danish M, Yoo GH, et al. Nasal alar reconstruction: a critical analysis using melolabial island and paramedian forehead flaps. Laryngoscope 1999;109:376–82.
43. Constantian MB. Indications and use of composite grafts in 100 consecutive secondary and tertiary rhinoplasty patients: introduction of the axial orientation. Plast Reconstr Surg 2002; 110(4):1116–33.
44. Karen M, Chang E, Keen MS. Auricular composite grafting to repair nasal vestibular stenosis. Otolaryngol Head Neck Surg 2000;122(4):529–32.
45. Kotzur A, Gubisch W, Meyer R. Stenosis of the nasal vestibule and its treatment. Aesthetic Plast Surg 1999;23(2):86–92.
46. Baker SR, Johnson TM, Nelson BR. The importance of maintaining the alar-facial sulcus in nasal reconstruction. Arch Otolaryngol Head Neck Surg 1995; 121(6):617.
47. Park SS. Nasal reconstruction in the 21st century: a contemporary review. Clin Exp Otorhinolaryngol 2008;1(1):1–9.
48. Bruschi S, Marchesi SD, Boriani F, et al. Galea-including forehead flap for lower one-third nasal reconstruction. Ann Plast Surg 2009;63(1):67–70.
49. Menick FJ. Restoring nasal lining – the folded forehead flap for lining; the Menick modified method. In: Menick FJ, editor. Nasal reconstruction – art and practice. Philadelphia: Saunders; 2009. p. 415–42.
50. Burget GC, Walton RL. Optimal use of microvascular free flaps, cartilage grafts, and a paramedian forehead flap for aesthetic reconstruction of the nose and adjacent facial units. Plast Reconstr Surg 2007;120(5):1171–207.
51. Zhang YX, Yang J, Wang D, et al. Extended applications of vascularized preauricular and helical rim flaps in reconstruction of nasal defects. Plast Reconstr Surg 2008;121(5):1589–97.
52. Boahene KD, Hilger PA. Alar rim grafting in rhinoplasty: indications, technique, and outcome. Arch Facial Plast Surg 2009;11(5):285–9.
53. Ayhan M, Sevin A, Aytug Z, et al. Reconstruction of congenital and acquired columellar defects: clinical review of 38 patients. J Craniofac Surg 2007;18(6): 1500–3.
54. Jung DH, Kim HJ, Koh KS, et al. Arterial supply of the nasal tip in Asians. Laryngoscope 2000;110:308–11.

Transposition Flaps in Nasal Reconstruction

Peter J.F.M. Lohuis, MD, PhD[a,b,*],
Willem P. Godefroy, MD, PhD[b], Shan R. Baker, MD[c],
Abel-Jan Tasman, MD[d]

KEYWORDS

- Nasal defect • Nasal reconstruction • Transposition flap
- Local flap • Forehead flap

ETIOLOGY

The challenge of nasal reconstruction is related to the complexity of the defect in an organ in which function, structural integrity, and contour are to be maintained. The differences in color, texture, and thickness between the nasal remnants and resources of skin available for the reconstruction pose aesthetic limits that are often difficult to overcome. The age, general health, and aesthetic goals of the patient should also be included in the decision-making process. These multifactorial problems can be approached with several reconstructive options, ranging from primary closure, healing by secondary intention, and skin grafting to the use of local or regional skin flaps. The decision as to which flap to use is based on a careful consideration of which tissue may be borrowed, how it can be repositioned, what the immediate- and long-term effects of moving that tissue will be, and how the scars may be hidden.

Flaps are the only reliable way to transfer bulk tissue for nasal reconstruction because their own source of nutrient blood makes them relatively independent of the vascularity of the recipient site for their survival. Flaps may therefore be used to cover nonvascular structures such as bare bone and cartilage. Nasal cutaneous flaps used to repair the nose provide excellent camouflage because of skin match in terms of texture, color, and thickness.[1,2] Excess skin in the cephalic two-thirds of the nose can be moved into adjacent defects. The alar region is less suited for local transposition flaps or rotation flaps because the alar crease is often distorted or obliterated by the flap.

This article discusses the major principles of nasal reconstruction and describes the local and regional transposition flaps for the reconstruction of nasal defects.

CONSIDERATIONS IN NASAL RECONSTRUCTION

Nasal units are covered by skin of a specific color, texture, and thickness. In addition, each unit has specific contours determined by soft and hard tissues. The decision-making process in reconstruction of nasal defects should include consideration of which tissue can be harvested for reconstruction, how it may be transferred to the nose, what the immediate- and long-term effects on the donor site will be, and how the scars may best be camouflaged. The nose must be restored

Financial disclosure: The authors have nothing to disclose.

[a] Department of Head and Neck Oncology and Surgery, The Netherlands Cancer Institute, Antoni van Leeuwenhoek Hospital, Plesmanlaan 121,1066 CX Amsterdam, The Netherlands
[b] Department of Otolaryngology-Head and Neck Surgery, Center for Facial Plastic Reconstructive Surgery, Diakonessen Hospital Zeist/Utrecht, Professor Lorentzlaan 76, 3707 HC Zeist, The Netherlands
[c] Section of Facial Plastic and Reconstructive Surgery, Department of Otolaryngology—Head and Neck Surgery, University of Michigan, 1500 East Medical Center Drive, 1904 TC, Box 0312, Ann Arbor, MI 48109-0312, USA
[d] Section of Facial Plastic and Reconstructive Surgery, Department of Otolaryngology—Head and Neck Surgery, Cantonal Hospital, Rorschacher Strasse 95, CH-9007 St Gallen, Switzerland
* Corresponding author. Department of Head and Neck Oncology and Surgery, The Netherlands Cancer Institute, Antoni van Leeuwenhoek Hospital, Plesmanlaan 121,1066 CX Amsterdam, The Netherlands.
E-mail address: p.lohuis@nki.nl

to as normal appearing and functioning structure as possible. The following are the 3 principles that form the basis for this reconstructive process[3–5]:

1. Replace missing tissue with like tissue.
2. Replace missing portions of the nasal skeleton with cartilage designed to precisely replicate the missing part.
3. Divide the topography of the nose into aesthetic units for planning incisions and flaps. For units with convex contours (alae, tip, columella), resurface the entire unit with a skin flap if most of the skin of the unit is lost.

Replace Missing Tissue with Like Tissue

Nasal skin varies in texture, color, and appearance within different areas of the nose. The nasal dorsum, sidewalls, columella, alar margins, and soft triangles are covered with thin smooth skin. The nasal tip and ala are covered with thick pitted skin because of the presence of sebaceous glands. The color of the skin may vary from pale with a matt texture on the side of the nose to a shade of red-pink with a shiny appearance over the nasal tip.

In an attempt to replace nasal skin with like tissue, cheek flaps (unlike skin grafts) are especially useful in thick-skinned zones of the nose because medial cheek skin has similar color and texture. Paramedian forehead flaps are used to repair larger deeper defects because they provide sufficient surface area to completely cover the defect and provide adequate vascularity to support structural framework grafts. Loss of internal nasal lining should be restored with septal mucosa or adjacent vestibular skin.

Replace Missing Portions of the Nasal Skeleton

Loss of cartilage support because of removal of the upper or lower lateral cartilages should be restored by replacing the missing portions of the nasal skeleton with septal or auricular cartilage. Defects extending to the alar margin may result in retraction or partial collapse of the nostril if the ala is not properly supported with a batten in the form of a cartilage graft. Structural alar grafts are usually obtained from the contralateral conchal cartilage. These grafts are positioned between the lateral crura and alar base.

Alar batten grafts give support to and prevent retraction of the nostril margin and prevent constriction of the external nasal valve. Auricular cartilage is usually used to replace missing portions of the alar cartilages. Septal cartilage is typically used to replace the upper lateral cartilage. When bone is missing, it is usually replaced with cranial bone grafts or costal bone and cartilage grafts.

Aesthetic Units

Strategic incision placement

Although there is no control over wound healing, the surgeon can select flap donor sites with preferred skin color, texture, and thickness. The surgeon also has control over the size, configuration, and placement of incisions used to harvest and transfer skin flaps so that scars are most ideally located for maximal camouflage.[6] Incisions are placed strategically so that they are parallel to relaxed skin tension lines (RSTLs) or are positioned at the junction of aesthetic facial regions (**Fig. 1**). When possible, skin flaps are positioned so that their borders lie along the ridges and valleys of the nasal aesthetic units.[7]

The unit principle

The aesthetic unit theory is important in nasal reconstruction. If a line of light or shadow (caused by scarring) crosses a smooth surface where it is not expected, it will be noticed at a glance (**Fig. 2**). A good scar remains hidden from view because it is perceived visually as a normal facial fold or contour line. If a scar is placed between nasal topographic units, where it follows the join of normal lighted ridges and shallowed valleys, it will also be taken as normal. Equally important, the bulge of a flap caused by trapdoor contractions will mirror the normal contour of convex nasal units.

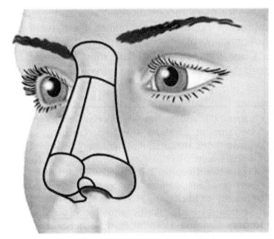

Fig. 1. The aesthetic unit principle in nasal reconstruction. Placing scars between topographic units, where they follow the join of the normal lighted ridges and shallowed valleys, will make scars less visible.

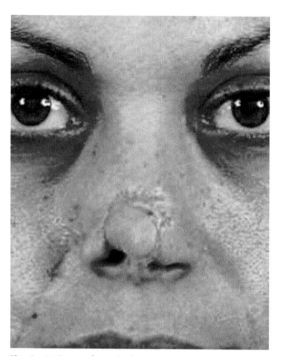

Fig. 2. Patient referred after reconstruction of human bite with a melolabial flap. Improper incision placement and improper use of the aesthetic unit principle resulted in a conspicuous scar.

The aesthetic unit principle suggests that if a defect encompasses more than 50% of a unit, excision of the residual normal tissue should be considered (**Fig. 3**).[8] This way, the entire unit is reconstructed with a flap instead of patching the original defect. Resurfacing the entire nasal aesthetic unit may position scars in joints between the 3-dimensional units, where they may be hidden and less visible. This maneuver is most effective in the reconstruction of the convex units of the tip and alae, which are surrounded with fairly abrupt distinct borders. In these locations, the unit principle uses the trapdoor effect to re-create a 3-dimensional convexity because many flaps have a tendency to pincushion and stand as a bulge above the adjacent skin.[7]

PRIMARY OR DELAYED NASAL RECONSTRUCTION

Especially in the caudal third of the nose, there is an intimate attachment between skin and lower lateral cartilages such that invasion of the cartilage occurs relatively early in the course of the disease. Studies have shown that the highest percentages of recurrent basal cell carcinomas are nasal, illustrating the difficulty of tumor control in this area. This may be because of a tendency toward narrow

excision margins in an effort to simplify reconstruction in this aesthetically important area and also because skin cancer of the midface is known to show subclinical tumor spread, which seems to be related to the embryonic fusion planes at this site.[9] Skin cancer invades deeply along these planes rather than crossing the borders of fusion planes.

Primary reconstruction of nasal skin cancer defects is safe in most cases under the conditions of proper patient selection and reliable histopathologic examination techniques. Delay of reconstruction should be considered, sometimes even after Mohs surgery, if there is doubt about the completeness of the tumor resection.[10] Particularly in large, recurrent, or aggressive skin tumors (eg, perineural growth, deep invasion of the bony or cartilaginous framework of the nose), the timing of reconstruction should be postponed until there is greater certainty that tumor regrowth has not occurred (**Fig. 4**).[11] Using a split- or full-thickness skin graft or allowing the wound to heal by secondary intention as an interim repair can offer surveillance for recurrence at the resected site.

NASAL RECONSTRUCTION TECHNIQUES

A variety of surgical techniques are available for reconstruction of the nose. The choice of technique is based on the size, depth, and location of the surgical wound as well as on the availability and condition of the surrounding tissue. Transposition flaps are reliable reconstructive tools for the reconstruction of nasal defects. A transposition flap is a random pattern skin flap that borrows skin from an adjacent area with relative skin laxity to fill a defect in an area with little or no skin laxity.[12] When the flap is transferred from the donor site to the recipient site, it is lifted over a segment of intervening tissue following a rotational pathway. When properly executed, an excellent redistribution and redirection of tension can be achieved. One of the biggest advantages of transposition flaps is that these flaps use adjacent skin, which provides a good color and textural match. The authors provide an overview of the most important local and regional flaps for nasal reconstruction in the following sections.

Local Flaps

Rhomboid flap
The rhomboid flap optimizes the distribution of wound tension by orienting the flap design according to the lines of maximum extensibility (perpendicular to the RSTLs). However, the geometric design of the rhomboid flap (with 8 possible variations) prevents placement of all necessary

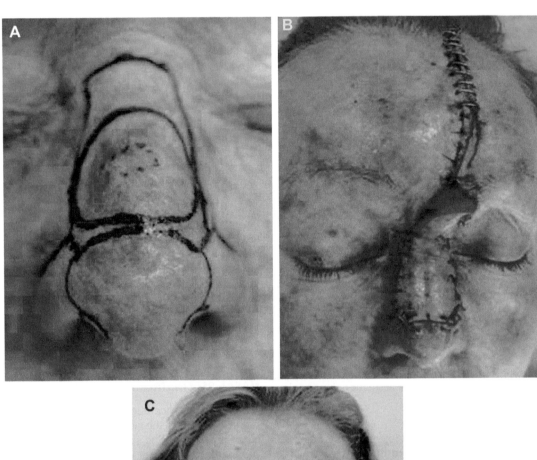

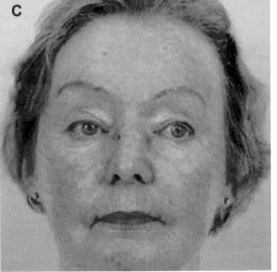

Fig. 3. (A) The aesthetic unit principle suggests that if a defect encompasses more than 50% of surface area of the unit, excision of residual normal skin of the unit should be considered. Patient shown had wide reexcision of superficial spreading melanoma. (B) Entire nasal dorsal unit reconstructed with paramedian forehead flap. The underlying cartilaginous hump was resected. (C) Postoperative result. (From PJFM Lohuis. Reconstruction of major nasal defects. In: JR Thomas, editor. Advanced therapy in facial plastic and reconstructive surgery. Connecticut: PMPH-USA; 2010; with permission.)

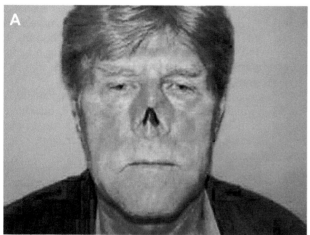

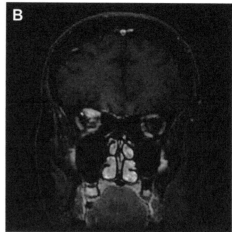

Fig. 4. Particularly in large, recurrent, or aggressive skin tumors, the reconstruction should be postponed until there is greater certainty that tumor regrowth has not occurred. (A) Patient awaiting reconstruction after resection of a desmoplastic melanoma. (B) Perineural growth towards the right side of the orbit after the initial cancer removal. (From PJFM Lohuis. Reconstruction of major nasal defects. In: JR Thomas, editor. Advanced therapy in facial plastic and reconstructive surgery. Connecticut: PMPH-USA; 2010; with permission.)

incisions in or parallel to the RSTL or aesthetic boundary lines. The possible exception is the lateral nasal sidewall and the glabellar region (Fig. 5).

Note flap

An elegant alternative to a rhomboid flap is a note flap. This flap avoids the need to sacrifice normal tissue at the margins of a circular defect to create the geometric pattern that is required for a rhomboid flap. The note flap is in essence a triangular transposition flap, which is capable of closing a circular defect with little donor site deformity. The simplest form of the flap is depicted in Fig. 6. It is extremely easy to design the flap in relation to the RSTL. For a circular defect, the surgeon draws 2 tangents approximately parallel to the RSTL of the nose. Then, 4 potential flaps are designed, and the surgeon selects the best of the 4 options. Ideally, the RSTL should parallel the final donor site wound closure line. One of the disadvantages of the note flap is that frequently there is a standing cutaneous deformity

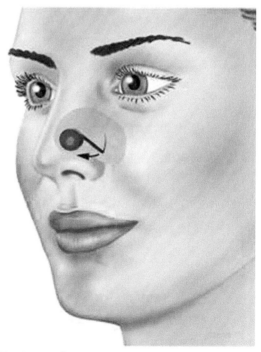

Fig. 5. Rhomboid flap from glabella. Closure of the defect with transposition of point A and B to A' and B' respectively.

Fig. 6. Note flap is an elegant alternative to rhomboid flap.

(SCD) at the base of the triangular flap, although usually no tailoring is required. A more important disadvantage is that the flap requires a certain degree of judgment based on experience. Because the note flap is somewhat smaller than the defect the surgeon must be sure that there is sufficient tissue laxity to allow wound closure.[13]

V-to-Y island subcutaneous tissue pedicle advancement flap

The V-Y island subcutaneous tissue pedicle advancement flap may be used to replace soft tissue of the caudal lateral nasal sidewall in select skin cancer defects. As a nasal cutaneous flap, its use is limited. This flap may be helpful in the reconstruction of small defects located in the region of the anterior alar groove and lateral nasal tip, including the nasal facet (**Fig. 7**).[5]

Bilobular transposition flap

The bilobed flap is a double transposition flap that allows movement of looser skin from the cephalic nasal area into small defects of the lateral caudal nose and adjacent tip.[14] The defect ideally should not exceed a diameter of 1.5 cm, and the bilobed flap is best based laterally. The primary flap or lobe is used to repair the nasal defect, and a secondary lobe is created to repair the donor site of the primary lobe (**Fig. 8**). The donor site of the secondary lobe is then closed primarily.[5] Wide

undermining beneath the musculature is essential. To prevent the development of an excessive SCD, the flap should not be pivoted more than 90° to 110°. Commonly, a Burow triangle is excised adjacent to the defect. The bilobed flap requires incisions that violate the boundaries of nasal aesthetic units but transfers skin of quality similar to that of the recipient site (**Fig. 9**). This advantage is more important than placing the borders of the flap along the aesthetic unit boundary lines.

Regional Flaps

When large areas of nasal skin are missing (>1.5 cm in diameter) or the underlying nasal support is absent, the cartilage framework must be restored with cartilage grafts. In such instances, a nasal cutaneous flap is not sufficient for wound closure. These circumstances require a local flap, which recruits skin from areas of the face immediately adjacent to the nose. Such flaps may take the form of a nasal dorsal glabellar flap, interpolated melolabial flap, or interpolated paramedian forehead flap. When defects extend to the paranasal region, such as the medial cheek or upper lip, cheek advancement flaps and subcutaneous tissue pedicled island advancement flaps may be required to repair cheek and upper lip soft tissue defects. These flaps remain distinct and separate from any flap used to repair the nose.

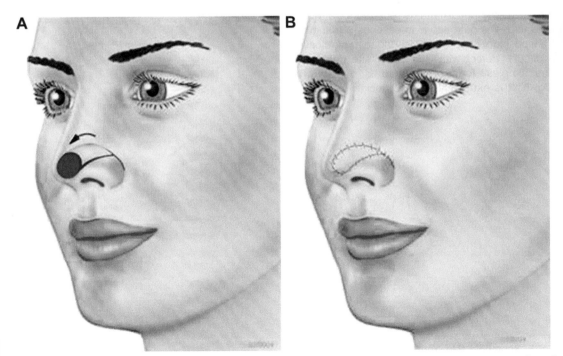

Fig. 7. (A) V-Y island subcutaneous tissue pedicle advancement flap can be used for the reconstruction of small defects of anterior alar groove and lateral nasal tip, including the nasal facet. (B) After advancement and closure.

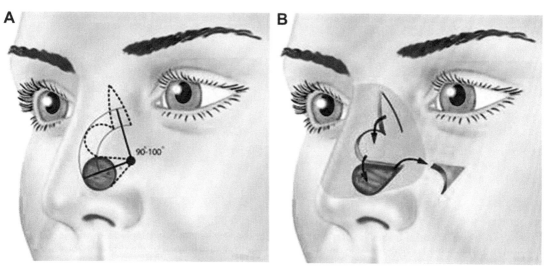

Fig. 8. (A) Preoperative markings of the flap. (B) Transposition of the bilobular flap.

Nasal dorsal glabellar rotation flap

The nasal dorsal glabellar rotation flap provides a 1-stage procedure to repair medium to large (1–2.5 cm in diameter) defects of the middle and caudal nose.[15] The flap, which is nourished by an axial blood supply from the angular artery, uses tissue from the lax glabellar skin. The design of the flap may seem unnecessarily large for the closure of a distal nasal or midnasal defect (**Fig. 10**). However, because the design of this flap is primarily that of a rotation flap (with a back cut in the glabellar region), the flap must be designed larger than the defect to maximize tissue movement and decrease wound closure tension at the donor site. The effective length of the flap diminishes progressively as the flap rotates about its pivotal point at the medial canthus. Dissection in the subcutaneous tissue plane of the glabellar portion of the flap is critical because the thicker glabellar skin is advanced to the medial canthus, where the skin is thinner. The nasal portion of the flap is dissected beneath the musculature (**Fig. 11**).

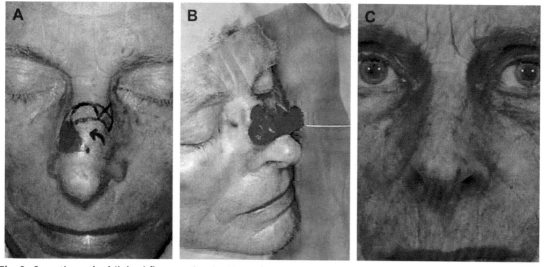

Fig. 9. Sometimes the bilobed flap requires incisions that violate the boundaries of the nasal aesthetic units, but this flap transfers skin of quality similar to that of the recipient site. (A) Nasal sidewall defect and flap markings. (B) Wide undermining beneath the musculature is essential. (C) The nose after 3 months. (*From* PJFM Lohuis. Reconstruction of major nasal defects. In: JR Thomas, editor. Advanced therapy in facial plastic and reconstructive surgery. Connecticut: PMPH-USA; 2010; with permission.)

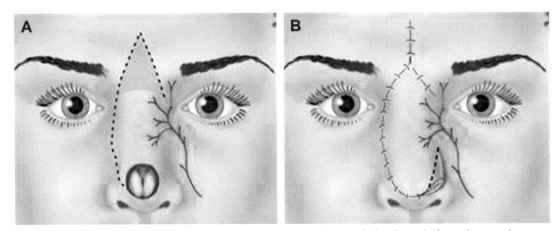

Fig. 10. (*A*) The Nasal dorsal glabellar rotation flap is nourished by axial blood supply from the angular artery, and uses tissue from the lax glabellar skin. In the glabellar portion, dissection is in the subcutaneous tissue plane, and in the nasal portion, it is beneath the musculature. (*B*) After rotation and closure.

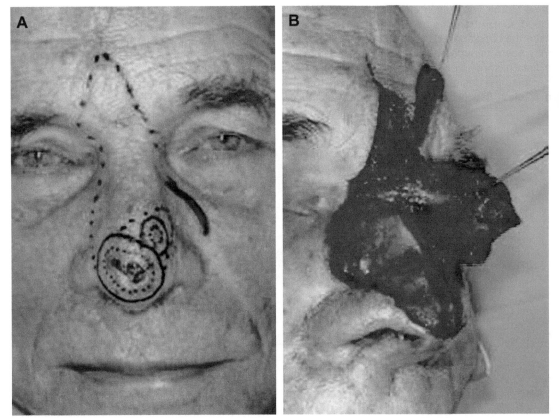

Fig. 11. (*A*) Excision of 2 primary basal cell carcinomas by Mohs surgery. (*B*) The nasal portion of the glabellar rotation flap is dissected beneath the musculature. (*From* PJFM Lohuis. Reconstruction of major nasal defects. In: JR Thomas, editor. Advanced therapy in facial plastic and reconstructive surgery. Connecticut: PMPH-USA; 2010; with permission.)

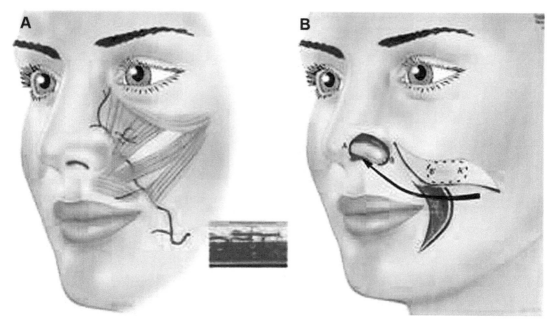

Fig. 12. (A) Melolabial flaps have a random vascularity based on directionally oriented subdermal plexus that courses parallel to melolabial crease and is derived from the angular artery. (B) Interpolated melolabial flap with points A and B corresponding with A' and B' when the defect is closed.

Melolabial flap

Melolabial flaps are used most frequently to repair large defects of the ala with or without extension to the lateral nasal tip and caudal sidewall. The flap provides skin of color and texture similar to that of the skin of these areas of the nose. The blood supply of the melolabial flap is not based on a specific named vessel but rather on a directionally oriented subdermal plexus that courses parallel to the melolabial crease and the angular artery, thus making it a random pattern flap (Fig. 12).

Two variants are described below: interpolated (2-stage) and superiorly based, cutaneous pedicled transposition (1-stage) melolabial flaps.

Interpolated melolabial flap The interpolated melolabial flap is a versatile flap for the reconstruction of a defect that remains within the aesthetic unit of the ala or columella. This flap is ideal for these sites because the skin of the flap tends to contract into a convexity that resembles the natural contours of these structures.

The flap is designed as an interpolation flap based on a cutaneous or subcutaneous tissue pedicle in which the final scar of the donor site closure line lies precisely in the melolabial crease (Fig. 13). The flap is dissected medially to the level of the orbicularis muscle and laterally to the level of the superficial musculoaponeurotic system (SMAS) fibers coursing to meet the former. The donor site is closed by undermining the adjacent

cheek skin and advancing it medially. After 3 weeks, the pedicle is divided and the flap inset in the second stage of the procedure.

Cutaneous pedicled transposition flap Defects of the ala may frequently be repaired with a superiorly based cutaneous pedicled transposition melolabial flap. If the defect does not involve the alar base and if the flap is thinned appropriately at the time of initial transfer, the procedure can be completed in 1 stage (Fig. 14). These flaps can remain edematous for a significant period and are prone to developing trapdoor deformity. Injection of steroids (triamcinolone [Kenacort], 10 mg/mL) and occasional second-stage debulking of the flap may be necessary. Reasonable results can be achieved, particularly in the elderly patient with large melolabial folds. The major disadvantage of the transposition flap is that its use frequently results in partial or complete obliteration of the alar crease and the more cephalic portion of the alar facial sulcus.

Paramedian forehead flap

The paramedian forehead flap is the keystone for nasal reconstruction and is ideal for reconstructing large or full-thickness defects of the caudal two-thirds of the nose, including the nasal tip, ala, columella, dorsum, and nasal sidewall.[16] This flap is far more preferred than its forerunner, the scalp flap, which is now more or less obsolete. The color and texture of the forehead skin provides an excellent

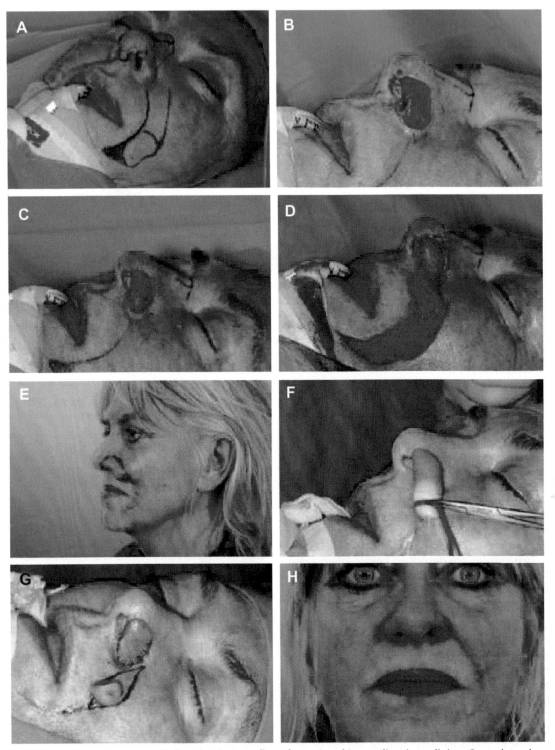

Fig. 13. (*A*) Alar automutilation defect. (*B, C*) Hinge flap of covering skin to adjust inner lining. Contralateral ear cartilage for contour and to avoid rim retraction. (*D–F*) Interpolated melolabial flap for external covering in 2 phases. (*G*) After cutting the pedicle, the alar defect is closed. (*H*) Postoperative result. (*From* PJFM Lohuis. Reconstruction of major nasal defects. In: JR Thomas, editor. Advanced therapy in facial plastic and reconstructive surgery. Connecticut: PMPH-USA; 2010; with permission.)

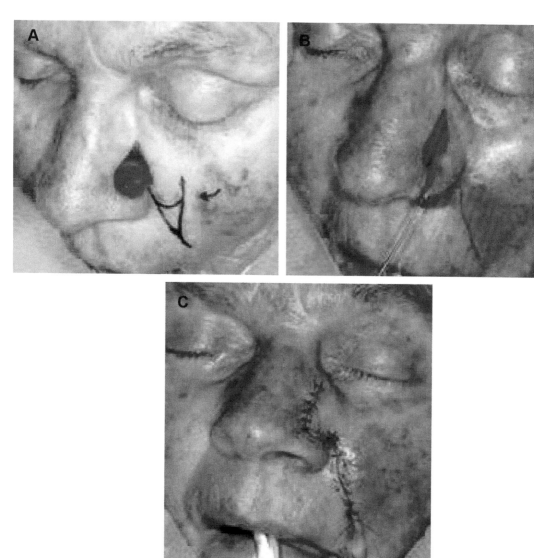

Fig. 14. Superiorly based cutaneous pedicled transposition (1 stage) melolabial flap. (*A*) Defect of the left ala and flap markings. (*B*) Flap transposition. (*C*) After closure. (*From* PJFM Lohuis. Reconstruction of major nasal defects. In: JR Thomas, editor. Advanced therapy in facial plastic and reconstructive surgery. Connecticut: PMPH-USA; 2010; with permission.)

match with native nasal skin, and the blood supply of the flap is extremely reliable. The majority of the blood supply to a paramedian forehead flap is from the supratrochlear artery (**Fig. 15**). This artery also has collateral circulation with the ipsilateral supra-orbital artery. Both arteries are terminal branches of the ophthalmic artery, which is derived from the internal carotid arterial system. The supratrochlear artery also richly anastomoses with the terminal branches of the angular artery supplied by the external carotid arterial system. Therefore there are 2 blood supplies: an axial pattern supply from the supratrochlear artery and a random pattern supply from the branches of the facial and angular arteries.

Because the paramedian forehead flap is the workhorse for nasal reconstruction, its designing and placement is described in detailed steps in the following section as a 2-stage procedure (**Fig. 16**). The first stage consists of elevation and transfer of the flap as well as closure of the donor site. The second stage consists of division of the pedicle, inset of the flap, and closure of the brow region.

First stage Care is taken to center the design of the flap over the supratrochlear vessels. The supratrochlear artery crosses the superomedial orbit vertically approximately 1.7 to 2.2 cm lateral to the

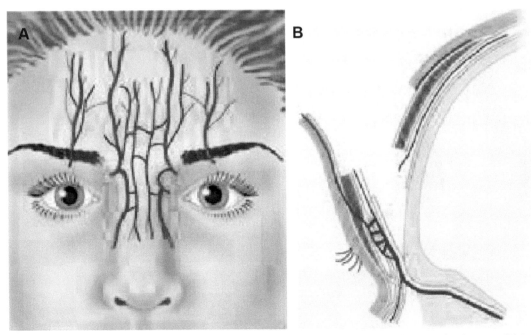

Fig. 15. (*A*) Blood supply of the forehead: the supratrochlear artery and ipsilateral supraorbital artery. (*B*) Transverse view of the supratrochlear artery, which provides the major blood supply of paramedian forehead flap, as it ascends the forehead. The artery passes from the orbit over the periosteum, through the frontalis muscle toward the subcutaneous tissue of the distal flap.

midline. It is helpful to identify the artery with a Doppler (see **Fig. 16C**) because this facilitates design of a narrow pedicle. The pedicle is centered over the vertical axis of the supratrochlear artery. A pattern is cut from foil of a suture pack to match the exact size of the defect or aesthetic unit. If the anterior hairline of a patient is low or if the flap is required for columellar reconstruction, the orientation of the flap may be designed to curve laterally to avoid the transplantation of hair-bearing skin. However, the design may also be extended into the hair-bearing scalp, if necessary. When extension is required, a secondary depilation procedure is necessary. The greatest portion of the flap is dissected in a supraperiosteal subfascial tissue plane. Approximately 2 cm above the supraorbital bony rim the periosteum is incised and the dissection carried inferiorly in a subperiostal plan. This step is done to safeguard the supratrochlear artery and allow the flap to be pivoted from a more inferior position in the periorbital area to lessen tension (see **Fig. 16E**). The excellent blood supply of the flap allows thinning of the distal portion of the flap, enhancing pliability and contouring, especially in cases in which the defect involves the nasal tip (see **Fig. 16F**). The flap is pivoted toward the nose and after limited undermining of the nasal skin, the flap is sutured in place with eversion of wound edges.

Closure of the forehead with wide supraperiosteal undermining, a subcutaneous mattress suture, and staples (see **Fig. 16H**), decreases wound tension and in most cases allows primary closure of the donor site with minimal scarring. In the hairline, a Burow triangle is usually removed to prevent SCD formation. Occasionally, particularly if part of the wound has been allowed to heal by secondary intention, it may be necessary to revise the forehead scar at a later date, most commonly after 6 months.

Second stage: dividing the pedicle and thinning of the flap The pedicle of the flap is divided and the flap inset approximately 3 weeks after the first procedure. As far as vascularity permits, this is also the time for appropriate debulking and contouring of the transferred skin flap. Alternatively, an intermediate stage at 3 weeks is performed before final pedicle division. This stage allows for more aggressive sculpturing and contouring of the flap. The pedicle division is then performed 3 weeks later. The unused portion of the forehead flap is amputated and discarded, except for a small triangle of the skin used to restore the normal

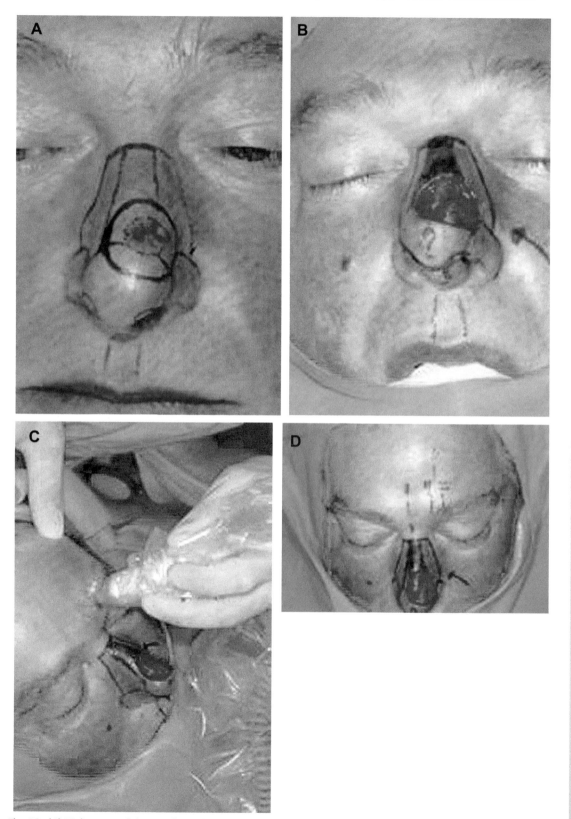

Fig. 16. (*A*) Melanoma of the nasal tip (*B*) Defect after removal of nasal tip after removal of melanoma. (*C*) Supra-trochlear artery identified with Doppler. (*D*) Paramedian forehead flap directed laterally because of shape and inferior position of anterior hairline.

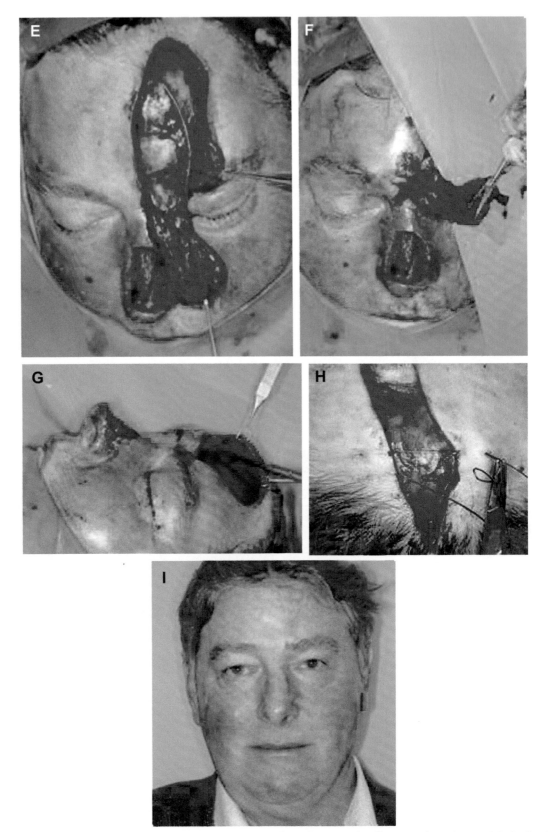

Fig. 16. (*E*) The nasal dorsal unit is further excised. About 2 cm above the supraorbital bony rim, the periosteum is incised and dissection carried inferiorly in a subperiosteal manner. (*F*) Thinning of the flap. (*G*) Undermining of the forehead skin. (*H*) The donor site is closed primarily. (*I*) The 3-month postoperative result. No additional contouring required. The eyebrows are restored to their natural anatomic relationship. (*From* PJFM Lohuis. Reconstruction of major nasal defects. In: JR Thomas, editor. Advanced therapy in facial plastic and reconstructive surgery. Connecticut: PMPH-USA; 2010; with permission.)

anatomic relationship of the medial aspects of the eyebrows. Closure of the brow region is performed with wide undermining and meticulous suturing to avoid a trapdoor deformity. The divided pedicle of the flap should not be replaced above the level of the eyebrow, because it will appear as a fingerlike peninsula on an otherwise smooth forehead.

Cheek and Cervicofacial Flaps

For larger wounds of the lateral nose, lateral upper lip, and cheek, the upper cervical and cheek areas can provide ample amounts of well-vascularized tissue for reconstruction. A variety of flap designs have been described in these areas and are primarily discussed in terms of the location or mode of transfer of donor tissue. There are 5 basic designs that are described in the following sections.

V-Y island subcutaneous tissue pedicle advancement flap

Subcutaneously, tissue pedicled V-Y flaps are most commonly used for soft tissue replacement of the lower lateral nasal sidewall, but they may also be used to repair small and deep skin defects of the ala. The flap is incised and freed from the adjacent cheek fat, but it remains attached in the deep plane. If the pedicle causes excessive fullness adjacent to the ala, a secondary procedure to contour this region is planned 2 to 3 months after the flap transfer.

Cheek advancement flap

Cheek advancement flaps are used for the closure of defects involving the lateral nose and adjacent cheek. Elevation of this flap should be performed in the midsubcutaneous tissue plane as far laterally as necessary to advance the flap to fill the nasal and/or cheek wound. The superior limb of this flap should be placed at the lower bony orbital rim or in a natural lower eyelid crease and carried to a more superior location at the lateral canthus to avoid postoperative ectropion. The inferior limb is usually placed in the melolabial crease.[17]

Cheek rotation flap

The cheek advancement-rotation flap has been proved to be useful for the repair of large and more complex defects involving the lateral nose and medial cheek. The flap is extremely vital, and the scars resulting from transfer of the flap are well concealed, especially in the elderly patient. The design follows the classic outline of the Mustarde flap (**Fig. 17**). If the superior border of the flap is located in the area of the infraorbital bony rim, the posterior extension of this limb should be carried superior to the level of the lateral

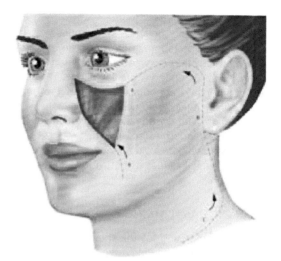

Fig. 17. Cheek advancement flap A that can be extended to a rotation advancement flap B and a cervicofacial flap C. For large wounds of lateral nose, lateral upper lip, and cheek, superior cervical and cheek areas can provide ample amounts of well-vascularized tissue for reconstruction.

canthus and then posterior toward the ear. After incision of the SMAS, undermining is continued below the plane of the SMAS and above the facial nerve branches. In its superior location, it is imperative to secure the dermis of the flap to the periosteum of the lateral bony orbital rim to avoid postoperative ectropion. Placing a back cut at the base of the flap or removing a Burow triangle of skin along the peripheral border of the donor site wound aid in improving the discrepancies in wound border lengths.

Cervicofacial flap

The cervicofacial flap (see **Fig. 17**) is an inferiorly based facial rotation advancement flap that has an extension into the neck for recruiting additional cervical skin to increase the size of the flap. Defects as large as 6 × 10 cm can be closed in 1 stage with this flap. Cervicofacial flaps have a random vascularity, relying entirely on the circulation of the subdermal plexus coming from the branches of the facial vessels. The blood supply and reliability can be improved significantly by dissecting the flap in a tissue plane below the SMAS. In the cervical region, undermining is beneath the platysma, which is transected transversely in the inferior cervical region to facilitate superior mobility and satisfactory transposition of the flap.[17] The cervicofacial flap offers excellent exposure for concomitant dissection of the parotid gland and cervical lymph node chains, if skin cancer has metastasized to the parotid gland or neck.

Extended Abbe flap

Defects extending beyond the confines of the upper lip may be reconstructed with an extended lip switch flap that is based on the inferior labial artery.[18] This extended Abbe flap allows functional and cosmetically acceptable repair of the upper lip, medial cheek, columella, and nasal sill. In combination with an advancement of cheek fat, using an extended Abbe flap can be of great help to restore both volume and skin in case of major paranasal defect without the use of a free flap (**Fig. 18**).

INTERNAL NASAL LINING

When reconstructing full-thickness nasal defects, the importance of ensuring adequate osseocartilaginous support and internal nasal lining cannot be overemphasized. Ensuring these can prevent scar formation and retractions resulting in deformity that is worse than the one to be concealed.[19] Reconstruction of a full-thickness defect involves 3 layers: external skin covering, nasal skeleton, and internal nasal lining (**Fig. 19**). Cartilage grafts are used to reconstruct the nasal skeleton to prevent retraction of the nostril margin, avoid collapse of the nasal valve, and maintain the 3-dimensional configuration of the nose (see **Fig. 19**).

The most common alternatives for the internal nasal lining are the prefabricated forehead flap, the staged sequential skin graft technique, and the intranasal lining flap. Intranasal lining flaps are preferred and include the bipedicled vestibular skin advancement flap and septal mucoperichondrial hinge flap. The former is a flap of residual vestibular skin based medially on the nasal septum and laterally on the nasal floor (see **Fig. 19**), whereas the latter is based on a 1.5- to 2-cm pedicle located in the area of the anterior nasal spine, supplied by the ipsilateral septal branch of the superior labial artery (see **Fig. 19**). For larger lining defects, a contralateral septomucoperichondrial flap based on the dorsum of the septum and supplied by the anterior ethmoid artery is also used. This flap is turned laterally to line the sidewall and middle vault.[20]

Although adjacent turnover flaps are somewhat thick, stiff, and limited in their size, they may be used for lining small full-thickness nasal defects. These flaps are based along the periphery of the defect.[20,21]

NEAR-TOTAL AND TOTAL NASAL RECONSTRUCTION

Reconstructing near-total and total nasal defects is a formidable project. If there is sufficient septum available, septomucoperichondrial hinge flaps are developed for internal lining. If a portion of the caudal or dorsal nose is missing, composite septomucoperichondrial flaps are turned outward from the interior of the nasal passages to provide lining and structural support. External covering is nearly always provided by a paramedian forehead flap.

Extensive defects of the bony pyramid are best reconstructed with a 3-dimensional structural framework of autologous bone, using sculpted plates of the tabula externa of the parietal bone. The bone segments are positioned to replicate the shape of the bony vault and are fixed to each other and the surrounding maxillary skull with mini AO-plates (**Fig. 20**).

Composite septomucoperichondrial pivotal flaps are not delayed when the caudal septum remains intact because of the ample blood supply provided to the flap by bilateral septal branches of the superior labial artery. However, when the caudal septum has been resected, it is prudent to delay the flap before pivoting it forward out of the nasal passage. The flap is large relative to the pedicle, which consists of 2 mucoperichondrial flaps based on the anterior floor of the nasal passages. It is also prudent to delay large composite septomucoperichondrial flaps for patients who use tobacco products and those who have received previous irradiation of the nasal passages.

The pedicles of interpolated forehead flaps used as a covering for the nose are typically divided 3 weeks after transfer of the flap of the nose. However, when reconstructing large full-thickness defects of the nose, there is less surface contact between the covering flap and vascularized tissue at the recipient site. In such cases, the ingrowth of vessels required to revascularize the covering flap is derived only from scar tissue along the border of the constructed nose and the caudal border of the lining flaps. This limited access for revascularization translates into a longer duration before anastomotic connections are sufficient between the forehead flap and adjacent cheek skin to adequately sustain the flap once the pedicle is divided. For this reason, delaying the detachment of covering flaps for 2 months after initial flap transfer is recommended in cases of total or near-total nasal reconstruction.

In most cases, the pedicle of an interpolated covering flap is divided and the flap inset before performing a contouring procedure. However, in the case shown in **Fig. 21**, the pedicle of the forehead flap remained attached while 2 contouring procedures were performed 1 month apart before pedicle division. The first procedure created a thinner covering flap for the entire nose. The

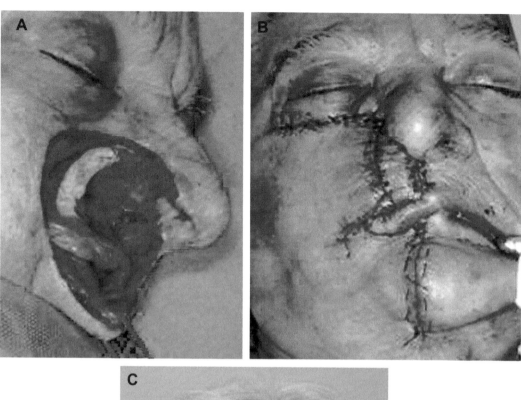

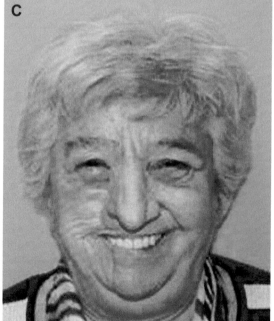

Fig. 18. Patient with a serious loss of volume in the medial cheek, upper lip, nasal sill, and premaxilla after removal of a recurrent basal cell carcinoma after radiotherapy. (*A*) An extended Abbe flap based on the inferior labial artery restored both volume and skin of the cheek and upper lip. (*B*) After closure of the defect. (*C*) Postoperative result after a 3 -layer reconstruction of the ala with a hinge flap of an earlier placed skin graft, ear cartilage, and forehead flap was also performed.

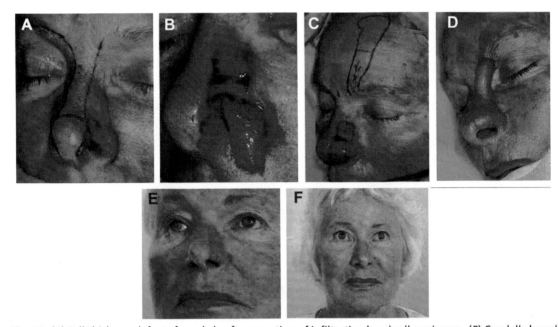

Fig. 19. (*A*) Full-thickness defect of nasal ala after resection of infiltrating basal cell carcinoma. (*B*) Caudally based ipsilateral septal mucoperichondrial hinge flap used for inner lining based on 1.5- to 2-cm pedicle located in the area of nasal spine and supplied by the ipsilateral septal branch of superior labial artery. (*C*) Contralateral auricular cartilage used as a graft to restore contour and to avoid retraction of nostril rim. (*D*) Flap in place, 5 weeks after transfer. (*E*) The 3-month postoperative result. (*F*) Final postoperative result. (*From* PJFM Lohuis. Reconstruction of major nasal defects. In: JR Thomas, editor. Advanced therapy in facial plastic and reconstructive surgery. Connecticut: PMPH-USA; 2010; with permission.)

second procedure created alar grooves. Maintaining the integrity of the flap's pedicle during these operations ensured the vascularity of the flap while achieving optimal flap contour. The total interval required to complete nasal reconstruction was approximately 5 months, excluding a minor office procedure that was performed 7 months later.

In cases of total and near-total nasal reconstruction, it is not always possible to construct the nose of ideal length. The limiting factor is the quantity of mucosa available for internal lining. As in the case presented, when a large portion of the nasal septum has been resected, the composite septomucoperichondrial flap used to line the lower vault may be of insufficient size to reach the ideal position for the nasal tip. In such instances, the constructed nose is short and the tip is cephalically rotated. In the case presented, the function and contour of the constructed nose are ideal; however, the nose is foreshortened and the tip is more cephalad than ideal.

The use of microsurgical transfer of skin to reconstruct the internal lining of extensive nasal defects has brought the evolution of nasal reconstruction to a further level. Because of its long pedicle, the thin and well-vascularized fasciocutaneous tissue of a transposed radial forearm flap can be used as internal nasal lining after connecting the radial artery and cephalic vein to vessels of the face or superior neck by microanastomosis. In this way, healthy tissue unsullied by prior irradiation, cocaine injury, or disease can provide a basis on which the nasal skeleton and external skin covering can be further reconstructed.

In selected cases, when aesthetic and functional demands are beyond the capacity of reconstructive efforts, a facial prosthesis may be a reasonable alternative. Osseointegrated dental implants can be connected with a gold bar or magnets to keep a nasal prosthesis (intrinsically pigmented silicone) in place (**Fig. 22**).

REFINEMENT TECHNIQUES

In nasal reconstruction, grafts mainly serve 3 functions: restoration, support, and contour. Restorative grafts replace defects of the nasal skeleton and may be made of bone or cartilage, depending on the missing framework. Support grafts (columellar strut, lateral alar batten graft, spreader grafts) provide reinforcement to the existing

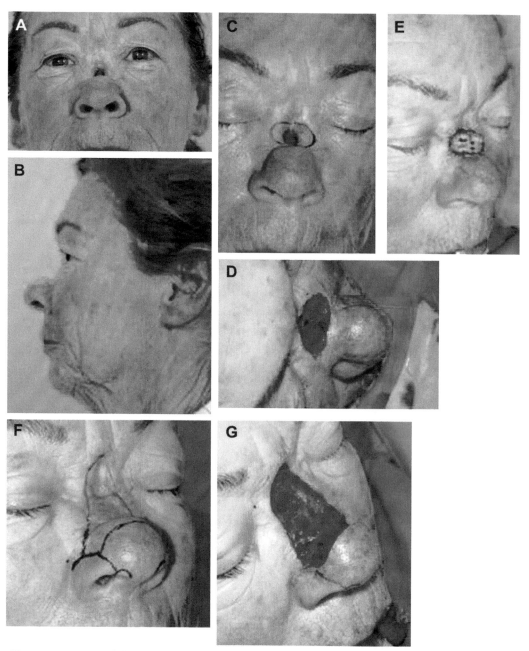

Fig. 20. Reconstruction of the nasal dorsum. (*A*) Defect as a result of sarcoma. (*B*) Lateral view. (*C*) Deepithelialisation of the defect. (*D*) Inner lining closure by 2 hinge flaps. (*E*) Skin graft covering the defect. (*F*) Preparation of the second stage of the reconstruction. (*G*) Deepithelialization of the aesthetic units.

skeleton. Contour grafts (shield graft, cap graft, onlay grafts) are used to enhance the shape of the nasal tip or to correct topographic irregularities.

Auricular cartilage grafts are mostly used to replace missing segments of alar cartilages and to support the ala. A columellar strut is designed from septal cartilage to provide structural support to the central tip and columella. By changing the angle of placement of this graft in the inferior columella, or the width of the strut, it can also be used to augment the nasolabial angle or increase the columellar prominence. Lateral crural struts composed of septal or auricular cartilage

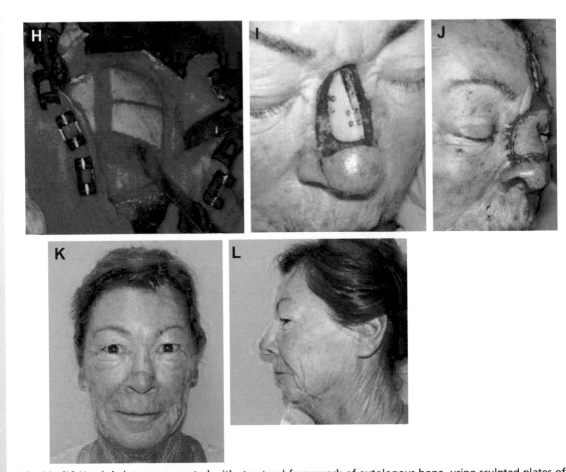

Fig. 20. (*H*) Nasal skeleton was created with structural framework of autologous bone, using sculpted plates of the tabula externa of the parietal bone. (*I*) The bone segments are positioned to replicate the shape of the bony vault and are fixed to each other and the surrounding maxillary skull with mini AO-plates. (*J*) External covering with paramedian forehead flap. (*K*) Postoperative frontal view. (*L*) Postoperative lateral view. (*From* PJFM Lohuis. Reconstruction of major nasal defects. In: JR Thomas, editor. Advanced therapy in facial plastic and reconstructive surgery. Connecticut: PMPH-USA; 2010; with permission.)

produces slight lateral flaring of the alar cartilage in the region of the internal and external nasal valves, increasing the nasal aperture. Spreader grafts are used to lateralize upper lateral cartilages and increase the aperture of the internal nasal valve. Shield grafts of septal or auricular cartilage are used to enhance tip definition, projection, and rotation. A cap graft of cartilage is used in single or double layers to enhance tip definition, projection, and rotation. Septal or auricular cartilage is also used to correct areas of contour depression on the surface of the nose.

Other modifications of the nasal skeleton include tip sutures to narrow the domes, hump resection to lower the nasal dorsum, and osteotomies to medialize the bony sidewalls. Second- or third-phase contouring procedures, which involve sculpting the subcutaneous tissues of the covering flap, are occasionally necessary and can be performed under local anesthesia.

Despite efforts to assemble a delicate nostril, the reconstructed ala may be too thick. Secondary contouring is then best performed through rim incisions. When the defect extends cephalic to the alar groove, a specific contouring procedure is required to create a new groove, which is often obliterated by the base of the covering flap. A template of the contralateral normal ala is made, reversed, placed over the reconstructed ala, and carefully traced with a marking pen.[5] Excision of soft tissue and cartilage is performed by incising the scar along the cephalic border of the flap or by creating a new incision in the flap along the superior border of the tracing. Dermabrasion of

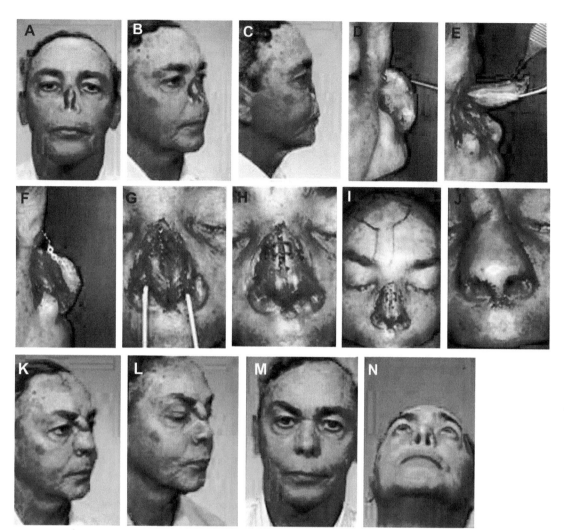

Fig. 21. Nasal reconstruction after removal of small cell carcinoma with adjuvant radiotherapy. (*A*) Frontal view. (*B*) Oblique view. (*C*) Lateral view. (*D*) Composite septal flap. (*D, E*) Composite septal flap is pivoted anteriorly and (*F*) the position was maintained by a fixation plate. (*G*) Septal mucoperichondrial flaps reflected to assist nasal lining. Bilateral mucoperiosteal flaps of the middle turbinate hinged on anterior attachments. Septal mucoperichondrial flap and middle turbinate mucoperiosteal flap sutured to close inner lining. (*H*) Upper two-thirds reconstructed with bone grafts connected with miniplates, lower one-third reconstructed with auricular cartilage. (*I*) Paramedian forehead flap markings. (*J*) External covering with interpolated paramedian forehead flap. (*K, L*) Contouring in 2 procedures before detachment of the flap from forehead. (*M, N*) Final results. (*From* PJFM Lohuis. Reconstruction of major nasal defects. In: JR Thomas, editor. Advanced therapy in facial plastic and reconstructive surgery. Connecticut: PMPH-USA; 2010; with permission.)

incisional scars may help smooth out any minor discrepancies in contour and texture. The thick skin of the nose and face lends itself well to dermabrasion.

POSTOPERATIVE CARE

Written instructions for postoperative care of the wound are to be provided to the patient and must be specific to each procedure. In general, after 24 hours, patients may remove their dressings and take a shower. Any crusts should be removed gently. Subsequently, suture lines are cleaned with soap or diluted hydrogen peroxide twice daily, after which a thin layer of antibiotic ointment is applied to the wound. Bolster dressings for skin grafts remain in place for approximately 4 days. In cases of an interpolated flap to improve epithelialization, the

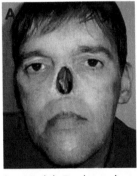
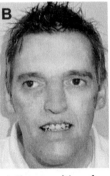

Fig. 22. (*A*) Total nasal amputation resulting from resection of recurrent SCC. (*B*) Silicone prosthesis in place.

pedicle is kept moist with gauze impregnated with ointment or simply with an antibiotic ointment.

SUMMARY

The aim of reconstructive nasal surgery is not only to rebuild all or part of the nose but also to blend and tailor the new and old tissues in such a way as to create the best possible result. Although a variety of reconstructive options exist, local or regional skin flaps are one of the most powerful reconstructive tools for the reconstruction of cutaneous nasal defects. This article describes the fundamentals of nasal reconstruction and focuses on transposition flaps for the reconstruction of nasal defects.

REFERENCES

1. Zitelli JA, Fasio MJ. Reconstruction of the nose with local flaps. J Dermatol Surg Oncol 1991;17:184–9.
2. Becker FF, Langford FP. Local flaps in nasal reconstruction. Surg Clin North Am 1996;4:505–15.
3. Menick FJ. Artistry in aesthetic surgery. Aesthetic perception and the subunit principle. Clin Plast Surg 1987;14:723–34.
4. Burget GC, Menick FJ. Aesthetic reconstruction of the nose. St Louis (MO): Mosby; 1994.
5. Baker SR, Naficy S. Principles of nasal reconstruction. St Louis (MO): Mosby; 2002.
6. Singh DJ, Bartlett SP. Aesthetic consideration in nasal reconstruction and the role of modified nasal subunits. Plast Reconstr Surg 2003;111:639–51.
7. Menick FJ. A 10-year experience in nasal reconstruction with the three-stage forehead flap. Plast Reconstr Surg 2002;109:1839–55, [discussion: 1856–61].
8. Burget GC, Menick FJ. The subunit principle for nasal reconstruction. Plast Reconstr Surg 1985;76: 239–47.
9. Panje W, Ceilley R. The influence of embryology of the mid-face on the spread of epithelial malignancies. Laryngoscope 1979;89:1914–20.
10. Evans GR, Williams JZ, Ainslie NB. Cutaneous nasal malignancies: is primary reconstruction safe? Head Neck 1997;19:182–7.
11. Goepfert H, Dichtel WJ, Medina JE, et al. Perineural invasion of squamous cell skin carcinoma of the head and neck. Am J Surg 1984;148:542.
12. Rohrer T, Bhatia A. Transposition flaps in cutaneous surgery. Dermatol Surg 2005;31:1014–23.
13. Walike JW, Larrabee WF. The note flap. Arch Otolaryngol 1985;111:430–3.
14. Flint ID, Siegle RJ. The bipedicled flap revisited. J Dermatol Surg Oncol 1994;20:394–400.
15. Dzubow LM. Nasal dorsal flaps. In: Baker SR, Swanson NA, editors. Local flaps in facial reconstruction. St Louis (MO): Mosby; 1995. p. 225–46, Chapter 14.
16. Park SS. Reconstruction of nasal defects larger than 1.5 cm in diameter. Laryngoscope 2000;110: 1241–50.
17. Kroll SS, Reece GP, Robb G, et al. Deep-plane cervicofacial rotation-advancement flap for reconstruction of large cheek defects. Plast Reconstr Surg 1994;94:88–93.
18. Naficy S, Baker SR. The extended Abbe flap in the reconstruction of complex midfacial defects. Arch Facial Plast Surg 2000;2:141–4.
19. Burget GC, Menick FJ. Nasal support and lining: the marriage of beauty and blood supply. Plast Reconstr Surg 1989;84:189–203.
20. Menick FJ. Lining options in nasal reconstruction. Operat Tech Plast Reconstr Surg 1998;5:65–75.
21. Park SS, Cook TA, Wang TD. The epithelial "turn-in" flap in nasal reconstruction. Arch Otolaryngol Head Neck Surg 1995;121:1122–7.

Bilobed Flaps in Nasal Reconstruction

Jacob D. Steiger, MD

KEYWORDS

- Bilobed flap • Nasal reconstruction • Local flap
- Nasal transposition flap

Bilobed flaps are local flaps useful for the reconstruction of nasal defects. These flaps are especially useful for defects of the caudal portion of the nose. Defects in this region pose a reconstructive challenge because the skin is thick, sebaceous, and lacks elasticity. Significant advancement, rotation, or transposition in this area can result in distortion of the nasal tip.

The bilobed flap is a double transposition flap whose basic principle relies on transposing mobile skin from the cephalic portion of the nose in order to close defects of the thicker immobile skin of the caudal portion of the nose. This double transposition flap distributes tension over an area greater than a single transposition, allowing for successful closure of defects in the inelastic skin of the nose.

The bilobed flap for nasal reconstruction was first described by the Dutch surgeon Esser[1] in the early twentieth century. He described a total transposition arc of greater than 180°. The large degree of rotation created large lobes that required the flap to extend into the glabella, resulting in significant standing cutaneous deformities. Later in the twentieth century, McGregor and Soutar[2] discussed the use of the bilobed flap with smaller pivotal arcs, which resulted in smaller standing cutaneous deformities and decreased pincushioning. Zitelli's[3] modification of the bilobed flap emphasized a total pivotal arc no greater than 90° to 110°, with an approximately 45° pivotal arc between each lobe. His results demonstrated the practical utility of this flap in nasal reconstruction.

FLAP SELECTION

Bilobed flaps are ideal for defects of the central or lateral nasal tip that range up to 1.5 cm in size.[4]

These flaps are best suited in the distal third of the nose, where most other skin flaps would cause significant distortion of the nasal tip. Defects that extend onto the nasal ala are generally not favorable for this type of repair because of a high likelihood for alar retraction. The defect should be at least 0.5 cm away from the nostril-free margin in order to reduce the risk of notching.

Bilobed flaps may also be used to repair more cephalically positioned nasal defects; however, size limitations exist as the donor site of the second lobe moves cephalad. In these cases, the second lobe donor site would be located at the medial canthus or glabella and donor site closure may lead to distortion of these structures, compromising the overall aesthetic and functional reconstructive outcomes. In these locations, alternative flap selection may lead to a more desirable outcome.

Bilobed flaps are especially advantageous for defects whose depth extends into and past the level of the subcutaneous fat, which is the main benefit of the bilobed flap over skin grafts when considering reconstruction of the nasal tip. Skin grafts placed over deeper defects often results in visible depressions over the nose and a less-than desirable aesthetic result. The depth of the nasal defect often dictates the use of a bilobed flap over a skin graft in this area.

FLAP DESIGN

Bilobed flaps are classified as random flaps whose blood supply originates at the base of the flap. The flap is most commonly based laterally, on the nasal sidewall, where there is a robust arterial supply to the nose. However, medially based flaps can also

The author has nothing to disclose.
Steiger Facial Plastic Surgery, 1001 North Federal Highway, Boca Raton, FL 33432, USA
E-mail address: jds@drsteiger.com

Facial Plast Surg Clin N Am 19 (2011) 107–111
doi:10.1016/j.fsc.2010.10.013

facialplastic.theclinics.com

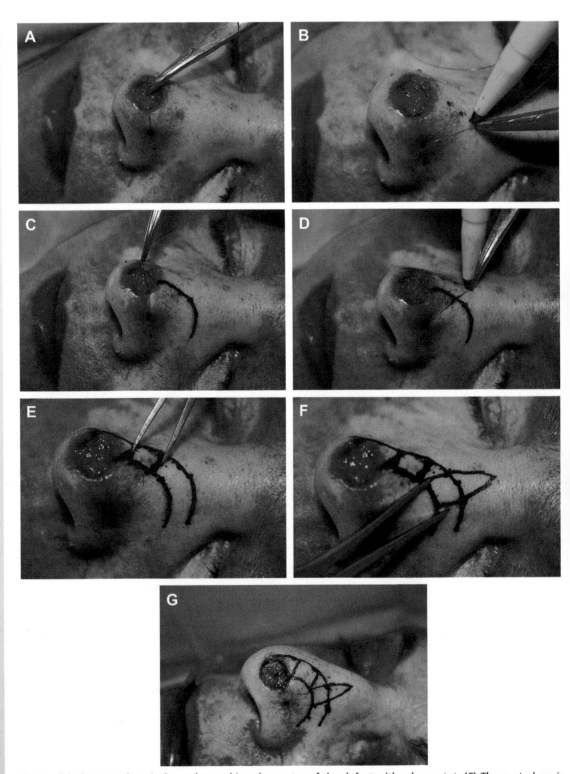

Fig. 1. (*A*) The central arc is drawn by marking the center of the defect with a hemostat. (*B*) The central arc is marked while rotating the hemostat 120° from the center point (*C*) The central arc has been drawn, and the distal point of the defect is marked with a hemostat. (*D*) The hemostat is once again rotated 120° and the distal arc is drawn. (*E*) The first lobe of the flap is drawn at 45° away from the defect and with a diameter equal to that of the defect. (*F*) The second lobe is designed at 45° away from the first lobe, with a diameter slightly smaller than that of the defect. The lobe is extended to remove a standing cutaneous cone to allow for primary closure of the donor site. (*G*) A bilobed double transposition flap marking is complete using a pivotal arc totaling 90°.

be placed successfully, if necessary, with little risk of flap necrosis. The high vascularity of this region makes the blood supply to the bilobed flap robust and provides for a high success rate of flap viability.

The design of the bilobed flap is based on a geometrically configured pattern that spans a 90° pivotal arc. The first step in the proper design of this flap is to mark the 2 arcsthat will define the boundaries of the flap and its proper angulations. In order to do so, the radius and diameter of the nasal defect are measured with calipers. A pivot point is selected 1 radius from the free edge of the defect and is placed in the region from where the standing cutaneous cone has to be removed. This pivot point is most commonly placed within the alar groove. A marking pen is used to mark the pivot point over which the arcs are based.

A suture is then passed full thickness through the nose at the pivot point, and a knot is placed within the suture itself to anchor it into position at the nasal vestibule (**Fig. 1A**). Next, the suture is marked at the center of the defect with a hemostat. The hemostat is then pivoted cephalad in a 120° rotation, using a marking pen at the level of the hemostat to draw the first arc (see **Fig. 1B**). The second arc is then configured by repositioning the hemostat at the center of the defect's distal edge (see **Fig. 1C**) and marking out the resultant arc using a similar 120° rotation (see **Fig. 1D**). Alternatively, a standard geometry compass can be used to perform these markings.

Once the 2 arcs are properly drawn, the 2 lobes of the flap are configured. The thick skin of the nasal tip has minimal elasticity and does not allow for significant advancement without distortion. Unlike bilobed flaps in the rest of the face and body, the first lobe of a nasal bilobed flap should have the same diameter as the defect itself (see **Fig. 1E**). The first side of the first lobe is drawn as a perpendicular line between the 2 arcs, 45° away from the defect. The second side of the first lobe is then drawn parallel to this line, 1 diameter away from the first side. The first side of the second lobe is then marked, 45° away from the adjacent lobe. A line marking this side of the second lobe is then drawn. The second lobe is then marked out to be similar or slightly smaller then the nasal defect (see **Fig. 1F**), which will depend on the elasticity of the skin in this region and can be judged by pinching the skin of the lateral nasal wall. Once again, the final side of the second lobe is marked, extending the planned incision past the arcs in order to allow for the excision of an additional triangle of skin for adequate donor site closure (see **Fig. 1G**).

When designing a bilobed flap, the standing cutaneous cone excision, at the base of the defect, is taken into consideration and preferably placed within the alar crease. The apex of the cone is positioned at the pivot point that was previously marked. However, one should not be too conservative as to the amount of skin to remove because small dog-ears in this area do not settle out well. A disadvantage of the bilobed flap is the amount of incision necessary, which cannot be placed within the relaxed skin tension lines. Despite this, incisions of the nose heal well when meticulously closed in layers.

SURGICAL TECHNIQUE

Incisions are made along the previously described markings, taking care to keep them perpendicular to the skin (**Figs. 2–5**). The proper plane of dissection is the one below the nasal superficial musculoaponeurotic system, just above the perichondrium of the nasal cartilage. Once this layer is reached, the flap is easily elevated with either sharp or blunt dissection.

Wide undermining in the supraperichondrial plane is then performed over the entire nose, including the lower lateral cartilages. Undermining may sometimes extend into the cheek and is essential to minimize wound tension, pincushioning of the flap, and distortion of the nose. The lobes should then easily transpose into their desired locations with minimal wound tension. If excessive tension exists, a wider undermining of the flap at the proper depth may be necessary.

Once hemostasis is achieved, a 5-0 absorbable monofilament suture is used to close the deep muscle layer. Closure is first performed in the

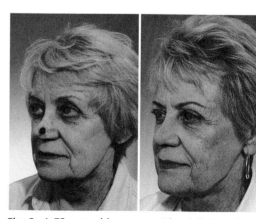

Fig. 2. A 72-year-old woman with a left lateral nasal tip defect measuring 1.2 × 1.1 cm. The defect extended down to the lower lateral cartilage (*left*). Bilobed flap repair was performed. Results shown are 6 months after surgery (*right*).

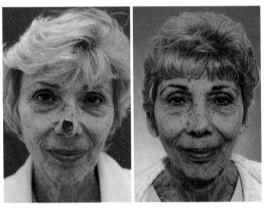

Fig. 3. A 74-year-old woman with a 1.5 × 1.6-cm defect of the central nasal tip. The defect extended to her lower lateral cartilage and was 0.5 cm away from the nostril margin (*left*). She is shown 4 months after operation (*right*).

regions of highest flap tension and then dispersed throughout the rest of the flap to distribute the tension evenly. The skin layer is then closed with a running polypropylene suture along the length of the incision. A compression dressing is then applied over the nose.

COMPLICATIONS

Risks and complications of the use of bilobed flaps are similar to those of other nasal skin flap procedures. The biggest concern and most common complication is the distortion of the nasal structure. Distortion of the nasal tip may occur when the defect is in close proximity to the free margin of the nose. Distortion is commonly seen as elevation of the nasal tip or nostril margin. Tension with

wound closure commonly elevates the tip; however, with proper flap selection, undermining, and design, the skin and soft tissue envelope redistributes and the distortion is minimized. Patients who have an inherently weak nasal structural support are noted to have a greater tendency for nasal distortion and elevation of the nostril-free margin.

In addition, the topographic appearance of the nose can be altered with a bilobed flap repair. Nasal flaps have an inherent tendency to form a convex surface. This tendency can be further exacerbated by the development of a trapdoor deformity. This property of the flap can be used to the advantage of the reconstructive surgeon for appropriately positioned defects. However, when considering bilobed flap repair over concave surfaces of the nose, such as the alar crease, the patient is counseled to the possible need for a secondary procedure to reestablish the contour of this unit.

Topographic changes may also occur in the region of flap transposition. The first lobe of the flap is inherently thicker than the second lobe because of the location of the donor site. This difference in thickness can lead to visible depressions at the sites of transposition. Differential sculpting of the flap is performed to minimize this. Care is taken to trim excess subcutaneous tissues from full areas of the flap, and this extra tissue may be used to fill in areas of potential depression.

Nasal obstruction is another potential complication of the bilobed flap. This condition is most commonly seen in patients with a combination of thin skin, weak cartilage, and large nasal tip defects. Although tension on the nasal framework

A   **B**

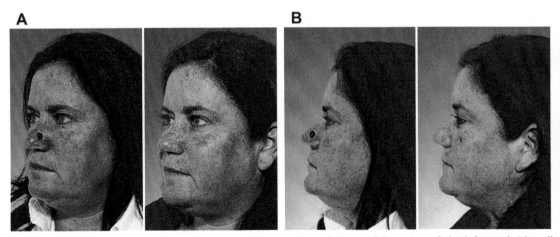

Fig. 4. (*A, B*) A 40-year-old woman with a 1.0 × 0.9-cm defect of the caudal portion of the left nasal sidewall (*left*). This defect is deep to the upper lateral cartilage. She has thick skin, and bilobed flap was used to repair this defect. She is shown 3 months after repair (*right*).

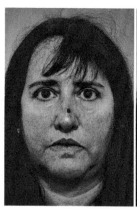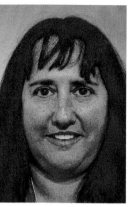

Fig. 5. A 49-year-old woman with a 0.7 × 0.6-cm defect of the left nasal dorsum. The defect extends into the subcutaneous fat (*left*). She has thick skin, and a bilobed flap was chosen to repair the defect. She is shown 3 months after repair (*right*).

is rare, it can lead to compromise of the internal or external nasal valve. When compromise occurs and is not resolved using conservative measures, repair of the nasal valves may be necessary with secondary procedures.

Additional potential complications of bilobed flaps are similar to those of other local flap procedures of the head and neck, including wound infections, hematoma, flap necrosis, and hypertrophic scarring. Although possible, these complications are uncommon. In some instances of noticeable scarring, flap revision and/or dermabrasion may be necessary.

SUMMARY

Bilobed flaps are an excellent choice for the repair of nasal defects. These flaps are especially useful for defects of the caudal portion of the nose and the nasal tip, where the skin is less elastic. Appropriate flap selection, design, and execution will lead to excellent aesthetic and functional results.

REFERENCES

1. Esser JF. Gestielte locale nasenplastik mit zweizipfligem lappen decking des sekundaren detektes vom ersten zipfel durch den zweiten. Dtsh Z Chir 1918; 143:385.
2. McGregor JC, Soutar DS. A critical assessment of the bilobed flap. Br J Plast Surg 1981;34:197.
3. Zitelli JA. The bilobed flap for nasal reconstruction. Arch Dermatol 1989;125:957.
4. Baker SR. Bilobe flaps. In: Baker SR, editor. Local flaps in facial reconstruction. Philadelphia: Mosby; 2007. p. 189–211.

Glabellar Flaps in Nasal Reconstruction

Cody A. Koch, MD, PhD, David J. Archibald, MD,
Oren Friedman, MD*

KEYWORDS

- Glabellar flap • Dorsal nasal flap • Medial canthus
- Rieger flap • Nasal reconstruction

The nose occupies the central third of the face and is bordered by important functional and aesthetic structures, such as the medial canthus and lacrimal apparatus. The ideal nasal structure does not draw focus on itself but rather blends with other facial structures, focusing attention on perioral and periorbital areas. Defects of the nose and surrounding structures occur most commonly as a result of malignancy but also as a result of infection, trauma, congenital anomalies, and prior surgery. These defects, if not properly addressed, lead to a potentially aesthetically displeasing form and potentially impaired function. The surgical correction of defects of the nose and surrounding structures can pose significant challenges to the reconstructive surgeon.

Nasal reconstruction was revolutionized by Burget and Menick,[1] who divided the nose into multiple subunits based on the multitude of differences of elasticity, color, contour, and texture of the skin. The repair of defects of the nose and surrounding structures requires the knowledge of these aesthetic subunits as well as a variety of surgical techniques. Generalized options for addressing nasal defects include primary closure, healing by secondary intention, skin grafting, and the use of local and distant flaps. Although multiple options exist, optimal results are obtained when "like is used to repair like." The use of tissues of similar color, texture, and thickness for the repair of defects usually requires various local flaps to recruit adjacent tissue into the defect.

The purpose of this article is to revisit the application of the glabellar flap and its modifications for reconstruction of defects of the external nose. We also review modifications of these flaps to provide inner lining of the nose as well as reconstruction of the medial canthus.

RELEVANT ANATOMY

The nose is a 3-dimensional structure consisting of 3 layers. The external layer contains the skin that drapes over the middle layer, which consists of the bony/cartilaginous skeleton. The nasal cavity is lined by the third layer, which is the nasal mucosa. According to the principles of Burget and Menick,[1] the nose can be divided into 9 aesthetic subunits. These include the paired lateral side walls; alar lobules; soft tissue triangles; and the singular nasal dorsum, nasal tip, and columella. The nasal subunits can be divided into concave and convex. The 4 concave nasal subunits include the lateral side walls and the soft tissue triangles, whereas the 5 convex subunits include the nasal tip, dorsum, columella, and paired alar lobules.

The nose may be further divided into 3 zones. Zone 1 covers the dorsum and side walls. The skin of Zone 1 is thin and does not contain sebaceous glands. Zone 2 typically begins approximately 1.0 to 1.5 cm above the supratip and covers the 3 nasal subunits consisting of the alar lobules and the nasal tip. The skin of Zone 2 is thicker than that of Zone 1 and contains sebaceous glands. Zone 3 is the most inferior skin that overlies the soft tissue triangles, columella, and infratip lobule. The skin is relatively immobile,

Financial Disclosure: none.

Conflicts of Interest: none.

Department of Otorhinolaryngology—Head and Neck Surgery, Mayo Clinic College of Medicine, 200 First Street SW, Rochester, MN 55905, USA

* Corresponding author.

E-mail address: friedman.oren@mayo.edu

smooth, and thin, and does not contain sebaceous glands.

The glabella is defined as the area between the eyebrows. The glabella lies directly above the nose and joins the superciliary ridges. The area is slightly elevated and contains a significant amount of redundant skin, which can be recruited for use in local flaps. The skin of the glabella is thicker relative to the skin of the nasal dorsum and this fact should be considered when designing local flaps for nasal reconstruction.

The musculature of the glabellar region consists of the frontalis, procerus, and corrugator supercilli (**Fig. 1**). The frontalis is the anterior portion of the occipitofrontalis. The frontalis arises from the epicranial aponeurosis and inserts into the skin of the eyebrows. It functions to elevate the eyebrows and produces the transverse wrinkles in the forehead. The frontalis is innervated by the frontal branch of the facial nerve. The procerus muscles are thin extensions of the frontalis muscles arising from the skin of the eyebrows and inserting over the dorsum of the nose. Contraction of the procerus produces transverse wrinkles over the radix of the nose and is supplied by the buccal branch of the facial nerve.

The corrugator supercilli muscles arise from the medial aspect of the superciliary arch beneath the frontalis muscles. They are small thin muscles of pyramidal shape that pass between the orbital and palpebral portions of the orbicularis oculi muscles to insert on the skin of the eyebrows. Contraction of the corrugator supercilli draws the eyebrow medial and downward, producing

vertical wrinkles in the glabellar region. The corrugator supercilli is innervated by the frontal branch of the facial nerve.

The vascular anatomy of the nose, and in particular that of the forehead, glabellar, and medical canthal regions, are pertinent to the design of local flaps in these regions. The blood supply to the forehead consists primarily of the supraorbital and supratrochlear arteries, which branch from the ophthalmic arteries arising as the first branch of the internal carotid arteries.

An extensive vascular arcade exists around the paranasal region that communicates via multiple branches with the supraorbital and supratrochlear arteries (see **Fig. 1**). The angular artery and its branches are the primary blood supply to the lateral nasal side walls and nasal dorsum. The angular artery arises from the facial artery after the latter gives rise to the superior and inferior labial arteries. The angular artery traverses the nasojugal groove giving off the lateral nasal artery, which communicates with a branch of the ophthalmic artery, the dorsal nasal artery. The extensive vasculature of this region allows axial pattern flaps to be developed in not only the glabellar, but forehead and medial canthal regions as well. For example, Kelly and colleagues[2] performed 9 cadaver dissections and radiologic studies of the arterial anatomy of the supraorbital and paranasal region and found that the flaps based in the glabellar and medial canthal regions receive blood supply from both the angular as well as supratrochlear arteries. McCarthy and colleagues[3] injected the facial arteries of 6 cadavers with blue dye and found blood flow to the forehead even after ligation of the supratrochlear and supraorbital arteries. These results exhibit the role of the dorsal nasal artery as a collateral circulation for the forehead with contributions from the angular artery.

GLABELLAR FLAPS IN NASAL RECONSTRUCTION
Glabellar Flap

Recruitment of redundant skin from the glabella was first reported by von Graefe in 1818 with subsequent reports by Joseph, Labott, Limberg, and others.[4] The glabellar flap has traditionally been described as a V-Y advancement flap based on a random blood supply for the reconstruction of defects of the upper third of the nose; however, multiple modifications of the procedure have been described (**Fig. 2**). For example, Field[4] described a modification of the V-Y advancement, which he called the glabellar transposition banner flap, in which the pedicle of the flap arises from the

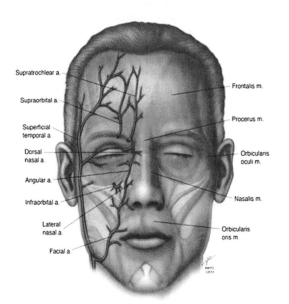

Supratrochlear a.
Supraorbital a.
Superficial temporal a.
Dorsal nasal a.
Angular a.
Infraorbital a.
Lateral nasal a.
Facial a.

Frontalis m.
Procerus m.
Orbicularis oculi m.
Nasalis m.
Orbicularis oris m.

Fig. 1. Relevant muscular and vascular anatomy of the face.

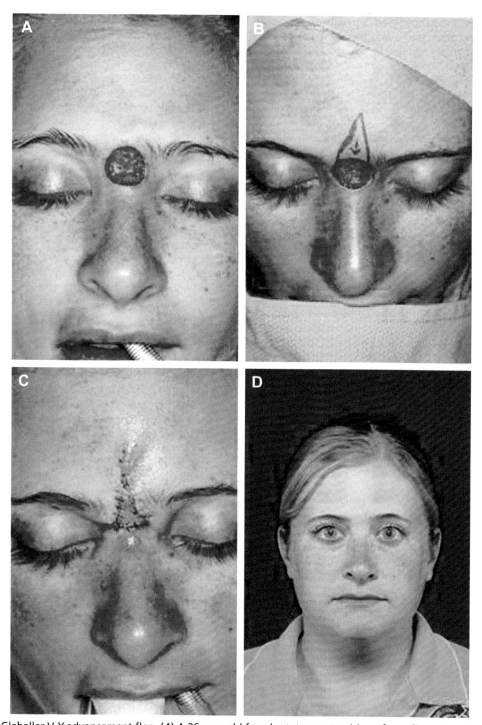

Fig. 2. Glabellar V-Y advancement flap. (*A*) A 26-year-old female status postexcision of a malignant melanoma in situ of the nasal dorsum. (*B*) Glabellar V-Y advancement flap outlined. (*C*) Flap inset and secondary defect closed in V-Y fashion. (*D*) Patient at 19-month follow-up.

lateral nasal side wall on the side opposite the defect. The glabellar skin is recruited into the defect by rotation, and the secondary defect created in the glabella is closed primarily with

excellent aesthetic results observed by the investigator. Field[5] also described a bipedicled modification of the glabellar flap for reconstruction of defects of the upper third of the nose. The defect is excised and a bipedicled flap, with each pedicle originating from the lateral nasal side walls and medial canthal region, is elevated in the subcutaneous plane. The flap is advanced inferiorly and a region of glabellar skin is undermined to advance inferiorly for closure. Field[5] reported excellent camouflage of the incisions as well as no distortion of the medial eyebrows.

Modifications of the glabellar flap have been described to address more distal defects involving reconstruction of the nasal tip, columella, alar lobule, and upper lip, generally relying on an axial blood supply rather than a random pattern. For example, Morrison and colleagues[6] described a reverse island glabellar flap based on the terminal branches of the angular artery to reconstruct defects of the nasal tip, alar lobule, columella, and even the upper lip. The investigators observed 2 complications in their series with both consisting of superior necrosis of the flap. Most of their donor site could be closed primarily or with local flaps; however, 5 donor sites required closure with full-thickness skin grafts from a postauricular donor site. Seyhan[7] reported a series of 10 patients undergoing reconstruction of Moh's surgery defects of the lower eyelid, nose, and medial canthal and malar region with a modification of the reverse island glabellar flap, which he called the "radix nasi island flap" based off of the dorsal nasal branch of the ophthalmic artery. The average defect size in greatest dimension in their series was 2 cm, and all 10 donor defects could be closed primarily.

Surgical Technique

The procedure can be done under either local or general anesthesia based on patient preference, comorbidities, and other planned procedures. First, an inverted V is outlined from the midpoint of the glabella just above the brow (less than 60° angle). Both segments of the flap should extend below the brow and the longer portion of the flap should join the lateral aspect of the defect (**Fig. 3**).

The outlined skin and subcutaneous tissue are incised with a #15 blade and undermined extensively in the subcutaneous plane. The flap is then rotated into the defect with its apex placed at the lateral edge and the point at the inferior tip of the defect. Once the tip of the flap is trimmed to fit the defect, the flap is secured with buried, interrupted, subcutaneous 6–0 Vicryl sutures. The skin is then closed with interrupted 6–0 nylon or silk sutures. The donor site is sutured in a V-Y closure, which may cause narrowing of the interbrow distance and, occasionally, require a secondary debulking procedure.

The flap may be thinned significantly at the time of harvest. Resection of most subcutaneous fatty tissues in approximately half of the distal side of the flap has been reported not to compromise the circulation to the flap. This thinning is possible because of its stable blood supply arising from the subcutaneous vascular network of the nose, consisting of the lateral nasal branch of the facial artery, the angular artery, and the dorsal nasal artery.

Advantages/Disadvantages

The glabellar flap can easily be performed under local anesthesia, leading to decreased risk to the patient and increased convenience. Additionally, glabellar flaps use local skin that is of similar texture, consistency, and color to that of the defect. The resultant secondary defect can be closed primarily in most cases, and the incisions and resultant scars are generally well camouflaged.

The disadvantages of the glabellar flap and its modifications include the thick skin of the glabella, which is frequently discrepant with the thickness of the skin of the defect; however, the glabellar flap generally tolerates thinning of the skin at the time of harvest such that this hurdle can be overcome. Although the scars are usually unnoticeable, there are reports of difficulty with pin cushioning, especially glabellar island flaps, leading to noticeable deformity and suboptimal cosmetic outcome.[6] Finally, closure of the secondary defect can lead to narrowing of the interbrow distance, especially when larger amounts of skin are needed for reconstruction.

DORSAL NASAL FLAP

The glabellar flap can address only defects of the middle and upper third of the nose. An extension of the glabellar flap to treat defects of the lower third of the nose is the dorsal nasal flap. The dorsal nasal flap was first described by Rieger[8] in 1967 as a rotation advancement flap, and subsequently by Marchac.[9] Rieger[8] described making an incision from the glabellar region down into the nasobuccal sulcus and undermining the entire nasal dorsum laterally to the canthal ligament on the side of the pedicle. The nasal skin was then advanced inferiorly with the resultant glabellar defect closed in a Z-plasty or V-Y fashion (**Fig. 4**). Rieger[8] reported satisfactory results in all 12 patients in which he used this flap. Marhac[9] described the dorsal nasal flap as an axial pattern flap based off of a branch from the angular artery in contrast to the random flap described by Rieger.

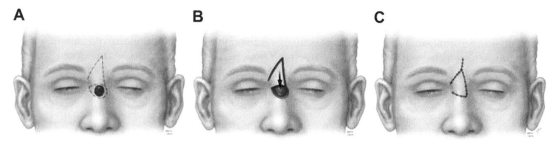

Fig. 3. Glabellar rotation advancement flap. (*A*) Defect marked for excision and proposed glabellar rotation advancement flap outlined. (*B*) Defect excised and flap being rotated into the defect. (*C*) Inset of the flap into the defect with closure of the secondary defect in a V-Y fashion.

Rigg[10] reported excellent results in a series of 32 patients with nasal tip defects reconstructed with the dorsal nasal flap and listed its advantages as the following: (1) adjacent tissue of similar color, texture, and consistency is used to reconstruct the defect; (2) the scars follow local contours and are well camouflaged; (3) the flap can be performed in one stage; and (4) complications are rare. Multiple other authors have reported their success with the dorsal nasal flap, citing the ease of the procedure and relatively rare complications.[11–13] The largest report on dorsal nasal flaps was by Bitgood and Hybarger,[14] who reviewed their experience with 61 dorsal nasal flaps to treat a variety of nasal defects. They noted 4 minor complications that consisted of 2 cases of stitch abscess and 2 cases of hypertrophic scar formation with

excellent cosmetic and functional outcomes in the series.

The vascular supply to the dorsal nasal flap is robust and if needed can be performed on both sides sequentially. Bray and colleagues[15] reported 2 cases in which a dorsal nasal flap had been used to reconstruct defects that result from excision of skin cancer. In both cases, the patients experienced recurrences on the nose that were subsequently reconstructed without any complications using a dorsal nasal flap based on the opposite side from the prior reconstruction.

Various modifications of the dorsal nasal flap exist to tailor the flap to specific defects. Cronin[16] modified the dorsal nasal flap to encompass only the skin on one side of the nose, rather than extending it across the entirety of the nose, to repair defects of the lateral nasal side wall, tip, and alar

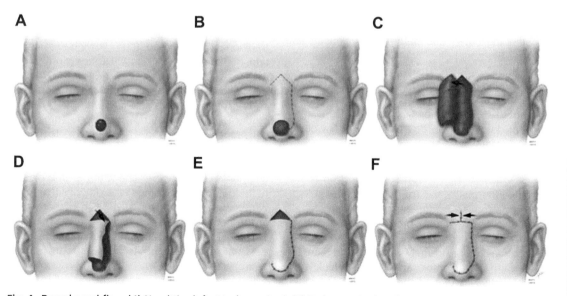

Fig. 4. Dorsal nasal flap. (*A*) Nasal tip defect to be excised. (*B*) Defect excised and proposed dorsal nasal flap outlined. (*C*) The flap is widely undermined. (*D*) The flap is rotated inferiorly into the defect. (*E*) The flap is inset within the defect and the resultant dog-ear deformity corrected. (*F*) The resultant secondary defect is closed in a V-Y fashion.

lobule. In addition to limiting the extension of the flap across the nose, he also incorporated excision of the dog-ear deformity that results from the rotation of the flap, which had not previously been described. Ducic and colleagues[17] described a series of 10 patients undergoing reconstruction of defects of the lower third of the nose using a modification of the dorsal nasal flap. The investigators describe a heminasal transposition flap on one side of the nose in combination with a glabellar flap. The heminasal transposition flap is rotated into place, leaving a secondary defect that can be repaired by rotation of the glabellar flap and primary closure of the inverted V defect superiorly. The investigators reported excellent cosmetic results without any cases of partial or complete flap loss.

Surgical Technique

Similar to glabellar flaps, the procedure can be performed under general or local anesthesia. The aesthetic subunits are drawn on the skin, and incisions should be kept within these borders whenever possible. The pedicle can be based on a random blood supply as traditionally described or via an axial blood supply from branches of the angular or infratrochlear artery, which allows a narrower pedicle. The pedicle is typically based on the ipsilateral side of the defect with an inverted V incision extending into the glabellar region but preferably not rising above the medial brow. The skin of the dorsum is undermined in a submuscular plane through the defect before incision. Incisions are made and meticulous hemostasis achieved. The flap is rotated into place and contoured, and the standing cutaneous deformity is excised as needed. The donor site is closed in a V-Y fashion in the glabellar region. The flap is sutured in place using buried, interrupted, subcutaneous 6–0 Vicryl sutures. The skin is then closed with interrupted 6–0 nylon or silk sutures. Consideration for dermabrasion can be given at 6 weeks postoperatively.[18]

Advantages/Disadvantages

Similar to the glabellar flap, the dorsal nasal flap can be performed under either local or general anesthesia as a 1-stage procedure. The dorsal nasal flap can be applied to a wide variety of nasal defects, making it extremely versatile, and recruits tissue with similar color, texture, and thickness characteristics to that of the defect. When incisions are limited to aesthetic subunits, the scars are well camouflaged, and although extensive undermining is required to mobilize the flap, partial or total flap necrosis is extremely rare.

Disadvantages of the flap include the need to elevate the entire skin of the dorsum of the nose. Additionally, unwanted nasal tip elevation and excessive tip rotation can ensue when the incisions are extended superiorly into the glabella, and it is not always possible to hide the incisions within the aesthetic subunits, which makes scars noticeable and may require additional procedures for refinement.

GLABELLAR FLAPS FOR MEDIAL CANTHAL RECONSTRUCTION

The medial canthus is an ill-defined region that exhibits the convergence of multiple adjoining areas, including the eyelids, brow, glabella, and nose that all possess different skin textures, colors, and thickness. Reconstruction of this area is challenging and has not been well described. The glabellar flap and its modification represent one frequently used local flap for reconstruction of this challenging region because of decreased scar contracture relative to full-thickness skin grafts (**Fig. 5**).

Multiple modifications of the glabellar flap exist for use in medial canthal reconstruction. Smaller defects can be reconstructed with traditional glabellar flaps or minor modifications. For example, Moretti and Gomez Garcia[19] describe a series of 14 patients undergoing medial canthal reconstruction with a modification of the glabellar V-Y advancement flap to be used for defects of the medial canthus smaller than 2 cm and not involving the canthal tendon or lacrimal apparatus. The investigators' modification consisted of rotating the V-Y design of the flap 90° from the traditional glabellar flap, thus allowing recruitment and transposition of tissue in a horizontal rather than vertical fashion, with V-Y closure. None of the patients developed epiphora postoperatively and all patients were satisfied with the cosmetic outcome without need for revision. Turgut and colleagues[20] described a "flap in flap" technique for using the glabellar flap in medial canthal reconstruction, in which the inverted V is divided into 2 segments via a diagonal line with the limb closest to the defect transposing to the defect site and the larger more superior limb advancing inferiorly to fill in the secondary defect, allowing a V-Y closure. One must be careful using this technique to ensure adequate blood supply to both flaps to prevent necrosis.

Potential disadvantages of the glabellar flap in medial canthal reconstruction is a bulky nasal dorsum secondary to the bulky skin and subcutaneous tissue of the glabella, or the unsightly diagonal scars needed for the flap to access the site of

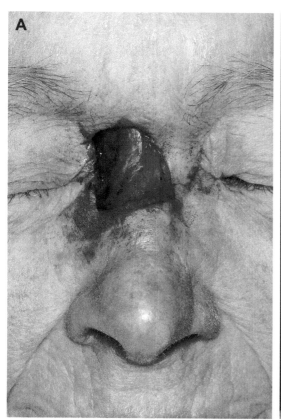
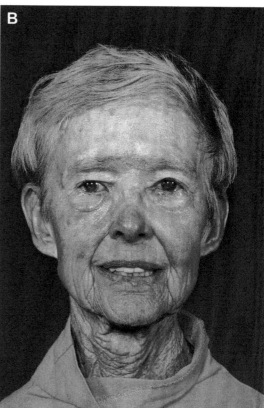

Fig. 5. Glabellar rotation advancement flap for medial canthal and dorsal nasal reconstruction. (*A*) A 74-year-old female with a medial canthal and dorsal nasal defect secondary to multiply recurrent squamous cell carcinoma. Defect is shown as well as adjacent areas of prior resection, reconstruction, and skin grafting. (*B*) Patient at 4-week follow-up after glabellar rotation advancement flap.

the defect. Multiple investigators have described modifications of the glabellar flap to improve cosmesis. Bertelmann and colleagues[21] described a modification of the glabellar flap for medial canthal reconstruction in which the flap was tunneled to the defect site to avoid a potential bulge over the dorsum of the nose. The investigators described their experience with 10 consecutive patients in which this technique was used, and observed that all patients were satisfied with the cosmetic outcome of this procedure without functional consequences. Of note, this modification required a second-stage procedure 4 weeks later to resect the pedicle, which was performed under local anesthesia. Emsen and Benlier[22] reported a series of 8 patients undergoing glabellar flap reconstruction of medical canthal defects, and advocate aggressive thinning of all associated musculature and subcutaneous fat while preserving all axial blood vessels to reduce bulk. The investigators reported excellent cosmetic outcomes without any incidence of flap necrosis.

Narrowing of the interbrow distance is one consequence of primary closure of the inverted V

following advancement of the glabellar flap. In an effort to decrease the narrowing of the eyebrows associated with this closure, Meadows and Manners[23] described a series of 10 patients in which the tip of the glabellar flap, which is usually trimmed and discarded during flap inset, was used to fill in the secondary defect rather than primary closure. The investigators report prevention of narrowing of the inter-brow distance and excellent cosmetic and functional results in all 10 patients.

Some defects involve not only the medial canthus but also the lower and/or upper eyelids. Traditional glabellar flaps are not suitable to address these defects without modifications. For example, Chao and colleagues[24] described the use of a combined glabellar and orbicularis oculi myocutaneous advancement flap for these more complex defects (**Fig. 6**). The flap was designed to have 2 limbs, one the traditional glabellar flap and the second extending onto the skin overlying the orbicularis oculi. The 2 limbs were then rotated and transposed to the upper and lower eyelid, respectively, and the inverted V deformity from the glabellar flap closed primarily. Satisfactory

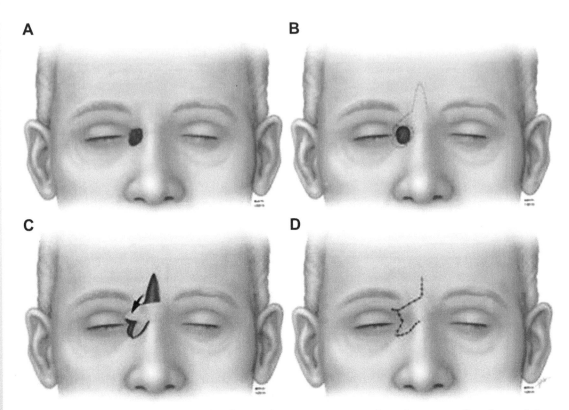

Fig. 6. Use of combined glabellar and orbicularis oculi myocutaneous rotation advancement flaps for medial canthal reconstruction. (*A*) Defect to be excised. (*B*) Defect excised and proposed flap outlined. (*C*) Flap rotated and advanced into defect. (*D*) Flap inset and sutured into defect.

cosmetic and functional results were reported in all patients. Onishi and colleagues[25] describe the use of the glabellar flap for reconstruction of large medial canthal defects. Because of the size of the defects and necessity for a large glabellar flap, the secondary defects were not amenable to primary closure and instead the investigators advocate the use of combined Rintala flaps to allow for closure with excellent cosmetic results (**Fig. 7**).

ALTERNATIVE USES OF GLABELLAR FLAPS

Multiple alternative uses of glabellar flaps have been described. One potential alternative use for glabellar flaps is obliteration of the nasofrontal duct following frontal sinus fractures. Disa and colleagues[26] reported the use of both bipedicled and unipedicled transverse glabellar flaps for the obliteration of the nasofrontal duct in 6 patients with comminuted frontal sinus fractures involving the nasofrontal duct. Access to the nasofrontal duct region was via a bone window created in the superomedial orbital wall or through the use of a preexisting fracture. The investigators reported a mean follow-up of 20 months with no

complications or evidence of mucocele and no contour irregularities of the glabellar region.

Other alternative uses of glabellar flaps include internal nasal lining for full-thickness defects of the nose. Park and colleagues[27] reported the use of the epithelial "turn-in" flap for reconstruction of internal lining of 18 patients with full-thickness nasal defects. Although multiple types of epithelial "turn-in" flaps were used, 1 patient described in the study had a full-thickness defect of the lower third of the nose because of recurrent basal cell carcinoma, and an epithelial "turn-in" flap recruited from the nasal dorsum and glabella was used to reestablish internal lining. Iida and colleagues[28] reported the case of a patient with an extensive basal cell carcinoma requiring resection of two-thirds of the external and right mala area leaving a full-thickness defect on the right side of the nasal cavity. The investigators successfully reconstructed this with the combination of a glabellar "turn-in" flap based on the infratrochlear artery for internal lining followed by an expanded paramedian forehead flap for external covering of the reconstructed cartilaginous framework. The patient underwent scar revision 6

A

B

C

D

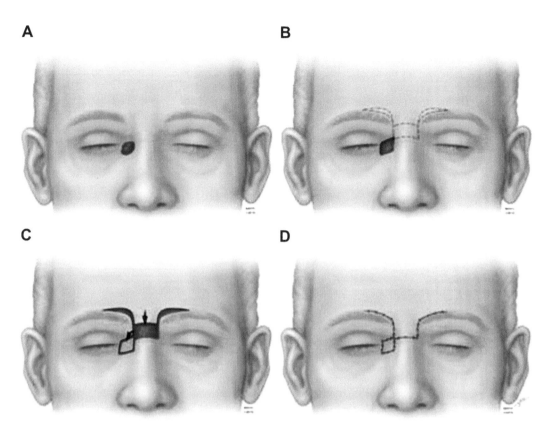

Fig. 7. Use of combined glabellar and Rintala flaps for medial canthal reconstruction. (*A*) Defect to be excised. (*B*) Defect excised and proposed flap outlined. (*C*) Rotation of the rectangular glabellar flap into the defect with advancement of additional glabellar skin through the use of the Rintala flap. (*D*) Glabellar and Rintala flaps inset and sutured in place.

months later but at last follow-up 5 years after the operation, the investigators report cosmetically acceptable results with no signs of functional deficit.

SUMMARY

The glabellar and dorsal nasal flaps are versatile local flaps that can be used to reconstruct a variety of defects of the nose, cheek, medial canthus, and upper lip with primary closure of the secondary defect that is created. In addition to defects of the external nose, these flaps have been modified to obliterate nasofrontal duct injuries as well as provide internal nasal lining in the case of full-thickness defects. Although easily performed in a 1-step procedure under local anesthesia, these relatively versatile flaps do not always produce optimal cosmetic results; however, the glabellar and dorsal nasal flaps should be considered for patients who desire a convenient and prompt reconstruction of their defect without committing

to multiple stages and who understand the potential trade-offs.

REFERENCES

1. Burget GC, Menick FJ. The subunit principle in nasal reconstruction. Plast Reconstr Surg 1985;76: 239–47.
2. Kelly CP, Yavuzer R, Keskin M, et al. Functional anastomotic relationship between the supratrochlear and facial arteries: an anatomical study. Plast Reconstr Surg 2008;121:458–65.
3. McCarthy JG, Lorenc ZP, Cutting C, et al. The median forehead flap revisited: the blood supply. Plast Reconstr Surg 1985;76:866–9.
4. Field LM. The glabellar transposition "banner" flap. J Dermatol Surg Oncol 1988;14:376–9.
5. Field LM. The use of a bipedicled flap for defects on the bridge of the nose. J Dermatol Surg Oncol 1980; 6:200–2.
6. Morrison WA, Donato RR, Breidahl AF, et al. Island inner canthal and glabellar flaps for nasal tip reconstruction. Br J Plast Surg 1995;48:263–70.

7. Seyhan T. The radix nasi island flap: a versatile musculocutaneous flap for defects of the eyelids, nose, and malar region. J Craniofac Surg 2009;20:516–21.

8. Rieger RA. A local flap for repair of the nasal tip. Plast Reconstr Surg 1967;40:147–9.

9. Marchac D. [The naso-frontal rotation flap]. Ann Chir Plast 1970;15:44–9 [in French].

10. Rigg BM. The dorsal nasal flap. Plast Reconstr Surg 1973;52:361–4.

11. Zimbler MS. The dorsal nasal flap for reconstruction of large nasal tip defects. Dermatol Surg 2008;34:571–4.

12. Fliss DM, Freeman JL. The nasal glabellar flap. J Otolaryngol 1994;23:6–7.

13. Wentzell JM. Dorsal nasal flap for reconstruction of full-thickness defects of the nose. Dermatol Surg 2010;36(7):1171–8.

14. Bitgood MJ, Hybarger CP. Expanded applications of the dorsal nasal flap. Arch Facial Plast Surg 2007;9:344–51.

15. Bray DA, Eichel BS, Kaplan HJ. The dorsal nasal flap. Arch Otolaryngol 1981;107:765–6.

16. Cronin TD. The V-Y rotational flap for nasal tip defects. Ann Plast Surg 1983;11:282–8.

17. Ducic Y, Hilger PA, Waters K. A new flap for reliable nasal reconstruction. J Otolaryngol 1998;27:327–31.

18. Zimbler MS, Thomas JR. The dorsal nasal flap revisited: aesthetic refinements in nasal reconstruction. Arch Facial Plast Surg 2000;2:285–6.

19. Moretti EA, Gomez Garcia F. Myocutaneous flap (V-Y design) from the nasal bridge for medial canthal reconstruction. Ophthal Plast Reconstr Surg 1998;14:298–301.

20. Turgut G, Ozcan A, Yesiloglu N, et al. A new glabellar flap modification for the reconstruction of medial canthal and nasal dorsal defects: "flap in flap" technique. J Craniofac Surg 2009;20:198–200.

21. Bertelmann E, Rieck P, Guthoff R. Medial canthal reconstruction by a modified glabellar flap. Ophthalmologica. Journal international d'ophtalmologie. International journal of ophthalmology 2006;220:368–71.

22. Emsen IM, Benlier E. The use of the superthinned inferior pedicled glabellar flap in reconstruction of small to large medial canthal defect. J Craniofac Surg 2008;19:500–4.

23. Meadows AE, Manners RM. A simple modification of the glabellar flap in medial canthal reconstruction. Ophthal Plast Reconstr Surg 2003;19:313–5.

24. Chao Y, Xin X, Jiangping C. Medial canthal reconstruction with combined glabellar and orbicularis oculi myocutaneous advancement flaps. J Plast Reconstr Aesthet Surg 2010;63(10):1624–8.

25. Onishi K, Maruyama Y, Okada E, et al. Medial canthal reconstruction with glabellar combined Rintala flaps. Plast Reconstr Surg 2007;119:537–41.

26. Disa JJ, Robertson BC, Metzinger SE, et al. Transverse glabellar flap for obliteration/isolation of the nasofrontal duct from the anterior cranial base. Ann Plast Surg 1996;36:453–7.

27. Park SS, Cook TA, Wang TD. The epithelial 'turn-in' flap in nasal reconstruction. Arch Otolaryngol Head Neck Surg 1995;121:1122–7.

28. Iida N, Ohsumi N, Tonegawa M, et al. Repair of full thickness defect of the nose using an expanded forehead flap and a glabellar flap. Aesthetic Plast Surg 2001;25:15–9.

Melolabial Flaps for Nasal Reconstruction

Seth A. Yellin, MD[a],*, Ajani Nugent, MD[b]

KEYWORDS

- Melolabial • Nasolabial • Interpolated • Facial • Nasal
- Mohs • Flap • Reconstruction

Nasal defects, particularly those created by Mohs surgery to eradicate locally invasive skin carcinoma, can leave the patient with a deformity of significant magnitude. The challenge for the reconstructive surgeon, as in all cases, is to recreate the patient's normal anatomy as accurately and naturally as possible with a minimum of additional noticeable scar. Regardless of the circumstance that leads to the nasal deformity, the reconstructive options selected, closely related to the skill and artistry of the surgeon, most often dictate the aesthetic and functional outcome of the reconstructive effort. Due to the critical function of the nose, nasal breathing must be maintained or in some cases improved during reconstruction. This functional challenge, in addition to the importance of nasal appearance to one's sense of identity and attractiveness, makes nasal reconstruction a particular challenge.

Defects of the nose that are too large to close using local nasal flaps, are not appropriately repaired with a skin graft or are unfavorable for healing by secondary intention, regional flaps present an important, available source of vascularized soft tissue for reconstruction. Although there are several important regional flaps available for nasal reconstruction, the melolabial flap is one of the workhorse flaps used by the nasal reconstructive surgeon. This article reviews the anatomy of the melolabial fold; the various designs, applications, advantages, and disadvantages of the melolabial flap; preoperative considerations, patient education, and photodocumentation; the types and size of nasal defects best addressed with these flaps; the technical aspects of surgical execution; and the postoperative measures required to obtain an optimal, aesthetic, and functional result.

ANATOMY OF THE MELOLABIAL CREASE AND FOLD

The melolabial crease is an important facial landmark, which grossly distinguishes the cheek from the lips. It is also recognized as the nasolabial crease because it provides a distinction between the caudal aspect of the nose and the cheek. However, the preferred terminology is the melolabial crease as it best describes this anatomic feature. Understanding the anatomy of the melolabial crease and corresponding fold is essential not only for fashioning the melolabial flap but also for a comprehensive appreciation of the changes that take place in the aging face. The anatomy of this crease and fold have been described extensively in prior publications; this article delineates the gross anatomy, histology, and pertinent vascular and neural anatomy of the melolabial region as they each are related to the creation of melolabial flaps.

Gross Anatomy

The mimetic muscles of the face are surrounded by a layer of fascia known as the superficial musculoaponeurotic system (SMAS). This fascial layer continues as the platysma in the neck and as the frontalis muscle in the forehead, eventually becoming the

[a] Division of Facial Plastic Surgery, Department of Otolaryngology—Head & Neck Surgery, Emory Healthcare, Emory University School of Medicine, Emory Facial Center, 5730 Glenridge Drive, Suite 230, Atlanta, GA 30328, USA
[b] Department of Otolaryngology—Head & Neck Surgery, Emory Healthcare, 1440 Clifton Road, NE Atlanta, GA 30322, USA
* Corresponding author.
E-mail address: yellins@bellsouth.net

Facial Plast Surg Clin N Am 19 (2011) 123–139
doi:10.1016/j.fsc.2010.10.010
1064-7406/11/$ — see front matter © 2011 Published by Elsevier Inc

galea aponeurotica of the scalp. Overlying the temporal region, this fascia continues as the temporoparietal fascia. The SMAS overlies the parotid gland, superficial to the parotidomasseteric fascia. In this region, studies have shown the SMAS to be thick and fibrous.[1] As the SMAS continues medially toward the melolabial fold, its fibrous connective tissue becomes progressively thinner because it envelops the mimetic muscles, including the zygomaticus major, zygomaticus minor, orbicularis oris, levator labii superioris, depressor labii inferioris, levator anguli oris, and depressor anguli oris. All these muscles surround the melolabial fold and send out vertically oriented fibrous septa to the dermal layer of the skin. This construct allows the face to express a broad spectrum of emotions, based on the relative contractions and actions of these mimetic muscles.

At the junction of the cheek and lip, there is a dense concentration of the fibrous mimetic muscular decussations. This consolidated area of fibrous extensions results in the melolabial crease. There is a thicker layer of subcutaneous fat lateral to the melolabial crease that facilitates a smooth gliding motion of the mimetic muscles in relation to the skin.[2] These fibrous extensions must traverse this fat layer, and thus, movement of the facial muscles moves both the skin and the thick fat layer below it. Medial to the melolabial crease, however, there is virtually no subcutaneous fat, and some studies suggest that the orbicularis oris fibers attach directly to the dermis in this region. The juxtaposition of the thick subcutaneous fat layer lateral to the crease compared with the subcutaneous tissues overlying the orbicularis oris, which is devoid of fat, creates what is clinically recognized as the melolabial fold. This lateral fat layer is clinically important because it provides adequate bulk and vascularity to the melolabial flap.

Histology

Evaluation of the microscopic anatomy of the melolabial area reinforces the findings of gross dissection. The following structures are encountered in sequence as the analysis moves from superficial to deep layers: epidermis, dermis, superficial adipose layer with vertically oriented fibrous septa, SMAS (a laminar layer of connective tissue), deep adipose layer with obliquely oriented fibrous septa, and deep (muscular) fascia (**Fig. 1**).[1] While moving from the lateral cheek to the melolabial crease, the superficial adipose layer and SMAS thin, whereas the deep adipose layer thickens. Additionally, the SMAS envelops the mimetic muscle of the medial face. Thus, the vertically oriented fibrous septa found within the superficial adipose layer connect the

SMAS to the dermis and transmit muscular movements to the skin. This transmission allows the facial skin to move and express emotions.

Vascular Anatomy

Unlike an axial flap that contains a named artery along its length, the melolabial flap is considered a random flap that is solely dependent on the microvascular anatomy of the melolabial region. Therefore, it is critical to understand the relationship of the blood supply to the superficial subcutaneous fat layer and the overlying skin when raising a melolabial flap.

The medial cheek is perfused primarily from branches of the facial artery and drained by the facial vein, with additional blood supply derived from the infraorbital artery and vein. The facial artery is a primary branch, and the infraorbital artery is a terminal branch of the external carotid system. Melolabial flaps are random flaps that take advantage of this rich vasculature via unnamed musculocutaneous arterial perforators that supply blood flow to the skin. Therefore, survival of this flap is contingent on perfusion pressure rather than being solely dependent on the flap's length to width ratio.[3]

Perfusion of the facial skin is facilitated by a horizontal arrangement of several vascular plexuses that lie in a parallel fashion and are distributed at different depths within the skin and its related soft tissue structures. The most superficial of these plexuses is the dermal plexus and the closely related subepidermal plexus. The dermal plexus is important for thermoregulation, whereas the function of the subepidermal plexus is to supply the skin with nutrients.[4]

The subdermal plexus is the vascular circuit encountered immediately deep to the subepidermal plexus. The integrity of this plexus is absolutely critical to flap survival because it is these vessels that are primarily responsible for the cutaneous blood supply. The abundance of the subdermal plexus is indicated by the bleeding encounterd along the skin edge after an incision is made. Histologically, this plexus is found between the reticular dermis and the SMAS, within the superficial adipose layer.[4]

The subcutaneous plexus and fascial plexus are then encountered sequentially, deep to the subdermal plexus. The fascial plexus is important when designing fasciocutaneous flaps, which are beyond the scope of this discussion.

Neural Anatomy

The infraorbital nerve, the second division of the trigeminal nerve, exits the infraorbital foramen approximately 2.5 cm from the midline and 1 cm

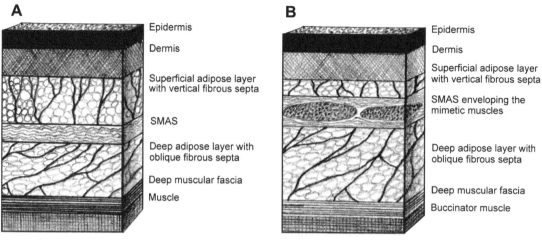

A

Epidermis

Dermis

Superficial adipose layer
with vertical fibrous septa

SMAS

Deep adipose layer with
oblique fibrous septa

Deep muscular fascia

Muscle

B

Epidermis

Dermis

Superficial adipose layer
with vertical fibrous septa

SMAS enveloping the
mimetic muscles

Deep adipose layer with
oblique fibrous septa

Deep muscular fascia

Buccinator muscle

Fig. 1. The organization of skin and subcutaneous tissues in the cheek (*A*) and melolabial fold regions (*B*).

below the inferior orbital rim and provides cutaneous sensation in the part of the face that involves the melolabial fold. This nerve has 3 main terminal branches: the lower palpebral, external nasal, and upper labial. These terminal branches have an average of 5.3, 7.0, and 7.3 end branches, respectively.[5] The external nasal and upper labial branches are most relevant to the melolabial fold. Most of the cutaneous endings of these branches are located medial to the melolabial fold. However, studies have demonstrated a tremendous redundancy and cross-innervation in this region, which explains why hypoesthesia and/or anesthesia is an infrequently encountered consequence of melolabial flaps.

ADVANTAGES AND DISADVANTAGES OF MELOLABIAL FLAPS

The melolabial flap is a cutaneous facial flap adjacent to the nose and lip, which takes advantage of the abundant, mobile, well-vascularized soft tissue mound of the medial cheek, and is commonly referred to as the melolabial fold. The skin of this region is appealing for nasal reconstruction because it provides reasonable skin color match, thickness, and texture. Because of the robust vascularity of the medial cheek skin, melolabial flaps lend themselves to several different designs. In each case, the flap takes advantage of the mobile and redundant skin of the medial cheek to correct a deformity of the lateral nasal sidewall or the lower one-third of the nose, depending on the flap's design. The nomenclature defining the different types of melolabial flaps is based on the mechanisms of movement of skin and soft tissue harvested from the melolabial fold region.[6]

The base of the melolabial transposition flap must be contiguous with the defect being reconstructed,

and the donor scar hidden within the melolabial crease. This flap permits the recruitment of lax tissue from the cheek to repair nasal sidewall defects in a single stage. Because the skin of the medial cheek remains attached, blood supply and lymphatic drainage remain intact. Unlike a skin graft, a circumferential scar is avoided, which can lead to a trapdoor deformity.[6] Although defects involving the nasal sidewall can be closed with this flap, the transferred skin matches best for defects of the lower one-third of the nose, which tends to have thicker and more sebaceous skin than the upper two-thirds of the nose. The most significant potential shortcoming of this flap design is that it can distort the alar facial sulcus because the flap must traverse this anatomic junction, which is critical to a normal appearance and is nearly impossible to completely correct once obliterated.

The second category of melolabial flaps avoids obliteration or distortion of the alar facial groove by crossing over the alar facial sulcus rather than going through it. The second category includes the interpolated subcutaneous tissue pedicle melolabial flap and the interpolated cutaneous pedicle melolabial flap. In each case, the flap is transferred across the alar facial sulcus with a pedicle of soft tissue that is removed in a second surgical stage several weeks after the initial flap transfer. Both types of interpolated flaps can be designed to reach, without tension, the lower half of the nose when rotated about their axis of attachment while providing full-thickness external soft tissue replacement. However, as with any interpolated flap, the need for at least 2 procedures is perhaps the most significant shortcoming. The initial procedure transfers the flap and closes the defect, followed by a second procedure after several weeks to sever the flap's pedicle and complete the inset. The theoretic advantage of the interpolated subcutaneous tissue pedicle melolabial flap is that the flap's nourishment is supplied by an attached mobilized subcutaneous fat pedicle, which may have improved vascular and lymphatic supply relative to the cutaneous pedicle flap. In addition, during pedicle division and flap inset, simply dividing and trimming the fat pedicle is often all that is needed, which create less distortion of the superior aspect of the melolabial crease and fold than the interpolated cutaneous pedicle melolabial flap. However, a significant shortcoming to the interpolated subcutaneous tissue pedicle melolabial flap design is that mobilizing the fat pedicle needs a wide dissection, placing the facial nerve branches to the zygomaticus major and minor muscles at risk. The interpolated cutaneous pedicle melolabial flap does not carry this risk, is better suited to thin faces with minimum subcutaneous fat, and reaches to the nasal supratip more easily. However, to optimize the flap's blood supply, at least 3 mm of fat should be preserved on its undersurface. An additional benefit of this flap is that if the distal aspect of the flap becomes necrotic and fails, because it is the most distal aspect of the flap and thus the most vulnerable, then the repair can sometimes be salvaged because vascularized skin is in abundance. If the pedicle is of sufficient length, the necrotic tissue can be debrided and the proximal aspect of the flap advanced distally into the wound bed, giving the reconstruction a second chance to heal. Lastly, in either interpolated melolabial flap design, a relatively thick subcutaneous fat layer may necessitate a future contouring procedure several months after the flap pedicle detachment.

Another flap design uses the superiorly based interpolated cutaneous pedicle melolabial flap as a hinge flap. When flipped 180° about its point of attachment, the skin of the melolabial fold can be used to replace nasal lining along the ipsilateral nasal sidewall. This staged flap design is helpful when other lining tissues are unavailable.

For most patients, regardless of the melolabial flap design used, the donor site scar can be well camouflaged in their existing melolabial crease. With time, the donor scar is often difficult to identify. An additional advantage of melolabial flap reconstruction is that it may be performed comfortably under local anesthesia. An infraorbital nerve block using lidocaine with epinephrine supplemented with a local anesthetic infiltration of the operative sites provides both anesthesia and hemostatic assistance. This method is particularly useful in the older ill patient in whom a general anesthetic may pose an unacceptable medical risk, possibly by delaying or preventing reconstruction.

Regardless of flap design, the most significant disadvantage is the random vascularity of the melolabial flap, which makes it less reliable than the similar axially based soft tissue flaps. The random blood supply, which relies on the subepidermal and subdermal vascular plexuses for flap viability, is at a particular risk in patients who smoke tobacco or have a disease that compromises the skin microvasculature. Additionally, for younger patients with good skin tone and a minimal melolabial crease, hiding the donor scar may be more challenging. However, with proper wound healing, sun protection, and time, these scars often do well even in this group of patients. Of course, the skin quality, which is less sebaceous than the lower one-third of the nose, is not a perfect replacement for nasal skin, and a line of demarcation between the flap and the native nasal skin is always discernable. However, no other skin is similar to that of the lower nose, and thus, this limitation is not unique to the melolabial flap. In addition, if the patient has abundant facial hair follicles, designing a flap for external nasal coverage may be challenging. If this flap is determined to be the best reconstructive option in spite of the issue of facial hair, depilatory techniques should be used postoperatively. However, this limitation is also seen in other regional flaps such as the forehead flap.

PREOPERATIVE CONSIDERATIONS, PATIENT EDUCATION, AND DOCUMENTATION

Nasal reconstruction, as with most surgical procedures, demands that we consider the overall health and life habits of the patient when selecting reconstructive options. Patients with medical conditions that may negatively impact healing, such as advanced cardiopulmonary or hepatic disease, diabetes, connective tissue disorders requiring steroid therapy or conditions requiring chronic anticoagulation, must be considered, and the impact of these conditions must be mitigated when possible. Smoking, perhaps the most deleterious condition of all, compromises the skin's microvasculature, which is critical when considering randomly supplied skin flaps such as the melolabial flap. Smoking cessation does not reverse the years of microvascular damage that already exists but may prevent possible nicotine-induced angiogenesis and wound healing mediated by nicotinic acetylcholine receptors.[7] Ironically, acute smoking cessation might in fact inhibit wound healing and may also make the patient's lungs more irritable during general anesthetic administration. However, additional study is needed before altering the standard preoperative admonition to stop smoking for at least 2 weeks before surgery, whenever practical. As with any surgical procedure, the patient is counseled to avoid aspirin products; nonsteroidal antiinflammatory drugs; vitamin E supplements; herbal products such as ginkgo, ginseng, garlic, and ginger supplements; and any other products known to inhibit clotting for 2 weeks preoperatively and 1 week preoperatively. If the patient is on prescription anticoagulants, a plan to normalize the patient's coagulation profile is determined preoperatively with the help of their primary care physician.

Wound size and location, perhaps more than any other factor, will determine the reconstructive option chosen to repair a particular nasal defect. For skin defects that are larger than 1 cm and involving the lower one-third of the nose, the melolabial flap offers an excellent option for replacing the skin component of the nasal defect. If the defect is full thickness and one must reconstruct the nasal lining, absent cartilage and skin of the nose, the melolabial flap can, in specific circumstances, provide nasal lining anywhere along the nasal sidewall or ala if other options such as the septal hinge flap, buccal flap or a forehead turn-in flap are unavailable or deemed to be less advantageous. The flexibility of this flap to provide either skin or nasal lining replacement makes it an attractive option for nasal reconstruction. Additionally, the donor site scar can be well hidden in the existing melolabial crease. The aesthetic impact of the donor site scar should not be underestimated, particularly in the younger patient. For this group of patients, aesthetic concerns are often paramount and a forehead flap donor site scar may be unacceptable to the patient. Of course if a larger skin paddle is required than can be provided by the melolabial flap, other reconstructive options such as the forehead flap must be seriously considered.

Given that most melolabial flaps require at least one additional procedure for flap takedown and inset and possibly additional contouring procedures in the future, the patient's tolerance for a staged reconstruction must be gauged. The patient must be counseled regarding the details of the planned staged procedures, the time frame for normal healing, and realistic expectations for both aesthetic and functional outcomes. Patients must understand that the lower one-third of the nose has skin that is more sebaceous with larger pores than any other skin of the face and that no perfect replacement skin exists. They must also understand the concept of aesthetic units. If the defect involves 50% or greater of a nasal aesthetic unit involving the lower one-third of the nose, it is generally aesthetically more advantageous to remove the remainder of the skin within the subunit and reconstruct accordingly. Finally, the patient must know ahead of time that a scar is permanent and takes many months to fully mature and that a line of demarcation at the junction of the transferred skin and the native nose will always be visible. The preoperative discussion must be explicit, and it must never be assumed that the patient knows these concepts.

Whenever a patient is to have a planned Mohs procedure, it is best to see the patient at least 2 weeks preoperatively to educate and prepare the patient for the reconstructive procedure. Because Mohs surgery is performed with the patient awake, the patient's anxiety regarding this fact must be gauged and accounted for. Because the reconstructive procedure is often more extensive than the Mohs procedure, it is best to explain this to the patient and decide at the initial visit what type of anesthesia is most appropriate. Even when a reconstructive procedure is safely performed under local anesthesia, many patients wish to have it done under general anesthesia to mitigate their anxiety relating to the surgery. It is important to review the various reconstructive options available and to remind the patient that the location, size, and depth of the final defect dictate the reconstructive options chosen. It is also important to inform the patient, based on the particular clinical circumstance, that the final defect may significantly larger than might be expected based on the appearance of the presenting lesion and that the ensuing reconstructive procedure may be extensive. Therefore, it is often advantageous to have a formal operating room environment available in case the final defect is larger and more complicated than anticipated.

If a patient is to have a tumor removed from the nose, photodocumentation of the patient's preoperative appearance, before any surgery is performed, is often helpful as a guide to reconstruction. The patient should also be informed that nasal reconstruction rarely returns the nose perfectly to its preoperative appearance, particularly when the defects are large or complex. One must set the patient's expectations at a realistic level and then try to exceed these expectations whenever possible. If a nasal deformity exists due to tumor resection, trauma, or congenitally, proper photodocumentation is critical both as a reminder to the surgeon and the patient as to the extent of the original deformity and as a legal document if such a need arises in the future. Finally, serial postoperative photodocumentation is critical as a means of tracking the patient's wound healing and as a guide to planning additional procedures.

SELECTION OF NASAL RECONSTRUCTIVE OPTIONS

The location, size, and depth of the nasal defect all play an important role when determining if a melolabial flap is the most appropriate reconstructive option. For full-thickness nasal skin defects larger than 1 cm and involving the lower one-third of the nose, where the skin is thicker, more sebaceous, and adherent to the underlying tissues, the interpolated melolabial flap provides an excellent source of vascularized tissue for reconstruction. This is particularly true if the defect lies within 5 mm of the alar rim because any local flap predisposes to alar retraction as it heals. By introducing adequate tissue for reconstruction, which is not subjected to the contractile forces of a local flap, this complication can be avoided. If the nasal defect requires cartilage grafting, which is often the case in the lower one-third of the nose even if the lower lateral cartilages are spared, a skin flap rather than a graft is required. This shift to graft is particularly true if the defect comes close to the alar margin and a cartilaginous rim graft is used to reduce the risk of alar malposition and external nasal valve collapse.

Another useful application of the melolabial flap is for columella reconstruction. The flap is folded to recreate this vital structure, and a cartilage strut is encased within the folded flap. Care must be taken, however, to avoid vascular compromise of the most distal aspect of the flap when reconstructing the columella. In some instances, bilateral melolabial flaps are required to avoid folding the flap at its most vulnerable aspect. Another option is to delay the melolabial flap to improve its vascularity. In any event, the melolabial flap can easily access the dependent position of the columella unlike other flaps such as the forehead flap, which often does not have the length to reach this area.

Lastly, melolabial flaps offer the reconstructive surgeon a good source of nasal lining when other tissue sources are unavailable and a full-thickness nasal defect is present. In this case, the flap may line an entire nasal sidewall if necessary. Once in place, either a skin graft or a second flap is used to recreate the external nasal skin.

MELOLABIAL FLAP SURGICAL TECHNIQUES

A patient's general health, smoking history, use of anticoagulants, and history of previous skin cancers are relevant when planning a nasal reconstruction. In addition to routine surgical preoperative instructions, if patients have facial hair, it is helpful to counsel them not shave the night before surgery to facilitate identification and avoidance of the hair follicles when designing the flap. If possible, it is always best to work closely with the Mohs surgeon and to see the patient several weeks before resection which permits time for adequate surgical planning and patient education. For a nasal skin cancer defect, reconstruction is typically performed the day after the resection. It is often helpful to communicate with the Mohs surgeon the evening before reconstruction, particularly when the defect is large or complex, to give the reconstructive surgeon adequate time to plan the definitive repair. The nasal defect is assessed regarding its location and size and the layers that are absent, that is, skin, cartilage, bone, and nasal mucosal lining. The surgeon must determine if the septum has been violated or if it is available for either cartilage grafts or mucosal flaps. The health, color match, and hair-bearing nature of the regional donor tissues are also determined. In general, the simplest reconstruction technique is chosen if a patient's general health is significantly compromised, otherwise the optimum reconstructive option is selected. The patient is shown the defect, and a frank and detailed discussion regarding the reconstruction is reviewed. If a melolabial flap is to be part of the reconstruction, the patient is reminded of the donor site scar and the need for multiple procedures.

The patient is then transferred to the operating room and anesthetized if the procedure is to be done under general anesthesia. If a melolabial flap is to be used, regardless of the type of anesthesia, an infraorbital nerve block is performed with 1% lidocaine with epinephrine 1:100,000. This nerve block decreases the requirements for other types of anesthesia and facilitates local hemostasis. If the surgical procedure is performed under local anesthesia exclusively, the local anesthetic is buffered with 8.4% sodium bicarbonate in a 9:1 ratio, which reduces the patient's discomfort and speeds the onset of the anesthetic's effects by neutralizing the pH of the lidocaine. For interpolated melolabial flaps, the outline of the anticipated defect size is then marked with a surgical pen and then this inked margin is transferred to a piece of reserved glove paper or foil from a suture pack as a template. If the surgeon will be enlarging the defect to respect a nasal subunit, this should be taken into consideration when creating a template of the defect. This template is trimmed to follow the inked margin and is then transferred to the donor cheek with the planned melolabial flaps medial border placed along the melolabial crease. When designing any flap to repair an existing skin defect, the intrinsic elastic properties of the skin cause the defect to be about 20% larger than the initial excision. In most cases, it is best to undersize the flap by about 20% to account for this discrepancy and to reduce the risk of excess flap bulk postoperatively. However, when defects extend to within 5 mm of the alar rim, it may be prudent to design the flap to the exact size of the existing skin defect and reduce the bulk later, if necessary. This is because the free alar margin is not a rigid fixed structure and may contract upward if the flap is undersized.

Melolabial Transposition Flap

Melolabial transposition flaps are best used to correct lateral nasal sidewall skin and soft tissue defects. When this type of flap is used, the typically circular defect resulting from a Mohs excision can be repaired with a modified rhombic transposition flap, with the final donor scar within the melolabial crease (**Fig. 2**). Since nasal sidewall defects do not routinely adhere to the strict subunit principle, because there are no clear lines of demarcation that exist as in the nasal tip and alar subunits, the initial defect is rarely enlarged to incorporate an entire nasal sidewall. To eliminate the need for removing normal tissue and unnecessarily enlarging the defect, the resultant circular defect is closed by first measuring its diameter. The first limb of the flap is designed to equal two-thirds of the diameter and is placed within the melolabial crease. The second arm of the flap is equal to the first and drawn at 60° from the first arm, at the flap's apex, extending laterally onto the cheek. The tissues are widely undermined circumferentially around the nasal defect in the supraperichondrial and supraperiosteal plane. The cheek flap is then widely undermined leaving approximately 3 mm of subcutaneous fat attached to the undersurface of the flap. Minimum undermining is done medial to the melolabial crease. The flap is handled carefully with hooks and rotated into position to close the defect. Once the flap is turned into position, the first suture is placed at the point of maximum tension where the 2 arms of the flap meet the defect. The rectangular flap is then distributed evenly across the circular defect, and the 2 corners of the flap are then sutured to the appropriate points of the defect to permit even distribution of flap tension. If the nasal-facial junction is involved in the defect, buried interrupted 4-0 polyglactin 910 sutures are placed on the undersurface of the flap at this junction to recreate this landmark. Typically, buried interrupted 5-0 polyglactin 910 sutures are used for the subcuticular closure, and vertical mattress sutures of 5-0 polypropylene supplemented with a running 6-0 fast-absorbing gut suture are used for the epidermal closure. Due to the elastic nature of skin, it is

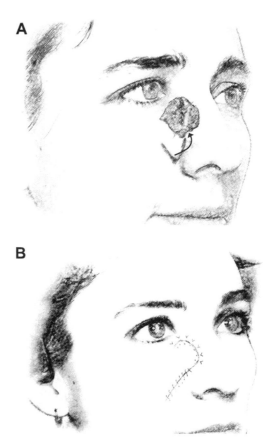

Fig. 2. The lateral nasal sidewall defect is repaired with a melolabial transposition flap. Note that the first limb of the flap is designed to equal two-thirds of the defect's diameter and is placed within the melolabial crease. The second arm of the flap is equal to the first and drawn at a 60° from the first arm, at the flap's apex, extending laterally onto the cheek (*A*). The flap is elevated in the subcutaneous plane and transposed into the defect. Skin elasticity permits the flap to be placed into the defect without modifying the shape of either the donor flap or the recipient wound. The flap is shown sutured into position and the donor site closed (*B*).

rare to tailor a flap corner to fit a circular defect. However, occasionally a standing cutaneous deformity is excised at the base of the flap, opposite the side of the melolabial donor site to complete the repair. With proper planning, no further touch-up procedures are required. If a touch-up procedure is required, it is done no sooner than 3 months after the initial surgery.

Interpolated Subcutaneous Tissue Pedicle Melolabial Flap

An interpolated subcutaneous tissue pedicle melolabial flap is frequently used to repair nasal alar defects that do not involve the alar facial sulcus

(Fig. 3). As mentioned, it relies on mobilizing a fat pedicle that is attached to an island of melolabial old skin, which is supplied by perforating branches of the angular artery and other facial artery perforators. The repair begins by first fashioning a template from glove paper or foil to mimic exactly the absent tissue. If the defect extends superiorly, beyond the alar subunit, the missing

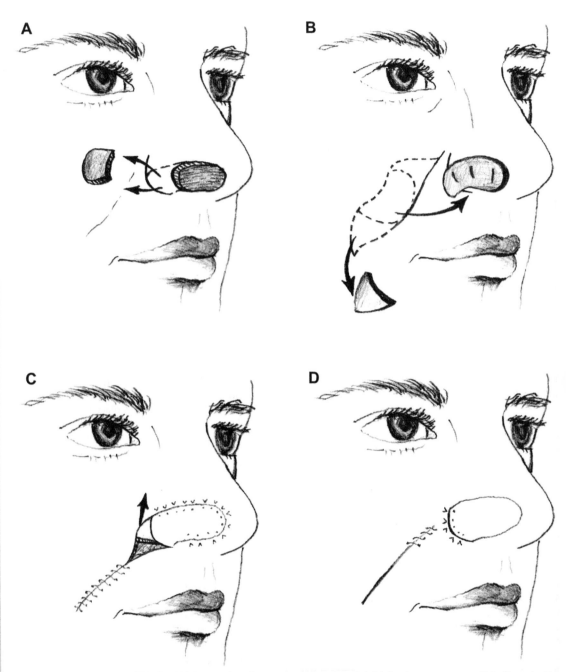

Fig. 3. The nasal alar defect is reconstructed with an interpolated melolabial subcutaneous pedicle flap. As the alar defect is greater than 50% of the nasal subunit, the subunit excision is completed (A). The skin is incised creating a cutaneous island, a fat pedicle developed, and the inferior triangle of skin excised to facilitate donor site closure. A cartilage graft is secured into the wound bed before flap transfer (B). The flap is inset, and the fat pedicle is left intact for 3 weeks. The superior triangle of skin is discarded during pedicle division (C). The completed second stage is shown with the pedicle divided, the lateral aspect of the flap contoured and inset, and the donor site closed (D).

skin in this area is replaced by undersizing this component of the flap by about 20% to account for the effect of wound distraction caused by the elastic properties of the skin. To check the appropriateness of the template's size and shape, it can be reversed and laid on the opposite side of the nose to determine the accuracy of the design. The template is then transferred to the ipsilateral melolabial fold, with the medial edge of the flap within the melolabial crease. The island cutaneous flap is placed in the center of the crease with a triangle of tissue drawn and excised superiorly and inferiorly to permit a straight-line closure within the crease. When designing the flap, care is taken to fall short of the alar sulcus superiorly to avoid distortion of this anatomic landmark.

First, the defect is widely undermined to permit tissue eversion and to evenly distribute wound tension on closure. Then complete excision of a nasal subunit can be performed, if required. If the alar subunit excision is being completed, care should be taken to spare the lateral most 1 to 2 mm to avoid involving the alar sulcus, which reduces the risk of a depressed scar and distortion of this anatomically sensitive area. For cases requiring nasal lining reconstitution or cartilage grafts, they are performed before skin flap inset. As a matter of routine, cartilage grafting, either from the nasal septum or ear, is routinely performed when defects are involving or within 5 mm of the alar rim margin. If cartilage is removed during the resection, the missing segments are recreated. However, the inferolateral alar is always reinforced with a cartilage graft before melolabial flap placement. The importance of over building the support in this area is critical to resist the contractile forces of healing and prevent nostril malposition and external nasal valve collapse.

The interpolated melolabial subcutaneous island flap is typically kidney bean shaped. It is incised circumferentially with elevation of the flap from inferior to superior in a subcutaneous plane leaving 1 to 2 mm of attached subcutaneous fat distally and getting deeper while developing a subcutaneous fat pedicle more superiorly. The inferior triangle of skin is excised to facilitate donor site closure. The superior triangle of skin is kept attached to the subcutaneous pedicle and discarded at the time of pedicle division. The fat pedicle is created by dissecting perpendicular to the skin incision down to the plane above the medial facial musculature. The wide blunt dissection, which minimizes risk to the facial nerve, then progresses superiorly to free the fat pedicle until the skin flap can reach the recipient site without tension. To reduce tension on the flap, a 4-0 polypropylene suture may be placed from the superior margin of the flap donor site to the alar sulcus, which in effect shortens the distance the flap has to travel and thus reduces tension on the closure. This dressing stitch is released during pedicle division.[6]

The donor site is then closed by undermining widely in a subcutaneous plane lateral to the melolabial crease. A distance of 2 cm is typically required; however, a greater dissection length does not provide additional benefit to reducing wound closure tension. Medial dissection is limited to a few millimeters to allow for tissue edge eversion. Providing wound traction with a single hook at either end of the donor site wound helps equalize the length disparity often encountered between the 2 sides of the donor site. Also, by closing the wound from superior to inferior rather than by serially halving the wound, the surgeon has more of an ability to compensate for the differences in length between the medial and lateral sides of the wound and can almost always avoid removing a Burow's triangle at the inferior aspect of the donor site. A layered wound closure is accomplished with 4-0 polyglactin 910 sutures for the subcuticular closure, and either a running 5-0 polypropylene suture or Dermabond (Ethicon, Somerville, NJ, USA) is used for skin closure. Dermabond is selected when the wound is a non–hair-bearing tissue that is dry and has a proper subcuticular closure with adequate wound edge approximation. If the patient has a deep melolabial fold, this can be recreated by placing the needle, during subcuticular closure, more superficially on the medial aspect and deeper on the lateral aspect of the wound. This asymmetric subcutaneous closure helps recreate the melolabial fold, thus creating a more natural appearance. The cutaneous flap is then sutured into position with interrupted vertical mattress sutures of 5-0 polypropylene supplemented with a running 6-0 fast-absorbing gut suture for epidermal approximation. Care is taken not to overly tighten the skin sutures and to have the knots on the side of the native nasal skin. If the flap is sewn to a mucosal lining flap at the edge of the alar margin, interrupted 5-0 plain gut sutures are routinely used.

The subcutaneous fat pedicle is typically divided, and the flap inset is completed at 3 weeks after the initial flap transfer procedure. The fat pedicle is transected at the cheek junction and then the superior aspect of the melolabial donor wound is incised, the edges freshened, and the subcutaneous tissue widely undermined and closed with the same technique used during the primary procedure. If the skin is redundant, resulting in a standing cone deformity, it is excised before closure.

The nasal wound is then addressed. The protruding fat is excised from the lateral aspect of the flap, which is then elevated for approximately 1 cm and the excess fat from the undersurface of the flap contoured. The excess skin left attached to the lateral aspect of the island flap is trimmed to fit exactly into the defect and closed with vertical mattress sutures of 5-0 polypropylene. All sutures are removed at 1 week after surgery.

Interpolated Melolabial Cutaneous Flap

The interpolated melolabial cutaneous flap differs from the subcutaneous island pedicle interpolated flap by maintaining a cutaneous attachment to the cheek superiorly (**Fig. 4**). This arrangement creates a peninsula of cutaneous tissue that is completely disconnected from the underlying fat and vascular attachments along most of its undersurface. Like

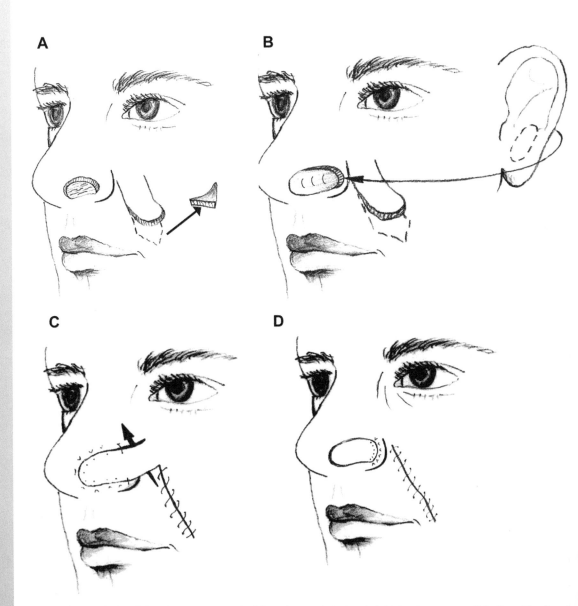

Fig. 4. The nasal alar defect is reconstructed with an interpolated melolabial cutaneous pedicle flap. The flap is designed to anticipate the complete excision of the alar subunit. The flap is incised, and the inferior triangle of skin is discarded to facilitate donor site closure (*A*). The defect is enlarged to complete the alar subunit excision because the original wound is greater than 50% of the nasal subunit. A conchal cartilage graft is then secured into the wound bed (*B*). The flap is inset and sutured into position, and the donor site closed (*C*). The completed second stage is shown with the pedicle divided, the lateral aspect of the flap contoured and inset, and the donor site closed (*D*).

the interpolated subcutaneous island pedicle flap, this flap crosses over the alar facial junction and does not distort this important anatomic feature. The flap's nourishment comes from the epidermal and subdermal vascular arcades that reside within the skin itself and in the fat layer left attached to the undersurface of the skin. To preserve the vascular supply, the flap must be of sufficient width and depth; thus, the flap is elevated in a plane similar to the subcutaneous dissection during a facelift, that is, fat up and fat down, leaving approximately 3 mm of fat on the undersurface of the skin flap. If the patient is a smoker or has other medical issues that may compromise the flap's microvasculature, such as advanced atherosclerotic disease or diabetes, or if the defect is particularly deep, a thicker fat layer can be incorporated into the flap. Like the subcutaneous pedicle flap, the flap design is based on a template that is created once the full extent of the defect is defined. After local anesthetic infiltration and appropriate skin preparation, the cheek flap is incised, elevated, rotated 90°, and transferred to the defect, with care taken to handle the tissues gently and to avoid excess torque on the pedicle. Thinning of the subcutaneous fat on the undersurface of the pedicle is not recommended during this initial procedure. The flap is sewn into position, and the donor site is closed similar to that of the subcutaneous island flap. The wound is dressed only with antibiotic ointment, and the flap's pedicle is wrapped loosely for protection with a xeroform gauze, which stays in place until the pedicle is divided.

Melolabial Cutaneous Hinge Flap

Nasal lining is ideally replaced by either a septal hinge flap or buccal flap, which are both thin and pliable. However, when these flaps are not available, a melolabial cutaneous hinge flap may be used as a mucosal replacement (**Fig. 5**). With time, the skin mucosalizes and is difficult to distinguish from native tissue. It is designed as a cutaneous peninsular flap with the aid of a template and elevated leaving 3 mm of fat on the undersurface. However, the flap is flipped 180° so that no twisting of the pedicle is required for inset. The advantage here is that the blood supply is optimized. Additionally, if hair-bearing cheek tissue is transferred intranasally, it does not present an aesthetic or functional issue, and thus, flap length and width can in some cases be larger than what can be harvested for external lining without the need for subsequent depilation. The flap is brought into the nasal defect through the most direct route available, and the skin edge is sutured to the existing intranasal mucosal lining with

interrupted 5-0 chromic gut sutures. Cartilage grafting is performed on top of this flap, and a second vascularized flap is placed on top of the cartilage for external skin coverage. Alternatively, a full-thickness skin graft can be placed directly on top of the cutaneous hinge flap and allowed to heal and if necessary, cartilage can be placed later.

For both the interpolated melolabial cutaneous flap and the melolabial cutaneous hinge flap, pedicle division and flap inset are typically performed 3 weeks after the first stage. If the patient is a heavy smoker or has underlying medical conditions that may compromise the development of collateral neovascularization of the flap, pedicle division may be delayed 1 to 2 additional weeks. The procedure is most often performed under local anesthesia. During this second stage, the cutaneous pedicle is divided, the proximal cheek component of the pedicle is discarded, and the donor site at the superior edge of the melolabial crease excised in a fusiform fashion, widely undermined, and then closed in layers in an identical manner to the closure of this area in the first stage. Alternatively, the pedicle edges and fat layer can be freshened, the superior aspect of the melolabial crease opened, and the pedicle remnant inset to preserve the tissue bulk in this area. However, the closure leaves a V-shaped scar at the apex of the melolabial crease, which can appear unnatural. The nasal aspect of flap inset mimics that of the interpolated melolabial subcutaneous pedicle flap discussed previously. It is appropriate at the time of flap pedicle division to partially debulk excess subcutaneous fat. However, to protect flap viability, over thinning of the flap must be avoided. If needed, a third procedure, under local anesthesia, is performed approximately 3 months after the second procedure to accomplish final tailoring and contouring of the flap. It is at this time that the wound may be partially reopened, the flap debulked of all excess subcutaneous fat, cauterization of individual hair follicles can be accomplished, and deep basting polyglactin 910 sutures placed to help recreate the alar crease or other concave nasal landmarks.

POSTOPERATIVE CONSIDERATIONS

Postoperative considerations following all surgical stages of a melolabial flap are focused on routine wound care and emotional support of the patient. As a general rule, all patients are counseled to keep the wound clean and free of dried blood and to cover the wound edges with mupirocin, 2%, ointment for the first 2 weeks following surgery. Polypropylene sutures are routinely removed on

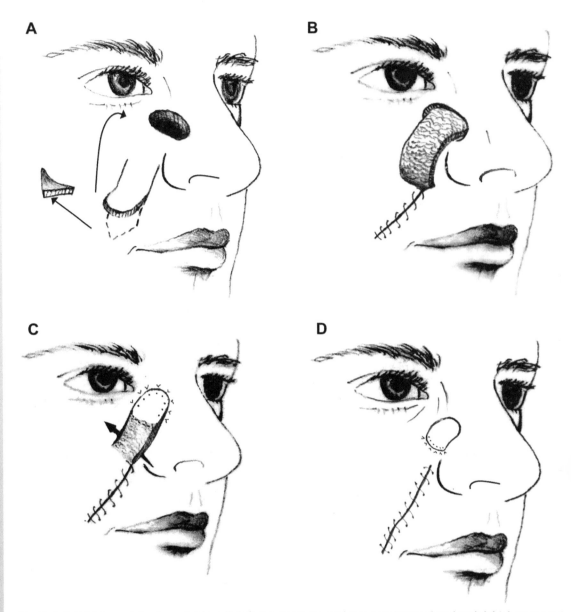

Fig. 5. A full-thickness lateral nasal sidewall defect is reconstructed using an interpolated melolabial cutaneous pedicle hinge flap as a replacement for nasal mucosal lining. The flap is designed to rotate 180° about its axis of attachment. The flap is incised, and the inferior triangle of skin is discarded to facilitate donor site closure (*A*). The flap is elevated in the subcutaneous fat plane and is then turned into the defect. The flap skin edge is sutured to the mucosa circumferentially except for the inferior aspect of the wound, to avoid compromising the flaps vascular supply (*B*). A full-thickness skin graft is shown covering the under surface of the flap and secured to the nasal skin (*C*). The completed second stage is shown with the pedicle divided, the inferior aspect of the flap contoured and inset, and the donor site closed (*D*).

postoperative day 7. All gut sutures are permitted to dissolve. If Dermabond is used for donor site skin closure, no specific wound care is required except not to manipulate the material until 2 weeks after closure, at which time the material can be peeled off. During the initial 2 weeks following each stage of the procedure, exposure to sun should be avoided, after which daily sunblock usage is encouraged. A physical block, such as a zinc oxide− or titanium dioxide−containing product, is routinely recommended. Four weeks after the second procedure and if needed the third procedure, the patient is encouraged to apply a moisturizer to the affected areas and deliberately massage the wound for 3 minutes, 3 times per day for 3 months.

If an additional flap contouring procedure is anticipated after pedicle division and inset, it is advisable to wait several months to allow the local edema to resolve and to permit normal wound healing to occur. Typically, no decision is made to undertake a third planned procedure until after 3 months. After which a reasonable estimate as to how well the flap contours are progressing is evident. From the beginning, the patient is advised that the final result will not be appreciated until approximately 1 year after the final surgical procedure. If during routine follow-up, which is done at 2 days; 1 week; and 3, 6, 12, and 18 months postoperation, the scar is found to be thickening, use of intralesional catabolic steroid injections and topical silicone liquid may be indicated. If required, triamcinolone acetonide at a concentration of 10 mg/mL, with an average dose of 1 to 5 mg per treatment is injected into the scar, starting as early as 6 weeks postoperatively. Several injections may be needed, spaced 4 to 6 weeks between treatments. However, this thickening is a rare occurrence because the midface generally heals well without hypertrophic or keloid scarring. If the wound edges remain clearly discernable or raised, dermabrasion or laser resurfacing may be appropriate at 1 year after the final procedure. Lastly, if hypervascularity and erythema persist after 12 to 18 months, a laser that targets the vasculature, such as a KTP (potassium titanyl phosphate) or pulsed dye laser or intense pulsed light therapy, may be recommended.

CLINICAL CASES
Case 1: Melolabial Transposition Flap for Nasal Sidewall Cutaneous Reconstruction

The patient is a 42-year-old woman who presented with a 2.2 × 2.1-cm cutaneous defect of the right lateral nasal sidewall and medial cheek following Mohs surgery for basal cell carcinoma (**Fig. 6**). She has a thin face with excellent skin tone and a minimal melolabial crease. Given this clinical reality, the melolabial fold was still thought to be the best flap donor site because the patient was concerned about any additional scar that would be created during the wound closure. Because the defect straddled the lateral nose and cheek, absorbable deep basting sutures at the nasal-facial junction were used to recreate this critical anatomic landmark during the repair. A single-stage procedure was performed, and the results at 13 months after surgery are shown. Notice that even with the patient's unfavorable

anatomy, the donor site scar is difficult to appreciate and facial balance is reasonably maintained.

Case 2: Interpolated Melolabial Subcutaneous Pedicle Flap for Cutaneous Alar Reconstruction

The patient is a 62-year-old man who presented with a 2 × 1-cm cutaneous defect of his left lateral ala following Mohs surgery for basal cell carcinoma (**Fig. 7**). The preoperative wound is filled with gel foam but represents a deep cutaneous defect. The wound is less than 50% of the alar subunit and thus was reconstructed without completing the subunit excision. An interpolated subcutaneous pedicle flap was chosen because the defect involved the lateral aspect of the nose and the patient had a full cheek with ample subcutaneous fat. Thus, the cutaneous island easily reached the defect with minimal tension. The flap pedicle division was performed at 3 weeks after the first surgical procedure. The postoperative result shown was taken 3 months after the initial surgery, and as can be seen, there is minimal distortion of the natural melolabial crease. The patient is pleased with the result and refused any additional contouring procedures.

Case 3: Interpolated Melolabial Cutaneous Pedicle Flap for Cutaneous Alar Reconstruction

The patient is a 62-year-old man who presented with a 3.2 × 2.2-cm full-thickness defect of the left alar subunit following Mohs surgery for basal cell carcinoma (**Fig. 8**). The absent alar margin and a hole through the portion of the nasal mucosa that remains can be appreciated. The repair required nasal mucosal replacement, which was accomplished with an anteriorly based septal mucosal hinge flap, cartilage reconstruction using a conchal cartilage graft, and an interpolated melolabial cutaneous pedicle flap for skin and soft tissue coverage. The second procedure was performed 3 weeks after the first procedure. The result shown is 4 months after the initial surgical procedure. The left alar has good contour but is subtly more full than the right side. However, the patient was pleased with the result and refused any additional contouring procedures at the time of his last follow-up visit.

Case 4: Interpolated Melolabial Cutaneous Pedicle Hinge Flap for Nasal Sidewall Intranasal Lining Reconstruction

The patient is a 68-year-old man who underwent reconstruction of a 1.8 × 1.7-cm full-thickness left lateral nasal sidewall defect and cranioplasty after

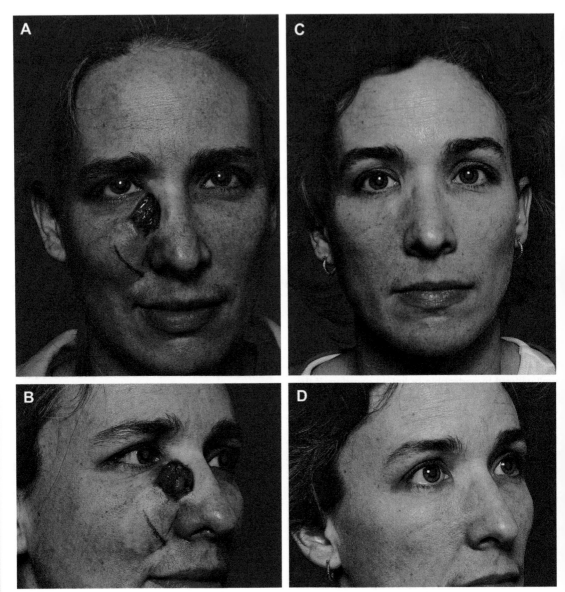

Fig. 6. (*A–D*) Melolabial transposition flap for nasal sidewall cutaneous reconstruction.

2 resections for a sinonasal squamous cell carcinoma, followed by radiotherapy, chemotherapy, and frontal bone flap removal for osteomyelitis (**Fig. 9**). The preoperative photograph shows a modified dorsal nasal flap, which was ultimately not used for the reconstruction. The concern was that it would complicate the cranial repair. Additionally, a septal hinge flap was unavailable due to partial surgical resection of the septum and previous irradiation to this area. The forehead flap was obviously unavailable as well. A buccal mucosal flap would neither be long enough to reach the nose nor provide adequate tissue volume.

Therefore, a melolabial cutaneous hinge flap was selected for internal lining, which was then covered with a full-thickness skin graft harvested from the patient's neck. No cartilage grafts were placed. Because the defect involved the superior nasal sidewall, the melolabial flap was placed into the defect without entering the nose and sutured circumferentially to the existing mucosa except for the pedicle portion of the flap. The flap division and inset procedure were scheduled 4 weeks following his initial surgery due to the history of radiotherapy. The figure shows the patient 11 months after the initial surgical procedure.

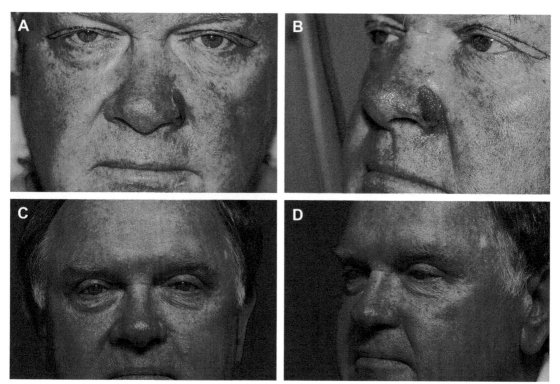

Fig. 7. (A–D) Interpolated melolabial subcutaneous pedicle flap for cutaneous alar reconstruction.

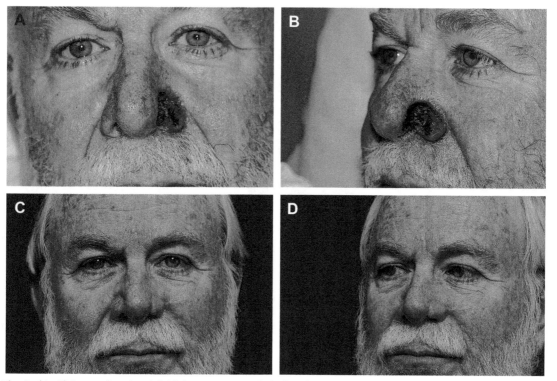

Fig. 8. (A–D) Interpolated melolabial cutaneous pedicle flap for cutaneous alar reconstruction.

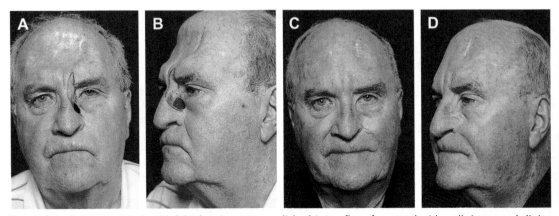

Fig. 9. (A–D) Interpolated melolabial cutaneous pedicle hinge flap for nasal sidewall intranasal lining reconstruction.

Case 5: Interpolated Melolabial Cutaneous Pedicle Flap for Columella Reconstruction

The patient is a 34-year-old man with a congenital facial deformity, deafness, and blindness corrected with corneal transplants, whose only concern was his inability to breathe through his nose (**Fig. 10**). His nasal columella had been completely eroded because his upper lip rubbed

against it throughout his life. His severe nasal tip ptosis led to complete nasal airway obstruction, which was corrected by manually elevating the nasal tip. The intraoperative photographs show the template constructed from a metal suture pack, the flap design, the conchal cartilage columella graft sutured into position, and the flap inset and closure. The undersurface of the interpolated melolabial cutaneous pedicle flap was skin grafted

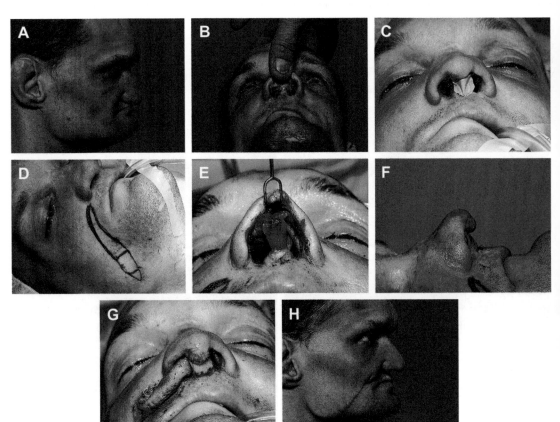

Fig. 10. (A–H) Interpolated melolabial cutaneous pedicle flap for columella reconstruction.

in this case because the pedicle was long and the exposed adipose tissue with its critical blood supply was vulnerable to desiccation and because the patient's handicaps made wound care more difficult. The flap takedown procedure was done at 4 weeks to give the wound more time to establish collateral blood flow because of the folding of the flap at its distal aspect. The patient is shown at 1 week following the flap takedown and inset procedure, immediately after suture removal. In this case, the cutaneous pedicle was salvaged, which accounts for the distortion of the superior melolabial fold. The flap was extended inferiorly to permit adequate length for wrapping of the cartilage graft and reconstructing the 3 sides of the columella requiring soft tissue coverage. The patient reported breathing well through his nose at the time of his last visit. Unfortunately, the patient has been lost to follow-up.

SUMMARY

The melolabial flap has proved to be a reliable workhorse flap for nasal reconstruction. The flap and its multiple variations rely on the robust vascularity and abundant subcutaneous fat of the melolabial fold to safely and reliably transfer skin and subcutaneous soft tissues to the lower one-third of the nose and the nasal sidewall and in some cases, as a replacement for nasal lining. All the flap designs share the ability to provide abundant vascularized soft tissue for nasal reconstruction while hiding the donor scar in the melolabial crease. Although no tissue has the exact skin characteristics of the nose, particularly the lower one-third, excellent reconstruction results are achievable with proper flap selection, surgical skill, and an artist's sensibility. The melolabial flap, in all of its iterations, when applied to properly selected nasal defects should enable the surgeon to achieve a final reconstruction result that closely approximates the preinjury state while producing limited donor site deformity.

REFERENCES

1. Macchi V, Porzionato A, Stecco C, et al. Histotopographic study of the fibroadipose connective cheek system. Cells Tissues Organs 2010;191:47–56.
2. Barton FE, Gyimisi IM. Anatomy of the nasolabial fold. Plast Reconstr Surg 1997;100:1276–80.
3. Cutting C. Critical closing and perfusion pressure in flap survival. Ann Plast Surg 1982;9:524.
4. Larrabee WF, Makielski KH, Henderson J, et al. Surgical anatomy of the face. 2nd edition. Lippincott Williams and Wilkins; 2003. p. 97–8.
5. Hwang K, Suh MS, Chung IH, et al. Cutaneous distribution of the infraorbital nerve. J Craniofac Surg 1997;15:3–5.
6. Baker SR. Melolabial flaps. In: Baker SR, editor. Local flaps in facial reconstruction. 2nd edition. Philadelphia: Mosby; 2007. p. 231–64.
7. Jacobi J, Jang JJ, Sundram U, et al. Nicotine accelerates angiogenesis and wound healing in genetically diabetic mice. Am J Pathol 2002;161:97–104.

The Midline Forehead Flap in Nasal Reconstruction

Kenneth K.K. Oo, MBBS, MSc[a], Stephen S. Park, MD[a,b],*

KEYWORDS

- Forehead flap • Nasal reconstruction • Aesthetic units
- Surgical technique

HISTORY

Nasal reconstruction originated almost 3000 years ago in India, where large cheek flaps were developed to reconstruct noses. Nasal amputation was a common form of social punishment for various crimes, from theft to adultery, thus giving rise to a large group of individuals in need of total or subtotal nasal reconstruction. A seventh century Indian medical document, the *Sushruta Samhita,* describes a technique of using a flap from the forehead for nasal restoration.[1] In the fifteenth century, Antonio Branca of Italy discovered an Arabic translation of the *Sushruta Samhita* and is believed to be the first to perform a similar procedure outside India. In Europe, Italian surgeons used a pedicled flap from the medial surface of the upper arm for nasal reconstruction.[2]

In the late eighteenth century, JC Carpue found a description of this Indian technique, giving rise to the modern era of nasal resurfacing with the use of a pedicled forehead flap.[3] Carpue first practiced these techniques on cadavers and later applied them to live patients, eventually publishing his results. His writings soon spread across Europe and to America, revolutionizing nasal reconstruction. Carpue's basic techniques laid the foundation for modern nasal reconstruction for the next century.

These techniques were modified further and popularized by other surgical giants. Kazanjian advanced the development of the forehead flap by advocating primary closure of the forehead donor site.[4] Millard,[5,6] in the 1960s and 1970s, used a characteristic gull-wing design with lateral extensions for alar reconstruction and extended the pedicle incisions below the brow to provide greater flap length.

Burget and Menick[7,8] made further contributions to the design by emphasizing aggressive thinning of the skin paddle, narrowing the pedicle base for easier rotation and length, and modifying defects to follow aesthetic subunits of the nose.

KEY PRINCIPLES

The use of the forehead flap in nasal reconstruction poses the challenges of restoring aesthetics in a prominent area on the face while preserving function. A full-thickness defect requires a multilayered reconstruction that addresses each of the 3 separate layers of the nose[9] (ie, cutaneous surface, structural support, internal lining). Once structural grafting is placed, its covering must be durable and of similar thickness and texture to native nasal skin and it must have its own blood supply. Ideally, this is accomplished with minimal donor site

The authors have nothing to disclose.
^a Department of Otolaryngology, Head and Neck Surgery, University of Virginia Health System, PO Box 800713, Charlottesville, VA 22908-0713, USA
^b Division of Facial Plastic and Reconstructive Surgery, University of Virginia Health System, PO Box 800713, Charlottesville, VA 22908-0713, USA
* Corresponding author. Department of Otolaryngology, Head and Neck Surgery, University of Virginia Health System, PO Box 800713, Charlottesville, VA 22908-0713.
E-mail address: ssp8a@virginia.edu

Facial Plast Surg Clin N Am 19 (2011) 141–155
doi:10.1016/j.fsc.2010.10.004
1064-7406/11/$ — see front matter © 2011 Elsevier Inc. All rights reserved.

morbidity and with reproducible dependability, which is best addressed with the forehead flap.

Facial and Nasal Subunits

At the core of any discussion about reconstruction of nasal defects is the concept of facial aesthetic units as popularized by Burget and Menick.[10] The face is divided into aesthetic units defined by subtle changes in contour and natural creases. These distinct topographic areas are characterized by their skin color, contour, skin thickness, hair density, skin texture, and mobility. The nasal subunits together with the eyes and lips form the central core of the facial aesthetic units. Our eyes tend to focus on this central core and therefore attaining adequate fidelity in our reconstruction ensures a successful result. Scars that traverse the subunit may result in an unfavorable scar. If greater than 50% of the subunit is involved, Burget and Menick[10] recommend completing the excision of the involved subunit before reconstruction. Nevertheless, this concept of aesthetic units has seen its fair share of critiques. Singh and Barlett[11] focused on local characteristics such as color, texture, contour, and actinic change that may override the traditional nasal subunits. Yotsuyanagi and colleagues[12] proposed a different set of nasal subunits for the Oriental face and used these for their reconstructions. Rohrich and colleagues[13] advocated reconstruction of the defect, not the subunit, seeking good contour as the aesthetic end point. Hence, it is important to know that there are limitations to this concept of aesthetic subunits. More recently, Menick[11] emphasized that the subunit principle can be helpful, but is only a single tool in a surgeon's armamentarium.

A more aggressive application of the subunit principle is used for the tip and alar regions where these subunits are convex, and can lead to a trapdoor effect following flap inset and healing thereby augmenting the effect of recreating the convex shape of the subunit. For the nasal dorsum and sidewalls, it is less applicable, because these relatively flat subunits blend indistinctly. The subunit principle is also less applicable when skin grafts are used for resurfacing because grafts do not pincushion.[11,14]

Therefore, reconstruction based on the principle of aesthetic subunits aims to maintain the normal segmentation of the face so that scars at the border of 2 units are inconspicuous to the casual observer. There are, however, certainly more factors involved before a successful nasal reconstruction is attained. Burget and Menick have both stressed that the aesthetic subunit principle should not be overemphasized.[12,14] Although it is

a useful concept in most instances, it should not be dogma and it should not replace the ingenuity and craftsmanship of the surgeon.

Form and Function

Internal lining

The internal lining is mentioned briefly as it is covered by other references.[15] A variety of strategies are available for reconstituting defects of the internal nasal lining. They can broadly be divided into

1. Grafts: typically chondrocutaneous grafts
2. Mucosal flaps: intranasal mucosal or intraoral mucosal flaps
3. Local flaps: nasal turn-in flaps, melolabial flaps
4. Free flaps: most frequently described would be the radial forearm flap and auricular ascending helical flap.

Specific to the forehead flap, the distal end may be turned in to provide internal lining over the lower third of the nose.

Framework

Reestablishing a framework in nasal reconstruction is of paramount importance for maintaining both form and function. It is an integral part of the 3-layer repair of any full-thickness defect of the nose. Structural grafts are used liberally and often in nonanatomic locations to prevent sidewall collapse, alar retraction, and maintain nasal projection. The current gold standard is an autogenous cartilage graft, typically harvested from the septum or auricle. Rib and split calvarial bone grafts are occasionally required in subtotal and total nasal reconstruction. Clinical success has also been reported with the use of irradiated homograft rib[16] as well as alloplastic[17] materials although we tend not to favor this approach.

Cartilage grafts in nasal reconstruction serve 3 primary roles[18]:

1. To provide rigidity to the sidewall and avoid lateral collapse during inspiration
2. To resist cephalic retraction of the alar margin
3. To establish nasal contour and projection.

The dimension of the cutaneous defect is not a direct indicator for the need of cartilage grafting. Many smaller defects, especially those involving the alar and supraalar crease may lead to sidewall collapse and hence nasal obstruction.

The auricle is ideally suited as a donor site for cartilaginous grafts to the nose and can be relied on with minimal donor site morbidity. Septal cartilage may be used in some circumstances, but there may be limited availability and the favorable curvature of the conchal bowl is often lost. When subtotal or total rhinectomy defects are encountered or when both septal and conchal cartilage is unavailable, rib grafts are the next material of choice.

Suture can be used to reshape existing cartilages, and their versatility is widely demonstrated in rhinoplasty techniques. Sutures can also be used to influence the position of the upper lateral cartilages and the corresponding internal nasal valve. The flaring suture[19,20] is a quick and noninvasive means of augmenting the cross-sectional area of the internal nasal valve. These flaring sutures are used even in patients without preexisting narrowing of the internal nasal valve as a prophylactic measure against sidewall collapse.

Cicatricial contracture along the vestibule is best prevented by repairing all linings meticulously and providing strong support to the rim. Secondary repair of this type of narrowing is more challenging.

Covering

Resurfacing of the nasal defect takes into consideration the previously mentioned concept of facial subunits. We use the forehead flap for larger nasal cutaneous defects. Its many virtues include abundant tissue availability, its excellent match in color and skin texture, low donor site morbidity, and its robust vascularity. Currently, we use the midline forehead flap, which harvests a skin paddle from the precise center of the forehead but is based on a narrow unilateral pedicle from the medial brow area. The pedicle can be narrow (1.5 cm) and extend below the level of the brow to facilitate flap rotation with less potential for vascular kinking. The oblique pedicle allows a slightly longer reach compared with the paramedian flap. The resultant scar from the midline forehead flap is in the exact center, which is consistent with the principle of aesthetic units.

ANATOMY

Forehead flaps are based on the robust vasculature to the forehead via the supraorbital, supratrochlear, and terminal branches of the angular and dorsal nasal vessels. The first anatomic point involves forehead flap terminology.

The median forehead flap is harvested from the mid forehead and has a wide pedicle based in the center of the forehead, which originally captured both supratrochlear vessels.

The paramedian forehead flap is designed around the medial brow area over the superior/medial orbital rim. The skin paddle and pedicle are aligned vertically over the supratrochlear notch. The resultant donor scar is oriented vertically and aligns with the medial brow.

The midline forehead flap is a hybrid of median and paramedian flaps, with the skin paddle harvested from the precise center of the forehead. The associated pedicle runs obliquely and is based on a unilateral supratrochlear vessel and collaterals from the medial brow area. Collateral flow from the angular artery can contribute to significant perfusion pressure at the pedicle base.[18] The body of the midline flap is harvested from the precise center of the forehead, allowing a less conspicuous donor scar that is more consistent with facial aesthetic units.[21,22] The pedicle may be based on either side, allowing choices between flap length and the arc of pedicle rotation.

The rich anastomosis between the supratrochlear, dorsal nasal, and angular arteries provides a robust perfusion pressure at the medial brow area,[23,24] thus driving the vascular design of the forehead flap. This zone, which contains the superior orbital plexus, extends 7 mm above the orbital rim as concluded by a study by Reece and colleagues[23] The pedicle base is usually narrow but captures this complex anastomosis at the superior/medial orbital rim. The pedicle can be safely brought down to the medial canthus if additional length is required.[24] A prominent central vein should be incorporated into the pedicle design.[25] The precise anatomic anastomosis between the named major vessels in the medial brow region remains variable. The supratrochlear artery exits at the superior and medial corner of the bony orbit, approximately 1.7 to 2.2 cm from the midline.[26] It passes superficial to the corrugator muscle and deep to the orbicularis, ascending in a paramedian position for approximately 2 cm before piercing the frontalis muscle. A periosteal branch extends beyond 3 cm above the supraorbital rim and sends additional perforators into the flap.

The supratrochlear artery then travels superiorly in the subcutaneous plane, above the galea/frontalis muscle, maintaining numerous anastomoses with the contralateral vessels. The terminal angular artery may ascend the forehead as a distinct vessel or communicate with the ipsilateral supratrochlear artery. The paired dorsal nasal arteries usually merge to form a single central artery of the forehead.

SURGICAL EVALUATION
Indications

Numerous techniques are available for nasal reconstruction but the forehead flap remains the standard technique for large cutaneous defects. Not only does it provide optimal color and texture match to the native nasal skin, but it carries its own vascular supply and can nourish underlying grafts and tenuous flaps. A single forehead flap can be used for resurfacing the entire nose, from ala to ala. Its dependability and consistent anatomy make the forehead flap a workhorse for major nasal restoration, setting the bar for an aesthetically inconspicuous reconstruction and restoration of function. The donor site on the forehead is similarly acceptable. No absolute indications for a forehead flap exist because patient considerations may override the selection of this flap. The forehead flap is more complex and involved than smaller local flaps, requiring a second stage at roughly 3 weeks after the original flap transfer. The overall health of the patient, including their surgical candidacy, must be considered.

Other considerations include the patient's aesthetic expectations. Some patients have little concern with their appearance and prefer the simplest intervention. This is particularly true with elderly men. Therefore, preoperative discussion with the patient, explaining the limitations of simpler methods is crucial. These simpler methods may leave contour problems, result in poor color match, or even some degree of alar base distortion and contraction. These outcomes are typically seen when skin grafts are used for a deeper defect or when pushing the limits of a local nasal flap (creating excessive tension). For most large or complex nasal defects, the forehead flap provides the most dependable and aesthetically acceptable reconstruction.

Generally, cutaneous defects involving the nasal tip fare poorly with skin grafts, even thicker ones, and either a local flap or a forehead flap is indicated. Conversely, native nasal skin of the upper third is much thinner and amenable to grafts. Defects larger than 1.5 cm may exceed the limits of a local flap and often do better with the interpolated forehead flap. Defect size is influenced by the consideration of the aesthetic nasal subunits that are often excised when involved with the primary defect. Any reconstruction that requires structural grafting necessitates a resurfacing flap that has its own blood supply.

Contraindications

Contraindication to the forehead flap may be anatomic issues relating to the axial blood supply to the skin paddle. The mid forehead area must be closely inspected, especially because most patients have a history of prior cutaneous malignancies (and are at risk for future recurrences). Incorporating a second cutaneous malignancy within the skin paddle is to be avoided. If the lesion lands in the pedicle, on the other hand, 1 might kill 2 birds with 1 stone. Small superficial scars crossing the pedicle may be acceptable, but scars that extend through the galea create a potential barrier to the blood supply and careful flap design is paramount.

A history of a previous forehead flap is not necessarily a contraindication. Certainly, the flap would be based on the contralateral side if a previous flap has been elevated. Even if both sides have been used, a third flap may be mobilized because of the robust collateral blood supply at the medial brow area and the angular artery.

Additional contraindications are based on the patient's comorbidities and their ability to tolerate surgery. Potential clotting problems or easy bruising indicates a potential surgical risk. In addition, the patient's general health status may indicate an anesthetic risk and should be fully considered.

The elaborate postoperative care should be clearly defined because it can have a substantial effect on decision making.

Preoperative Workup

Defect analysis
Defect analysis is based on the key principles discussed earlier. The size and shape of the defect is described based on its relation to the aesthetic units of the nose and if the defect extends to other facial subunits such as the cheek or lip. Variations in nasal topography must be noted and in certain instances a prominent dorsal hump, a twisted nose, or a bulbous tip may be corrected before designing the forehead flap to cover the defect. Depth and layers of tissue missing are broken down into deficiencies of the cover, framework, or lining. Function of the nose is then assessed, specifically for lateral nasal wall collapse or external nasal valve deficiency. The estimated length of the pedicle required to reach the defect is made with respect to the location of the defect as well as the patient's hairline.

Laboratory studies
Laboratory testing follows standard preoperative evaluation and screening. A history of clotting problems or easy bruising indicates that hematologic studies or bleeding times may help identify potential surgical risks. If general anesthesia is used, other testing, such as electrocardiograph (ECG), chest radiographs, and chemistry panels, may be indicated depending on the patient's particular health status and anesthetic risk.

Other preoperative preparations include various methods of optimizing surgical outcome depending on specific medical history. Patients with diabetes should have tight glucose control to improve healing. Occasionally the nutritional status of malnourished patients needs to be optimized.

If a patient's skin has excessive comedones, a brief presurgical course with tretinoin may reduce severity. Dermabrasion may be used to minimize the degree of rhinophyma and improve recipient site contour.

Patients who use tobacco products may be counseled at this time about the significant deleterious effects of nicotine, including compromised flap viability. Based on our previous data[27] showing a significant association between smoking and partial flap necrosis, we continue to enforce smoking cessation 2 months prior and 1 month after surgery. This is not always practical given the nature in which patients may present to us.

Photography
Preoperative photography is essential to document the defect, allow outcome review and comparison, and educate the patient regarding the condition before surgery.

Others
No specific radiographic imaging studies are required. Confirmation of the supratrochlear artery location and its path up the forehead can be achieved using Doppler studies, angiography, or palpation. These are not typically necessary because the anatomy in this region is consistent.

Consent
A comprehensive consent is obtained detailing the indications and possible alternatives we may take intraoperatively. We also obtain consent for conchal cartilage harvest and stress to the patient the possible complications and postoperative inconveniences they may encounter with a forehead flap.

The frequently cited complications include flap loss, nasal obstruction, alar notching and nasal asymmetry. We also inform our patients that revision procedures may be required at times.

SURGICAL TECHNIQUE
Intraoperative

Lining
The more common techniques used to reconstruct the internal lining are summarized briefly, focusing more on the details of the forehead flap. Deficits of the internal lining require meticulous repair. Very small punctate defects can be closed primarily, whereas an independent flap is required to repair larger full-thickness nasal defects. If left unrepaired, the area will heal secondarily, but not before significant wound contracture, alar distortion, and nasal obstruction. There are several different flaps available for reconstituting the internal lining and the surgeon must be familiar with them.

The ipsilateral septal mucosal flap can be based on the septal branch of the superior labial artery. The entire septal mucosa can be elevated and mobilized. This flap is rotated laterally to provide internal lining to that side of the nose and can be performed bilaterally.[28]

The bipedicled bucket-handle intranasal flap[18] is an excellent means of repairing lining defects along the caudal margin. Wide undermining is necessary superiorly as well as medially onto the septum and laterally toward the turbinate. A relaxing incision is created far intranasally to facilitate caudal mobilization of this mucosal flap. Once the mucosa is mobilized inferiorly, there should be no tension or retraction in the cephalic direction. Often, any tendency of the flap to pull superiorly continues after reconstruction and ultimately creates small degrees of alar notching. The hinged composite septal flap[29] is an excellent means of providing simultaneous internal lining and structural support to the middle third of the nose. The septum is based dorsally and hinged as a composite flap of cartilage and contralateral septal mucosa to repair internal lining defects. The ipsilateral septal mucosa can be replaced, although it often breaks down and leaves a septal perforation.

Folding the distal tip of the resurfacing flap can repair caudal defects of the internal lining. This must be planned at the outset and designed accordingly, extending the distal border of the flap. The alar border tends to be unnaturally thick but can be revised.

The inferior turbinate flap[30] is a source of intranasal lining and can be used when the septum has been significantly violated. The entire inferior turbinate is delivered extransally and the inferior conchal bone removed. The mucosal flap is based anteriorly and used for caudal lining repair.

The epithelial turn-in flap[31] uses external nasal skin to be turned over and faced intranasally. It is flipped 180° and has been shown to be a dependable alternative for reconstituting internal lining. The flap is elevated from a superior to inferior direction and based on a subcutaneous pedicle inferiorly. The skin can be thinned aggressively, but an adequate subcutaneous pedicle must be preserved.

Whichever is chosen, a viable inner cutaneous lining must be available to permit reliable healing, facilitate a patent nasal passage, and support the placement of structural graft.

For very large nasal defects without adequate septal mucosa, the radial forearm flap provides a reliable alternative; there are with various studies describing unique flap designs to reestablish the internal nasal lining.[32,33]

Framework

Defects of the lateral and inferior nose are often reinforced with autogenous cartilage grafts to prevent sidewall collapse, as well as cephalic soft tissue retraction. Existing cartilage and normal nasal anatomy have little to do with the need for structural grafting; defects of the alar lobule and sidewall that are moderately deep must be reinforced, despite not resecting any native cartilage. The alar lobule and tip are usually reinforced with conchal cartilage, and the middle one-third and sidewall are repaired with septal cartilage. The grafts are placed in a nonanatomic location because normal nasal anatomy does not have cartilage in these areas. The intention of these grafts is to reinforce the native fibroareolar tissues, and they are secured with a through-and-through suture to the internal nasal lining. A flaring suture is often placed from the caudal/lateral border of the upper lateral cartilage to either the dorsal septum or contralateral upper lateral cartilage.

Cover

The nasal aesthetic subunits are drawn directly on the nose at the onset of surgery. Great attention is given to creating straight lines and sharp corners at the junction of subunits. Then the defect is modified in 2 ways. First, the aesthetic subunits are often completed so that the resultant scars lie along the borders of these subunits (Fig. 1A, B). This typically involves enlarging the existing defect although the entire subunit is not uniformly excised. In midline defects some opportunity exists to reduce the size of the defect by advancing the skin flaps on either sides of the defect. Second, the depth of the defect is modified such that the whole defect is of the same depth and the edges of the defect are perpendicular, or if appropriate beveled away. It is useful to note that defect enlargement in the cephalad direction does not change the length of the forehead flap unlike caudal extension of the defect where a longer flap design may be needed. Subunits of minimal involvement (eg, <10%) are usually handled more conservatively by incorporating the defect into the adjacent unit. An exception to the aesthetic subunit principle is a midline vertical scar of the upper two-thirds of the nose; although this bisects the dorsal subunit, the casual observer also sees the face and nose as 2 halves making a vertical line between the 2 halves relatively inconspicuous (Fig. 2A, B).

A template is made of the defect using a suture packet, taking care to cut straight borders with crisp corners (see Fig. 1C) that is then transferred to the exact midline of the forehead for tracing (see Fig. 2). We find that the suture packet allows a well conforming template to be made in the three-dimensional spatial orientation. It is then converted into 2 dimensions as a tracing for the flap. The vertical position of the template is determined by measuring from the medial aspect of the brow, recognizing that the length-limiting point is not always the most inferior aspect of the wound but may be the proximal contralateral corner. Doppler study of the supratrochlear artery, although described, is not performed as we have found the vascular supply of the midline forehead flap to be very consistent. With the template positioned in the midline, the pedicle is designed to be based on the medial brow (see Fig. 2B, C), capturing the supratrochlear artery as well as collaterals from the angular artery. We tend to favor taking a contralateral flap because of less arc of rotation, hence less kinking of the pedicle and less visual obstruction. Ipsilateral flaps are used when we need a slightly longer design (as in the case example).

The incision over the forehead is made inside the tracing to match the defect, and elevation of the forehead flap then begins in the subcutaneous plane rather than the subgaleal plane as described elsewhere (Fig. 3A, B). The skin paddle is dissected off the frontalis muscle and galea, and then selective thinning is performed to match the native nasal skin thickness. The pedicle of the forehead flap is elevated in the subgaleal plane and runs obliquely toward the medial brow (see Fig. 3B). Often, the periosteum at the base of the pedicle is incorporated with the flap to provide more length and rigidity to this region. If more length is required, the pedicle can easily extend below the level of the brow, toward the medial canthus. For patients with extremely thick skin or significant small-vessel risk factors, the skin paddle can be elevated in the subgaleal plane with a planned intermediate stage for debulking.

The forehead flap is secured with a few polydioxanone sutures to its deep layer and the epithelial surface is closed with fast-absorbing gut (see Fig. 3C, D). Occasionally a temporary telfa bolster is used to eliminate a potential dead space between the flap and the framework. This bolster is secured with a stitch sewn through and through the skin flap, alar batten graft, and internal lining. The forehead defect is closed primarily after wide undermining of the subgaleal plane. The standing cutaneous defect at the apex of the donor site is excised and a series of vicryl sutures are used to close the galea before the skin is closed (see

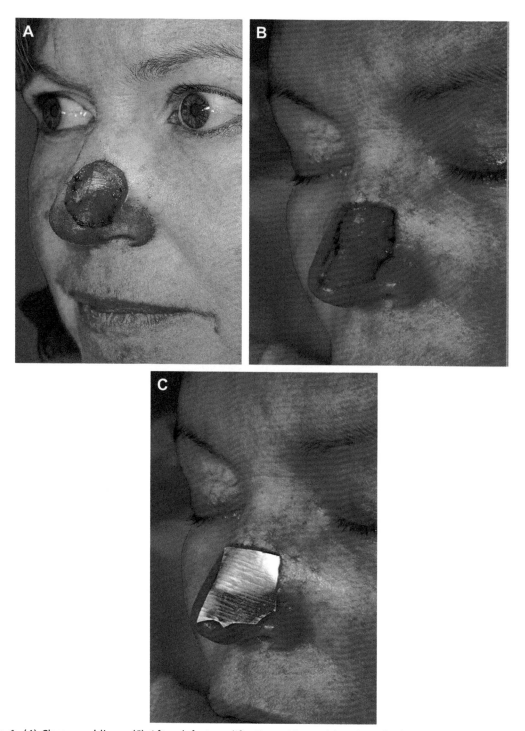

Fig. 1. (*A*) Close-up oblique. (*B*) After defect modification with consideration of subunits principle. (*C*) Precise template from the foil wrap of a suture package.

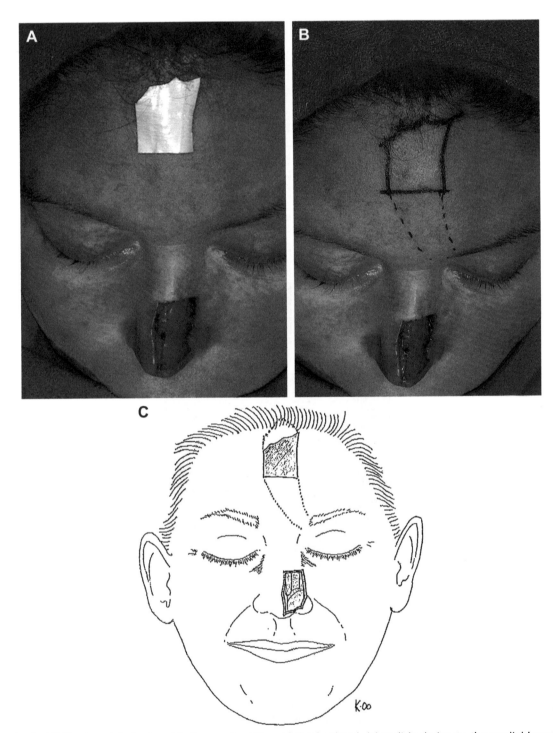

Fig. 2. (*A*) The template is placed in the exact midline of the forehead. (*B*) Pedicle design to the medial brow, narrowing to a maximum width of 1.5 cm, usually closer to 1.3 cm. (*C*) Line diagram showing the defect and template. Planned excision of the standing cutaneous deformity is marked out.

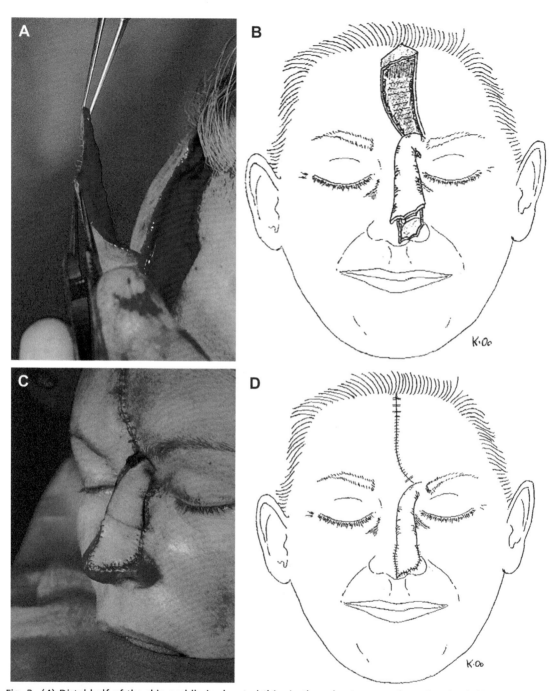

Fig. 3. (*A*) Distal half of the skin paddle is elevated thin, in the subcutaneous plane. Proximal skin paddle and entire pedicle is elevated in the subgaleal plane. (*B*) Line diagram showing flap transfer. (*C*) Immediate postoperative picture with the forehead flap in situ. (*D*) Line diagram showing the resultant midline forehead closure. Medial brow is typically pulled inferiorly and rotated medially.

Fig. 3D). Petrolatum gauze with 3% bismuth tribromophenate dressing is used to wrap the pedicle and pressure dressing placed over the forehead. Skin grafts are not used for the undersurface of the pedicle and we have found no issues with postoperative bleeding or excessive granulation. Transcutaneous quilting stitches to the flap are also not used.

Pedicle division

Pedicle division takes place after a 3-week interval, at which time the proximal portion of the flap is first elevated in the subcutaneous plane (**Fig. 4**C) before the rest of the pedicle is divided (see **Fig. 4**D). The scars along each side of where the flap was previously inset are included in the initial elevation so that they may be subsequently excised (**Fig. 5**A, B). A wedge of subcutaneous

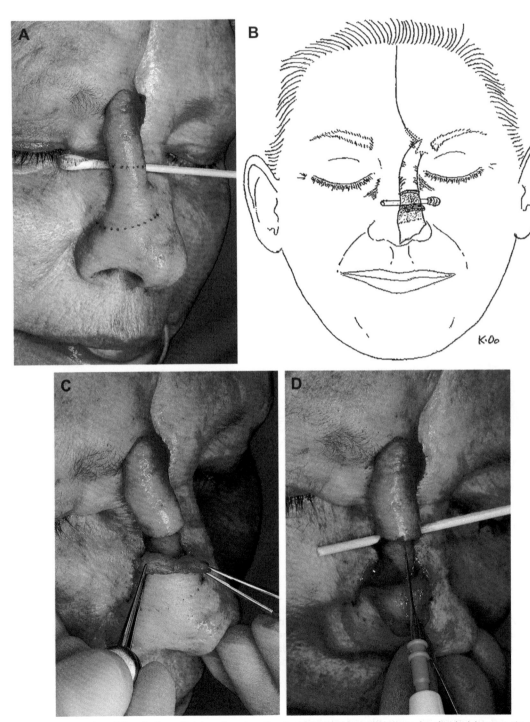

Fig. 4. (*A*) A forehead flap before division showing the line where the pedicle is to be divided (cotton tip applicator) and the more inferior dotted line indicating the inferior most extent of undermining. (*B*) Line diagram showing the skin paddle reflected inferiorly before complete division. (*C*) The flap is elevated in the subcutaneous plane initially before division. (*D*) The subcutaneous portion of the pedicle being divided.

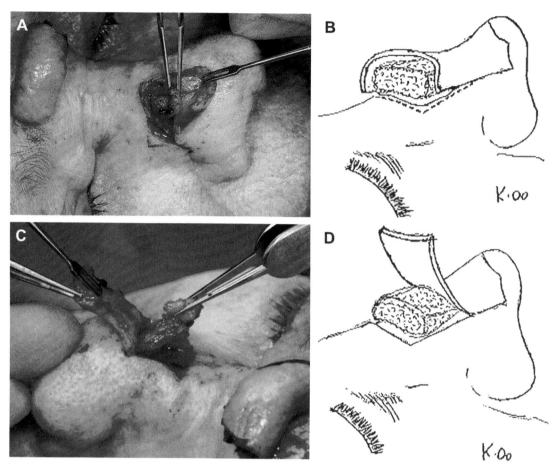

Fig. 5. (*A*) The wedge of subcutaneous tissue excised starting thicker superiorly and becoming progressively thinner caudally. (*B*) Line diagram showing planned incision and the excision of existing scars. (*C*) The wedge of subcutaneous tissue before removal. It is thin inferiorly to allow the skin paddle to drape evenly, without creating a step-off of soft tissue. (*D*) Line diagram showing the wedge and trimmed skin paddle.

tissue, broad cephalad and narrow caudally (see **Fig. 5C, D**), is removed to recontour the flap to match the thin native skin of the upper nose and the thicker skin of the lower nose. The edges of the superior and lateral aspects of the defect are freshened and beveled accordingly before the flap is trimmed. A few polydioxanone sutures are used to close the deep layer and the skin is then closed with fast-absorbing gut.

The remnant of the pedicle is then replaced by making an inverted V incision near its base and carrying the incisions superiorly, where they meet at the inferior aspect of the midline scar over the forehead (**Fig. 6A–D**). The triangle of tissue is then thinned aggressively before inset to avoid pin-cushioning. The inferior aspect of the lower glabellar scar is excised just deep to the epidermis (see **Fig. 6E, F**) to leave the deeper scar in place and serve as a platform for wound closure and maximize skin eversion. The tendency is for this area to invert as it heals. The apex of the triangular

pedicle base is then inset while ensuring that brow symmetry is restored. This often means that the triangle of tissue needs to be suspended medially and superiorly (see **Fig. 6G**). Standing cutaneous deformities on either side of the base of the triangle are addressed and the wound is closed.

Postoperative

Patients are seen the next day where the pressure dressing over the forehead is removed. The suture lines are cleansed regularly, followed by the liberal application of petroleum ointment. Patients often fall into a certain amount of depression and frustration during this time and it is important reassure them.

Follow-up

After the initial postoperative visits, our patients are seen several months later to assess for potential long-term complications and to assess their longer-term results. As well as evaluating the

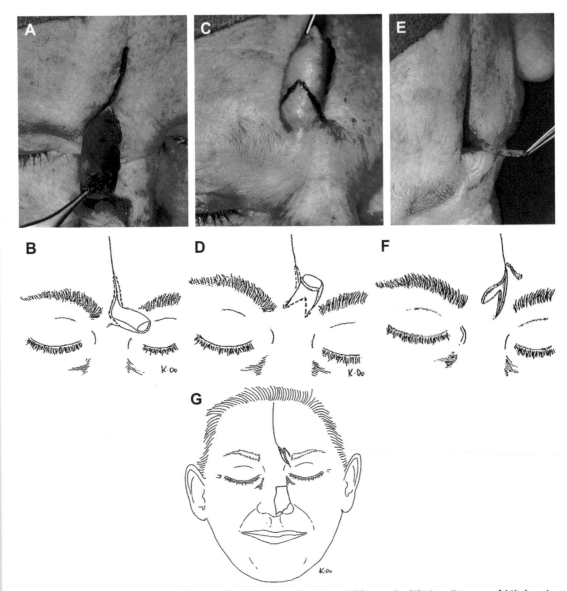

Fig. 6. (*A*) Base of pedicle with markings indicating where incisions will be made. (*B*) Line diagram of (*A*) showing where the incisions are to be made at the base of the pedicle. (*C*) Base of pedicle with marking indicating where incision will be made over its anterior aspect. (*D*) Line diagram of (*B*) showing the planned anterior incisions. (*E*) Sliver of epidermis excised over the lower glabellar scar. The deep scar is left in situ to augment the contour in this area and promote eversion. (*F*) Line diagram showing the resultant skin flap to be inset. The sliver of epidermis and dermis over the midline forehead scar is about to be removed. (*G*) Line diagram showing pedicle inset and the superior/medial vector needed to restore brow symmetry.

external appearance of the reconstruction, assessment of nasal airflow and dynamic nasal valve collapse is performed.

Pin-cushioning may be addressed with injection of some steroids. It is imperative for all patients who have had cutaneous malignancies to maintain regular follow-up with their dermatologist for regular surveillance.

OUTCOMES AND COMPLICATIONS

Surgical results with the forehead flap for nasal reconstruction remain very encouraging. Even large and complex defects of the nose are often repaired to a standard of excellent nasal function (nasal airway), acceptable donor site (forehead scar), and an inconspicuous nasal reconstruction (**Fig. 7**B; **Fig. 8**).

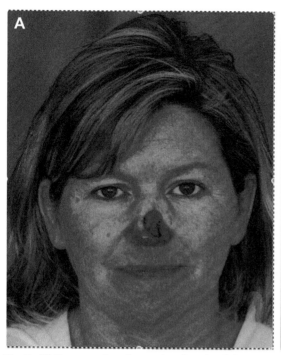
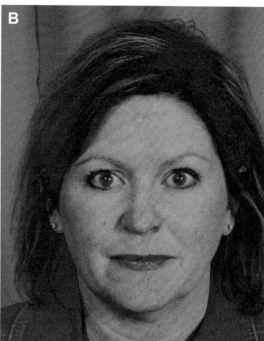

Fig. 7. (*A*) Preoperative picture showing the defect involving the tip, dorsum, and lateral nasal wall subunits. (*B*) Postoperative picture, 1 year after reconstruction. Brow symmetry has been reestablished and nasal aesthetics are acceptable.

Until recently, there has been little information with regard to complications and factors associated with suboptimal outcomes. Based on a retrospective chart review of 205 patients who had forehead flap reconstruction in a 13-year period, Little and colleagues[27] described this institution's experience. 16.1% developed a complication (defined as partial flap necrosis, nasal obstruction, or alar notching) at some point in their postoperative period. Full-thickness defects were significantly associated with major complications and, not surprisingly, smokers had higher odds of developing flap necrosis. Age, vascular disease, or diabetes were not significantly associated with higher rates of major complications. The authors advocate consideration of supportive measures

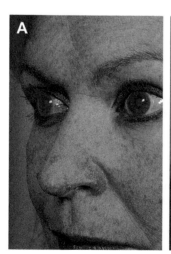
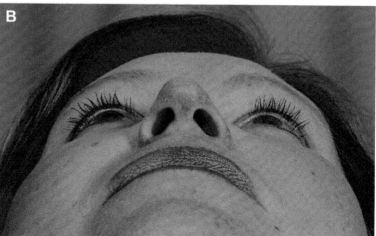

Fig. 8. (*A*) Close-up of the patient in **Fig. 7**A, 1 year after surgery showing resultant scars and brow. (*B*) Close-up of the basal view of the patient in **Fig. 7**A, 1 year after surgery showing nasal alar symmetry and airway.

for patients most at risk (ie, smokers with full-thickness defects). This group might require a delayed (3-stage) flap, or other simpler flaps or grafts.

Although no reports exist on its use in a compromised forehead flap, hyperbaric oxygen (HBO) therapy may also be considered in select cases where conservative debridement might have failed. HBO has shown some promise in various animal models where pedicled flaps were subjected to vascular compromise.[34]

Other options for salvaging a compromised forehead flap include debridement followed by a second flap or graft. The forehead flap may also be elevated again and the viable proximal portion advanced to cover the devitalized area.

SUMMARY

The forehead flap remains a workhorse flap for resurfacing of large nasal defects. As with many other tried and tested surgical techniques, it is reliable and provides predictable long-term results. The key principles of managing the defect based broadly on the aesthetic units must be maintained and the form and function of each of the different layers of the nose appreciated.

Forehead flap surgical technique: pearls and pitfalls

1. Midline placement of the skin paddle leaves a more aesthetically pleasing scar
2. Aggressive thinning of the skin paddle down to the immediate dermal plexus can be performed during the initial flap elevation or at an intermediate stage but is paramount for the appearance of a slender nose
3. The curved narrow pedicle designed from a midline forehead flap allows a greater range of movement with less chance of kinking of the vascular pedicle
4. Two-stage operations are appropriate for most patients requiring reconstruction unless they are smokers or have full-thickness defects
5. Scars are reexcised during the second stage of pedicle division and meticulous approximation of flap edges are essential to restore optimal cosmesis
6. Nasal contour is reestablished by aggressive thinning of the flap and excising the wedge of soft tissue during pedicle division
7. To restore brow symmetry, the medial brow needs to be brought medially and superiorly during the pedicle inset

REFERENCES

1. Sankaran PS. Sushurtua's contribution to surgery. Varanasi (India): Indological Book House; 1976.
2. Mazzola RF, Marcus S. History of total nasal reconstruction with particular emphasis on the folded forehead flap technique. Plast Reconstr Surg 1983; 72(3):408–14.
3. Carpue JC. An account of two successful operations for restoring a lost nose. Plast Reconstr Surg 1969; 44(2):175–82.
4. Kazanjian VH. The repair of nasal defects with a median forehead flap: primary closure of forehead wound. Surg Gynecol Obstet 1946;83:37.
5. Millard DR Jr. Reconstructive rhinoplasty for the lower half of a nose. Plast Reconstr Surg 1974;53(2):133–9.
6. Millard DR Jr. Reconstructive rhinoplasty for the lower two-thirds of the nose. Plast Reconstr Surg 1976;57(6):722–8.
7. Burget GC, Menick FJ. Nasal reconstruction: seeking a fourth dimension. Plast Reconstr Surg 1986;78(2):145–57.
8. Burget GC. Aesthetic reconstruction of the tip of the nose. Dermatol Surg 1995;21(5):419–29.
9. Menick FJ. A 10-year experience in nasal reconstruction with the three-stage forehead flap. Plast Reconstr Surg 2002;109(6):1839–55.
10. Burget GC, Menick FJ. The subunit principle in nasal reconstruction. Plast Reconstr Surg 1985;76(2): 239–47.
11. Singh DJ, Bartlett SP. Aesthetic consideration in nasal reconstruction and the role of modified nasal subunits. Plast Reconstr Surg 2003;111(2):639–48 [discussion: 649–51].
12. Yotsuyanagi T, Yamashita K, Urushidate S, et al. Reconstruction based on aesthetic subunits in Orientals. Plast Reconstr Surg 2000;106(1):36–44 [discussion: 45–6].
13. Rohrich RJ, Griffin JR, Ansari M, et al. Nasal reconstruction—beyond aesthetic subunits: a 15-year review of 1334 cases. Plast Reconstr Surg 2004; 114(6):1405–16.
14. Menick FJ. Defects of the nose, lip, and cheek: rebuilding the composite defect. Plast Reconstr Surg 2007;120(4):887–98.
15. Taghinia AH, Pribaz JJ. Complex nasal reconstruction. Plast Reconstr Surg 2008;121(2):15e–27e.
16. Murukami CS, Cook TA, Guida RA. Nasal reconstruction with articulated irradiated rib cartilage. Arch Otolaryngol Head Neck Surg 1991;117(3): 327–30.
17. Romo T, Sclafani AP, Sabini P. Reconstruction of the major saddle nose deformity using composite allo-implants. Facial Plast Surg 1998;14(2):151–7.
18. Park SS. Reconstruction of nasal defects larger than 1.5 cm in diameter. Laryngoscope 2000;110(8):1241–50.
19. Park SS. The flaring suture to augment the repair of the dysfunctional nasal valve. Plast Reconstr Surg 1998;101(4):1120–2.
20. Schlosser RJ, Park SS. Surgery for the dysfunctional nasal valve. Arch Facial Plast Surg 1999;1:105–10.

21. Tardy ME Jr, Sykes J, Kron T. The precise midline forehead flap in reconstruction of the nose. Clin Plast Surg 1985;12(3):481–94.
22. Thomas JR, Griner N, Cook TA. The precise midline forehead flap as a musculocutaneous flap. Arch Otolaryngol Head Neck Surg 1988;114(1):79–84.
23. Reece EM, Schaverien M, Rohrich RJ. The paramedian forehead flap: a dynamic anatomical vascular study verifying safety and clinical implications. Plast Reconstr Surg 2008;121(6):1956–63.
24. Kelly CP, Yavuzer R, Keskin M, et al. Functional anastomotic relationship between the supratrochlear and facial arteries:an anatomical study. Plast Reconstr Surg 2008;121(2):458–65.
25. Kleintjes WG. Forehead anatomy: arterial variations and venous link of the midline forehead flap. J Plast Reconstr Aesthet Surg 2007;60(6):593–606.
26. Shumrick KA, Smith TL. The anatomic basis for the design of forehead flaps in nasal reconstruction. Arch Otolaryngol Head Neck Surg 1992;118(4):373–9.
27. Little S, Hughley BB, Park SS. Complications with forehead flaps in nasal reconstruction. Laryngoscope 2009;119:1093–9.
28. Millard DR Jr. Hemirhinoplasty. Plast Reconstr Surg 1967;40:440–5.
29. Burget GC, Menick FJ. Nasal support and lining: the marriage of beauty and blood supply. Plast Reconstr Surg 1989;84:189–203.
30. Davinder J, Murukami CS, Kriet D, et al. Nasal reconstruction using the inferior turbinate mucosal flap. Arch Facial Plast Surg 1999;1:97–100.
31. Park SS, Cook TA, Wang TD. The epithelial "turn-in" flap in nasal reconstruction. Arch Otolaryngol Head Neck Surg 1995;121:1122–7.
32. Burget GC, Walton RL. Optimal use of microsurgical free flaps, cartilage grafts, and a paramedian forehead flap for aesthetic reconstruction of the nose and adjacent facial units. Plast Reconstr Surg 2007;120(5):1171–207.
33. Moore EJ, Strome SA, Kasperbauer JL, et al. Vascularized radial forearm free tissue transfer for lining in nasal reconstruction. Laryngoscope 2003;113(12): 2078–85.
34. Ulkür E, Yüksel F, Açikel C, et al. Effect of hyperbaric oxygen on pedicle flaps with compromised circulation. Microsurgery 2002;22(1):16–20.

Microvascular Reconstruction of Nasal Defects

Marcelo B. Antunes, MD, Ara A. Chalian, MD*

KEYWORDS

- Nasal reconstruction • Free flap • Microvascular
- Nasal lining • Radial forearm

The nose is perhaps the most complex structure in the face, and its 3-dimensional structure and function makes it one of the most challenging areas for reconstruction. A common saying in surgery is that availability of multiple options usually means that none of them work well in every situation. This is true in nasal reconstruction. The surgeon must consider many variables when planning for reconstruction and decide on the approach based on the individual patient.

The enthusiasm for microvascular reconstruction must be neutralized by the fact that local flaps provide excellent color and texture match without the technical difficulties and morbidity of free tissue transfer. Matching those qualities from the available donor sites of free flap are less than optimal for nasal resurfacing, which is why the forehead flap is usually considered the primary option for reconstruction of the nasal skin. On the other hand, there are instances in which microvascular reconstruction becomes an attractive option or even necessary. The use of free flaps for nasal reconstruction is usually limited to total nasal defects, defined as bilateral through-and-through loss of nasal skin, cartilage, bone, and lining mucosa,[1] defects with a lack of lining options, and defects that involve the upper lip or the cheek because of the limitation of recruitment of local tissues without distorting the facial units. Moreover, previous exposure to or the anticipation for postoperative radiotherapy can make the local tissues a more fragile form of reconstruction.

Reconstruction of total nasal defects must consider separately each of the 3 nasal components: skin, osteocartilaginous framework, and mucosal lining. The external envelope can be reconstructed with a variety of flaps and grafts, including free flaps. A few options include osteocutaneous or chondrocutaneous free flaps such as dorsalis pedis, radial forearm (prelaminated or not), and auricular helical rim that could potentially reconstruct the skin (or the nasal lining) and the framework simultaneously. However, the reconstruction of the nasal lining is the most difficult and possibly the most important. The likelihood of scarring and contracture need to be taken into consideration when choosing the lining reconstruction method because it can collapse the nose, obstruct the airway, and compromise the result of the entire effort. Options include mucosal grafts or flaps and skin grafts or flaps. Mucosal grafts usually provide good results, but in several situations their availability is limited, as in the case of loss of the nasal septum. Skin grafts are usually subject to contracture that leads to stenosis and nasal obstruction, dryness, and crusting. Free flaps have been used with success in nasal lining reconstruction, with radial forearm, lateral arm, dorsalis pedis, and first dorsal metacarpal[2,3] being the most used flaps.

Different types of free flaps have been used for nasal reconstruction, each one with its own advantages and disadvantages. However, these flaps share a few common features. Generally, they are thin and are also covered by thin skin, which helps to create the contour around the nasal framework or provide adequate lining without obstructing the nasal airway. The flap should

Department of Otorhinolaryngology—Head and Neck Surgery, University of Pennsylvania, 3400 Spruce Street, 5 Silverstein, Philadelphia, PA 19104, USA
* Corresponding author.
E-mail address: ara.chalian@uphs.upenn.edu

Facial Plast Surg Clin N Am 19 (2011) 157–162
doi:10.1016/j.fsc.2010.10.014
1064-7406/11/$ – see front matter © 2011 Published by Elsevier Inc

incorporate bone or cartilage for structural reconstruction or at least provide a well-vascularized bed for the bone and cartilage grafts, allowing them to survive and minimizing their resorption. The free flaps have a long pedicle because the vessels used for anastomosis are usually from the facial artery and vein, considering their location and caliber. In a few reports, surgeons have used vessels from previous free flaps for anastomosis[2] or other vessels in the face, such as the angular artery.[4]

Microvascular reconstruction of nasal defects is nearly always a staged procedure. The first step is to create a lining and support, the foundation for creating a patent nasal airway. The second stage usually involves refining the structural support and thinning of the flap. A third stage is usually done to refine the nasal contour.

TYPES OF FREE FLAPS FOR NASAL RECONSTRUCTION
First Dorsal Metacarpal Flap

The first dorsal metacarpal free flap gets its name from the name of its arterial supply, the first dorsal metacarpal artery. This vessel comes from the radial artery, usually at the level of the snuffbox, and has a consistent anatomic course along the first interosseous muscle, supplying the skin over the first dorsal web space and the radial aspect of the dorsum of the index finger.[5] The donor site skin paddle is small, which restricts its use (Fig. 1). The donor site can usually be closed with a skin graft. Even though this prevents minimal functional impairment, it is highly visible.

Despite its consistency, this flap has not been used frequently for facial reconstruction. It was reported to be used for eyelid[6] and nose[7] reconstruction. The major advantages of this flap are its thin skin and the possibility of a double skin island. One of its shortcomings, besides the skin paddle size, is the vessel caliber. Often, the size is about 1 mm, making the microvascular anastomosis technically challenging, and at times is less than 0.5 mm, making these flaps too small for microvascular transfer.[7,8]

Dorsalis Pedis Flap

The dorsalis pedis flap was initially described by McGraw and Furlow.[9] These flaps provide one of the thinnest skin sources, with minimal bulk and fat, and offer the possibility of incorporating the metatarsal bone, creating an osteocutaneous free flap.[10] The flap is based on the dorsalis pedis artery, which can provide a long pedicle that helps when used in head and neck reconstructions.[11] The amount of tissue is variable, depending on

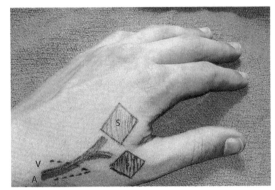

Fig. 1. First dorsal metacarpal flap. The artery (A) runs along with the vein (V) coming off the radial artery at the level of the snuffbox (*broken line*). The skin paddle (S) is small but provides thin skin.

the cutaneous distribution of the artery.[12] This flap was described as proximal or distal, depending on where the skin island is harvested in relation to the ankle (**Fig. 2**).[13,14]

Even though most reports describe an overall successful result, the donor site still carries the chance of significant morbidity. One of the major drawbacks of this flap is the questionable presence of collateral circulation to the foot. This situation becomes even more important when considering the elderly population, who are prone to atherosclerotic disease.

Auricular Helical Flap

The ascending portion of the helix of the ear has a peculiar structure that resembles the nasal alae: thin skin anterior and posterior surrounding a layer of thin cartilage. The first description of a free flap from the auricle to the nose used an accessory auricle, a cartilage fragment covered by skin right anterior to the tragus.[15] Shortly after, a formal description of a free flap from this region, pedicled on the superficial temporal vessels, was made to reconstruct the nose.[16,17] The pinna has a rich vascular network with extensive collateral circulation supplied from the superficial temporal and the postauricular arteries, and some investigators argue that most portions of the ear could survive as a flap based on either vessel.[18]

The center of the flap is the ascending helical rim, but it can be extended superiorly or inferiorly (**Fig. 3**).[19] Superiorly, advancing to the horizontal portion of the helix, the flap can be used to reconstruct the alae along with the columella. Inferiorly, to include the crus of the helix, the flap can be used to reconstruct the nostril sill. This flap has excellent color match and gives the reconstructed nose a similar contour. The dimensions of the flap

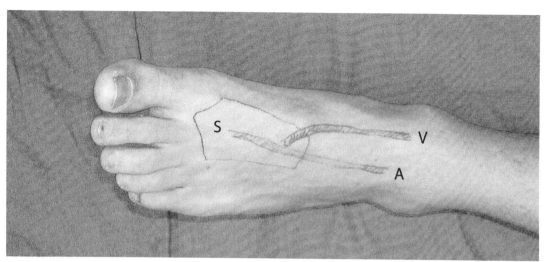

Fig. 2. Dorsalis pedis flap. The dorsalis pedis artery (A) and the long saphenous vein (V) coming from the dorsal arch pedicles the skin paddle (S), which can incorporate almost the entirety of the dorsal skin of the foot.

can be customized depending on the extent of the defect; however, this flap carries the limitation of reconstruction of only a unilateral defect. This limitation is because of the resulting deformity of the donor ear. Often, the donor site can be closed primarily with rotation and advancement of the helical rim,[20] which produces a smaller but acceptable ear. However, if the flap is very extensive, to reconstruct bilateral nasal alae defects, the donor ear may become unacceptably deformed.

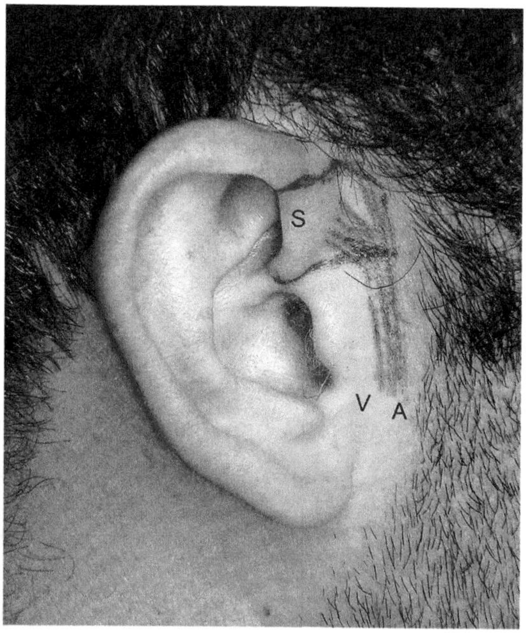

Fig. 3. Auricular helical flap. Based on the superficial temporal artery (A) and vein (V). The skin paddle (S) covers a thin layer of cartilage.

Microvascular reconstruction of the nasal alae means a substantial effort to reconstruct a small defect. Nonetheless, the reconstruction provides a well-vascularized tissue with a predictable result for the patient, unlike the composite grafts from the ear, and does not have variable survival or significant atrophy.

Radial Forearm Flap

The radial forearm free flap[21] was described in 1982 and since then became the workhorse in head and neck reconstruction. The flap is based on the radial artery. It is contraindicated in patients who do not have a palmar arch, which happens in about 15% of the population[11] and is assessed by the Allen test, which evaluates palmar recirculation when the radial artery is occluded by manual pressure. In this scenario, the ulnar artery flap can allow for harvest of nearly the same skin. The radial forearm flap provides thin and hairless skin similar to the dorsalis pedis flap (**Fig. 4**). However, the vessels in the forearm are not usually involved by atherosclerotic changes, and the donor site morbidity, functionally and cosmetically, in the upper extremity is much lower, with only the need of a skin graft to replace the forearm skin and a forearm splint to facilitate the skin graft success. The forearm flap is usually further thinned by a process called lipopluction, whereby the capsule of each lobule is punctured with a needle and the contents gently suctioned.[2,22]

Most reports involving the radial forearm flap use the skin paddle for reconstruction of the nasal lining,[1–3,23] because the tissue chosen for nasal lining reconstruction must remain viable and prevent contracture, which leads to distortion of

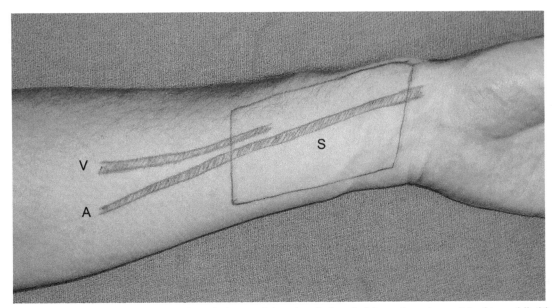

Fig. 4. Radial forearm flap. Based on the radial artery (A) and cephalic vein (V), confers a large, thin skin paddle (S).

the external skin cover, and must be thin enough to not obstruct the airway.

The radial forearm flap was also described as an osteocutaneous flap[4,24] with a split bone graft for the radius that was further divided and plated in place to provide nasal support. Winslow and colleagues[25] described the use of a radial forearm fascial flap for reconstruction of the intranasal lining. They harvested the flap in the subcutaneous plane, elevating the skin and harvesting the underlying fascia attached by the pedicle. The flap is thin and well vascularized, providing a good option for reconstruction of the intranasal lining as well as the vascular bed for the bone and cartilaginous grafts.

The radial forearm with its robust vascular supply; long pedicle; vessels with large caliber, which facilitates the transfer; and relatively thin skin and subcutaneous tissue provides one of the most attractive options for nasal reconstruction.

Prelaminated Flap

Prelamination consists of a multistage procedure in which additional tissues are introduced into a flap without interfering with its blood supply.[22] A prelaminated flap consists of a fabricated composite flap, with the layers specific to a reconstructive site, such as skin and cartilage or skin and bone, which are done remotely. Prelamination was introduced by Pribaz and Fine[26] in 1994 and since then has been used experimentally and clinically with a variety of tissue layers and forms[27,28] and proved to be a promising technique for reconstruction of the intranasal lining. The forearm is the most common site for prelamination (**Fig. 5**).[2,22,27,29]

The major advantage of prelamination is to allow for a precise configuration of the 3-dimensional tissue construct and predict contractive forces before implanting the tissue. Wound contracture takes place in an expendable soft tissue area. This procedure also provides availability for recruitment of additional tissues for adjacent defects on the upper lip or cheeks in a more predictable manner. Tissue expanders can be used in the first stage to increase the surface and provide some thinning to the skin. One of the drawbacks of prelaminated flaps is the need for multiple procedures. However, most of the regular free flaps to the nose require some sort of staging for thinning and adjustment of contour. Nevertheless, this is considered not to be a major problem given its benefits.

Moreover, in the case of nasal reconstruction, when space is limited and intranasal lining reconstruction is a challenging operation, the remote fabrication of the construct eliminates a significant amount of the technical difficulties.

PRACTICAL ASPECTS OF THE PROCEDURE

The most important aspect of microvascular reconstruction of nasal defects is a thorough analysis of the defect. The surgeon must consider the following questions:

- How much nasal septum is left? A remnant of nasal septum, if any, can provide a source for mucosal flap and support for reconstructed nasal framework.

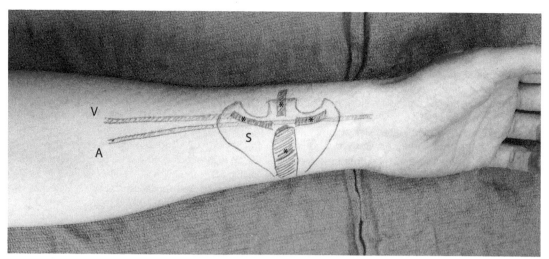

Fig. 5. Prelaminated flap. If harvested from the forearm, carries the same vessels as described previously. The skin paddle (S) is designed according to the defect to be repaired, in this case intranasal lining. The shaded area (*asterisk*) represents the areas the bone and cartilage graft will be implanted.

- What is the status of the columella? An absent columella is probably the most challenging portion to reconstruct. Failure to appropriately reconstruct the columella leads to difficulty in projecting the nose and to obstruction of the airway and results in a nasal reconstruction that has an amorphous structure.
- Does the defect extend into adjacent facial subunits such as the upper lip and cheek? The extent of the defect determines the total amount of skin needed for reconstruction.
- Is there a history of previous or plan for future radiotherapy? Radiotherapy makes local flaps vascularity more tenuous.

After the defect analysis, the choice of the appropriate flap is based on the patient's needs. As pointed out previously, the surgeon should keep in mind that the vascular pedicle should be long enough to allow a tension-free anastomosis with the facial vessels. The planning as to where the pedicle is going to be placed is the first step in harvesting any free flap. The pedicle is usually passed through a subcutaneous tunnel until it reaches the facial vessels, more commonly at the level of the jaw line. From there, the surgeon can design the skin paddles for the columella, the intranasal lining, and possibly the nasal external cover. The skin paddle size for the nasal lining needs to take into consideration the 3-dimensional structure of the nose and the forces of scar contracture. Some surgeons advocate the use of an intranasal stent that would be draped by the skin paddle, whereby the shape of the skin can be designed around the stent, ensuring a satisfactory nasal

projection. The construction of the columella can be done in the first stage, or a separate skin paddle can be placed remotely with cartilage or bone incorporated to it. The latter approach allows time for scar contracture and reabsorbs portion of the structural graft, making the columella reconstruction more predictable. These 2 steps, intranasal lining and columella reconstruction, are the most critical when performing a reconstruction of a total nasal defect. The framework, nasal dorsum, and alar cartilages can be reconstructed in several ways. The grafts are more commonly free-bone or cartilage grafts that are placed in the well-vascularized bed of the free flap or that, in some instances, can be incorporated with the flap as described previously. Along the same lines, the external cover can be obtained in different forms. It can be obtained from the free flap that provided the intranasal lining, when it is folded on itself, from a skin graft that is temporary until a second stage, or from the paramedical forehead flap. The details regarding this local flap were described by Oo and Park elsewhere in this issue.

COUNSELING THE PATIENT REGARDING THE APPROACH

When performing microvascular reconstruction of nasal defects, patient counseling assumes an important role. At this point, usually the other options such as prosthetics and local flaps were already exhausted. If not, they should be reviewed and offered when possible. The psychological state of the patients is crucial to understand the process, including their perception of self and body (body image), their medical and psychological ability to undergo a multistage reconstruction, and their perceived anatomic and cosmetic goals and outcomes. Any significant discordance should be further explored. Often a psychological/psychiatric evaluation can aid in both diagnostic clarity and support for the patient.

The patient should be counseled about the different approaches for microvascular reconstruction and the use of prelaminated or nonlaminated free flaps and the consequences. Both procedures have a multistage nature and take time to achieve the final result. Both the patient and the family, together with the surgeon, need to review the evolution of the nasal shape over time as the structures may fracture, shift, or contract.

SUMMARY

Microvascular reconstruction of nasal defects is an extremely complex procedure, requiring both experience and skill of the surgeon. There are multiple approaches possible, and each patient should be addressed individually.

REFERENCES

1. Cannady SB, Cook TA, Wax MK. The total nasal defect and reconstruction. Facial Plast Surg Clin North Am 2009;17(2):189–201.
2. Walton RL, Burget GC, Beahm EK. Microsurgical reconstruction of the nasal lining. Plast Reconstr Surg 2005;115(7):1813–29.
3. Moore EJ, Strome SA, Kasperbauer JL, et al. Vascularized radial forearm free tissue transfer for lining in nasal reconstruction. Laryngoscope 2003;113(12):2078–85.
4. Koshima I, Tsutsui T, Nanba Y, et al. Free radial forearm osteocutaneous perforator flap for reconstruction of total nasal defects. J Reconstr Microsurg 2002;18(7):585–8.
5. Earley MJ, Milner RH. Dorsal metacarpal flaps. Br J Plast Surg 1987;40(4):333–41.
6. Yap LH, Earley MJ. The free 'V': a bipennate free flap for double eyelid resurfacing based on the second dorsal metacarpal artery. Br J Plast Surg 1997;50(4):280–3.
7. Beahm EK, Walton RL, Burget GC. Free first dorsal metacarpal artery flap for nasal lining. Microsurgery 2005;25(7):551–5.
8. Germann G, Hornung R, Raff T. Two new applications for the first dorsal metacarpal artery pedicle in the treatment of severe hand injuries. J Hand Surg Br 1995;20(4):525–8.
9. McCraw JB, Furlow LT Jr. The dorsalis pedis arterialized flap. A clinical study. Plast Reconstr Surg 1975; 55(2):177–85.
10. Ohmori K, Sekiguchi J, Ohmori S. Total rhinoplasty with a free osteocutaneous flap. Plast Reconstr Surg 1979;63(3):387–94.
11. Swartz WM. Microvascular approaches to nasal reconstruction. Microsurgery 1988;9(2):150–3.
12. May JW Jr, Chait LA, Cohen BE, et al. Free neurovascular flap from the first web of the foot in hand reconstruction. J Hand Surg Am 1977;2(5):387–93.
13. Evans DM. Facial reconstruction after a burn injury using two circumferential radial forearm flaps, and a dorsalis pedis flap for the nose. Br J Plast Surg 1995;48(7):471–6.
14. Bayramiçli M. The distal dorsalis pedis flap for nasal tip reconstruction. Br J Plast Surg 1996;49(5):325–7.
15. Lin SD, Lin GT, Lai CS, et al. Nasal alar reconstruction with free "accessory auricle". Plast Reconstr Surg 1984;73(5):827–9.
16. Parkhouse N, Evans D. Reconstruction of the ala of the nose using a composite free flap from the pinna. Br J Plast Surg 1985;38(3):306–13.
17. Shenaq SM, Dinh TA, Spira M. Nasal alar reconstruction with an ear helix free flap. J Reconstr Microsurg 1989;5(1):63–7.
18. Park C, Lineaweaver WC, Rumly TO, et al. Arterial supply of the anterior ear. Plast Reconstr Surg 1992;90(1):38–44.
19. Pribaz JJ, Falco N. Nasal reconstruction with auricular microvascular transplant. Ann Plast Surg 1993; 31(4):289–97.
20. Antia NH, Buch VI. Chondrocutaneous advancement flap for the marginal defect of the ear. Plast Reconstr Surg 1967;39(5):472–7.
21. Song R, Gao Y, Song Y, et al. The forearm flap. Clin Plast Surg 1982;9(1):21–6.
22. Taghinia AH, Pribaz JJ. Complex nasal reconstruction. Plast Reconstr Surg 2008;121(2):15e–27e.
23. Burget GC, Walton RL. Optimal use of microvascular free flaps, cartilage grafts, and a paramedian forehead flap for aesthetic reconstruction of the nose and adjacent facial units. Plast Reconstr Surg 2007;120(5):1171–207.
24. Kobayashi S, Yoza S, Sakai Y, et al. Versatility of a microsurgical free-tissue transfer from the forearm in treating the difficult nose. Plast Reconstr Surg 1995;96(4):810–5.
25. Winslow CP, Cook TA, Burke A, et al. Total nasal reconstruction: utility of the free radial forearm fascial flap. Arch Facial Plast Surg 2003;5(2):159–63.
26. Pribaz JJ, Fine NA. Prelamination: defining the prefabricated flap—a case report and review. Microsurgery 1994;15(9):618–23.
27. Pribaz JJ, Fine NA. Prefabricated and prelaminated flaps for head and neck reconstruction. Clin Plast Surg 2001;28(2):261–72.
28. Ahn KM, Kim MJ, Lee JH. Prelaminated fasciomucosal flap using tongue mucosa in a rat model. J Reconstr Microsurg 2003;19(3):195–201.
29. Costa H, Cunha C, Guimarães I, et al. Prefabricated flaps for the head and neck: a preliminary report. Br J Plast Surg 1993;46(3):223–7.

Options for Internal Lining in Nasal Reconstruction

Stephen M. Weber, MD, PhD*, Tom D. Wang, MD

KEYWORDS

- Mohs • Skin cancer • Nasal defect • Nasal reconstruction
- Nasal lining • Vestibular advancement flap
- Inferior turbinate flap • Septal mucoperichondrial flap
- Composite septal pivotal flap • Forehead flap

CAUSE

Nasal reconstruction has been refined to the point that its goals should include full restoration of form and function in addition to an aesthetically pleasing result. Contemporary facial plastic surgeons have all the tools available in their armamentarium to repair the complex composite structure of nasal lining, structure, and skin cover. Nasal defects most often result from oncologic surgery (Mohs,[1] wide local, or square[2] excision) or nasal trauma. Of paramount importance in the reconstruction of oncologic defects is the confirmation of clear resection margins before undertaking reconstruction. Failure to confirm clear margins risks tumor recurrence, rendering moot the successful nasal reconstruction. Mohs micrographic surgery[3,4] lends itself to immediate confirmation of clear margins. Wide local excision, on the other hand, relies on frozen-section analysis of a representative sample of the defect margin or delayed reconstruction, allowing time to confirm negative margins of permanent pathologic specimens.

Although this article focuses on reconstruction of oncologic defects, the principles discussed can be effectively applied to reconstruction of nasal-lining defects resulting from any cause. Restraint should be exercised in the initial management of traumatic, or otherwise contaminated, defects to allow elimination of potential wound contamination before repair. In many cases, expectant management results in sufficient healing by secondary intention to either reduce the significance of the required reconstruction or preclude surgical intervention.

DEFECT ANALYSIS

Critical analysis of a nasal defect should precede reconstruction of even the smallest wound. The primary goal of this exercise is to identify viable options on the reconstructive ladder and to choose the optimal modality among those in the reconstructive surgeon's armamentarium. At the most basic level, nasal tissue may be divided into cover (skin, subcutaneous tissue, and nasalis muscle), structure (upper and lower lateral cartilages, septum, and nasal bones) and internal lining (vestibular skin and nasal mucosa). This article focuses on reconstruction of nasal-lining defects.

Unrepaired nasal-lining defects create two potential issues in nasal reconstruction. First, even small nasal-lining defects are subject to secondary intention healing. The resulting cicatricial contractile forces can result in distortion of the nasal framework. Second, unrepaired lining defects can expose overlying structural grafts. Exposed cartilage or bone grafts are susceptible to bacterial colonization and/or infection and lack the robust blood supply necessary for survival. Most nasal-lining defects occur in the context of a composite loss of full-thickness nasal tissue. Failure to restore continuity in the nasal lining

The authors do not have a financial interest in any aspect of the topic being discussed.
Division of Facial Plastic and Reconstructive Surgery, Department of Otolaryngology and Head & Neck Surgery, Oregon Health & Science University, 3181 SW Sam Jackson Park Road, Portland, OR 97239, USA
* Corresponding author.
E-mail address: weberst@gmail.com

facialplastic.theclinics.com

risks wound infections, graft exposure, graft extrusion, and suboptimal functional and aesthetic results. Thus lining defects, especially of the lower third of the nose, must be meticulously repaired with primary closure, bipedicled vestibular advancement, inferior turbinate mucoperiosteum, septal mucoperichondrium, or septal composite pivotal flaps.[5,6] Although additional options exist and are discussed in this article, these reconstructive modalities are ideal because they replace nasal mucosal lining with similar intranasal mucosal flaps. These methods maintain or replace the thin, supple, functioning nasal mucosal tissue to support nasal mucociliary clearance, humidification, and temperature regulation of inspired air.

Nasal-lining defects most often occur as part of a defect involving nasal structure and skin cover. Thus, in the context of discussing nasal-lining defects it is important to consider several basic principles of full-thickness nasal reconstruction. First, composite defects should be reconstituted with like tissue. In addition to reconstruction of the skin cover, discussed elsewhere,[7] robust structure must also be provided using structural cartilage (concha, septum, rib) or bone (perpendicular plate, split calvarium) grafts. Structural grafts are used both to support the nose and to fine-tune the contour of reconstructed nasal unit(s). To achieve these goals, autogenous grafts are placed in both anatomic and nonanatomic locations, as described later.

PATIENT FACTORS

Of the numerous patient factors to consider, one of the most important and modifiable risk factors is use of tobacco products. Current smokers are at risk for skin flap and graft failure.[8–11] Nasal-lining flaps are particularly at risk in tobacco users given the thin, delicate nature and tenuous blood supply of commonly used flaps. If patients are unable to curtail use of tobacco products before reconstruction they must be counseled about the increased risk of graft or flap failure. These risks can be mitigated by eschewing skin grafts, raising thicker cutaneous flaps (recruiting a more robust subdermal vascular plexus) and minimizing wound closure tension (optimizing flap perfusion). Regardless of the precision of nasal skin and structure replacement, a deficit of nasal lining caused by flap loss or poor surgical planning results in impressive contraction of the reconstructed nasal unit(s), with the expected nasal deformity and impairment in nasal breathing.

A history of previous skin cancer or nasal surgery should be elicited. In some instances this might include a history of head and neck irradiation. In many cases, a pattern of alopecia in the beard or neck region delineates the area of previous cutaneous irradiation and potentially compromised skin vascularity. Both head and neck irradiation and intervening scars may be expected to compromise skin flap vascularity and viability. Specifically with regard to use of nasal-lining flaps, previous septoplasty, rhinoplasty, or turbinate surgery should be investigated to determine whether intranasal flaps are viable reconstructive options. Septal perforations should be identified because their location might preclude ipsi- and/or contralateral septal mucoperichondrial hinge flaps.

RECONSTRUCTIVE LADDER

Nasal reconstruction requires careful composite reconstitution of missing nasal lining as well as structure and/or cover with like tissue. Given the diverse options for replacement of nasal lining, it is helpful to compartmentalize the options into a reconstructive ladder (**Fig. 1**) that stratifies reconstructive modalities from least (secondary intention) to most complex (free-tissue transfer). Secondary intention healing can be successful for carefully selected small defects limited to the nasal lining. Some nasal-lining defects of 5 mm or less can be closed primarily with careful undermining. However, most nasal-lining defects require repair with pedicled soft-tissue flaps such as bipedicled vestibular advancement, inferior turbinate mucoperiosteum, septal mucoperichondrial hinge, septal composite pivotal, or paramedian forehead flaps. In rare cases, microvascular free-tissue transfer is required for recreation of nasal lining. Detailed discussion of free-tissue transfer is beyond the scope of this article but is well described elsewhere.[12]

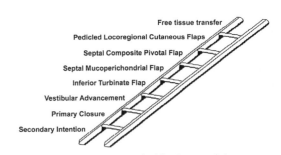

Fig. 1. The reconstructive ladder is a useful construct to organize reconstructive modalities from least (secondary intention) to most complex (free-tissue transfer).

SECONDARY INTENTION

Secondary intention is the most simple, and infrequently used, method of managing nasal-lining defects. No intervention beyond proper local wound care and monitoring the wound-healing process is required. General wound-healing principles to be observed include minimizing the bacterial burden and keeping the wound clean and moist. Nasal-lining defects most often occur as part of a full-thickness nasal defect, requiring composite reconstruction of nasal cover, structure, and lining. Nasal-lining defects, especially in the lower one-third of the nose, tend to contract, resulting in distortion of the tip and alar unit(s) and compromise of the nasal airway. For these reasons, lining defects are most often repaired using one of the methods detailed later.

GENERAL PRINCIPLES OF NASAL-LINING RECONSTRUCTION

- Confirm negative oncologic margins
- Determine size and location of nasal-lining defect
- Determine whether defects in nasal structure and/or cover are present
- Rule out preexisting septal incisions, septal perforation, or evidence of previous inferior turbinectomy that might preclude intranasal local flap repairs of the lining defect
- Inject nose, nasal septum, and/or turbinates with local anesthetic (typically 1% lidocaine containing epinephrine)
- Inject regional donor sites or involved adjacent facial aesthetic units in subcutaneous tissue plane, as necessary
- Consider conservative undermining for small (≤5 mm) lining defects to facilitate tension-free primary closure.
- Ensure that all nasal-lining defects are repaired and that composite defects are

reconstituted with robust structure to resist contractile effects of wound healing.

PRIMARY CLOSURE

Primary closure is suitable for small (≤5 mm) nasal-lining defects. This technique is best suited for repair of a linear, vertically oriented lining defect (**Fig. 2**) that lends itself to closure without elevation of the alar margin. Conservative undermining of the nasal lining away from surrounding cartilage or subcutaneous tissue can facilitate tension-free closure. If initial attempts at primary closure result in shortening the nasal lining, elevation of the alar margin or distortion of the nasal valve region another method should be used to repair the nasal lining.

SKIN GRAFTS
Full-thickness Skin Graft

Historically, full-thickness skin grafts (FTSGs) have been used for replacement of nasal lining. However, their use in nasal-lining reconstruction is limited by the inability to use FTSGs to cover structural cartilage grafts. FTSGs also have a predilection toward moderate amounts of contraction, which is problematic. Replacement of nasal mucosal lining with skin can interfere with nasal functions, including filtering of pollutants, humidification of inspired air, and mucociliary clearance.

The main indication for use of FTSGs involves reconstruction of the donor site for the bipedicled vestibular advancement flap (see later discussion). The bipedicled flap is used to reconstruct nasal-lining defects of the lower one-third of the nose, creating a nasal-lining defect cephalad to the scroll region/intercartilaginous incision. An FTSG is placed on the perichondrium of the upper and/or lower lateral cartilage(s) to repair the donor site and to prevent contraction and distortion of the reconstructed lower third of the nose.

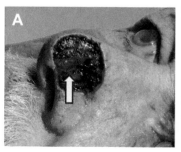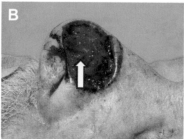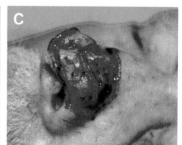

Fig. 2. (*A*) Primary closure is suitable for vertically oriented, linear nasal-lining defects 5 mm or less in width (*arrow*). (*B*) Care must be used to ensure that primary closure (*arrow*) does not result in retraction of the tip and/or alar unit(s). (*C*) Adequate support of the reconstructed unit(s) must be provided by autogenous graft material, in this case conchal cartilage grafts.

In theory, FTSGs can be used to reconstitute nasal lining when juxtaposed to the undersurface of a well-vascularized pedicled flap used to replace the nasal cover. This strategy does complicate composite reconstruction because structural cartilage grafts cannot be placed between pedicled cutaneous flaps and an FTSG. Division of the supratrochlear vessel into distinct branches that supply the skin/subcutaneous tissue and the frontalis muscle enables division of the forehead flap into 2 distinct vascularized units. Thus, it is possible to secure FTSGs to the galea/frontalis muscle of a paramedian forehead flap and simultaneously place cartilage grafts into precise pockets between the frontalis muscle and subcutaneous fat of the forehead flap.[13] This method does require secondary/tertiary procedures to debulk the cutaneous flap and add additional structural cartilage grafts to the cephalad portion of the reconstructed nose. In our experience this technique is highly complicated, technically challenging, and risks early contraction of the reconstructed nasal unit(s). Further, large lining defects repaired with this method rely on the blood supply of the frontalis muscle being able to adequately supply both the muscle and the underlying FTSG to ensure survival of the nasal lining and, by extension, the entire reconstruction. Secondary repair of a contracted nasal reconstruction resulting from a nasal-lining deficit can be challenging.

FTSGs consist of the epidermis and variable amounts of dermis. Although FTSGs are subject to less contraction than split-thickness grafts, their higher metabolic demand makes FTSGs survival more tenuous[14] than split-thickness grafts. Skin grafts obtain their nutrition through 3 distinct stages. During the initial 24 to 48 hours, FTSGs obtain nutrients and oxygen via plasmatic imbibition by drinking from the surrounding extracellular fluid. Next, blood vessels in the graft and donor site align and begin to penetrate the graft during the stage of inosculation. Last, vascular ingrowth proceeds and the entire periphery of the graft becomes vascularized. During this critical phase of graft survival, infection and small-vessel compromise (smoking) limit FTSG survival. Thus, antibiotics and smoking cessation are routinely recommended and have been shown to result in improved FTSG survival.[15]

Commonly used FTSG donor sites include pre- and postauricular skin, supraclavicular skin, and the melolabial fold. We prefer to use the preauricular donor site because it provides generous amounts of skin with similar color and texture match with nasal skin. Using the contralateral preauricular donor site allows 2 surgeons to work simultaneously on graft harvest and closure of the donor site and lining defect.

Split-thickness Skin Grafts

Split-thickness skin grafts (STSGs) have higher survival rates as a result of a lower metabolic demand than FTSGs. However, because of their greater predilection toward contraction, STSGs have had limited use in replacement of nasal lining. Nasal-lining defects amenable to skin graft repair tend to be small and thus can be accommodated using common FTSG donor sites with lower risk of contracture.

CUTANEOUS HINGE FLAPS

Cutaneous hinge flaps are based on a subcutaneous pedicle composed of scar tissue located at the defect margin. The most common donor sites for cutaneous hinge or turn-in flaps are the medial cheek and/or nasal sidewall as well as the cephalic edge of an alar defect (**Fig. 3**). The hinge flap in the latter case most often consists of the remaining skin of the alar unit, which would otherwise be discarded as part of the cutaneous alar reconstruction. The fact that the vascular pedicle is based on scar tissue at the defect margin limits the potential vascularity of this flap. Delay of the flap, wherein its borders are incised before being re-inset, can improve survival of the cutaneous hinge flap. However, this strategy adds an additional procedure and 3-week delay until definitive

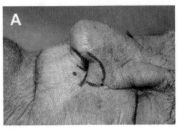
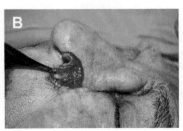
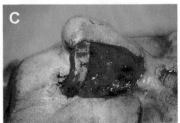

Fig. 3. (*A*) The cutaneous hinge flap based on the cephalic edge of a healed alar defect is marked out. (*B*) After elevation and inset of this flap, conchal cartilage (*C*) is used to buttress the shape and position of the reconstructed alar unit.

reconstruction. Delaying the cutaneous turn-in flap does create an opportunity to inset an FTSG for later use in replacement of nasal lining and/or cover. However, the ability of turn-in flaps resurfaced with an FTSG to adequately cover and nourish structural cartilage grafts is limited. Thus, the use of cutaneous hinge flaps should be reserved for defects in which other options are unsuitable.

BIPEDICLED VESTIBULAR ADVANCEMENT FLAP

Full-thickness defects of the ala and/or hemitip that have a vertical height of 1 cm or less can be lined by a bipedicled vestibular skin advancement flap. This skin-only flap is based on the floor of the vestibule laterally and nasal septum medially. An ipsilateral intercartilaginous incision is made from the nasal septum to the lateral floor of the vestibule. For a taller advancement flap, the incision may be placed more cephalad on the undersurface of the upper lateral cartilage. Attachments of the advancement flap to the overlying upper/lower lateral cartilages are released by careful dissection to prevent perforating the thin but well-vascularized flap. The flap is mobilized to allow tension-free advancement to the level of the nostril margin or most caudal extent of the lining defect (**Fig. 4**). Adequate structure is provided by a conchal cartilage graft, to which the vestibular advancement flap is secured with judicious horizontal mattress sutures. The donor site for the vestibular advancement flap is resurfaced with a thinned FTSG, which is inset on the intact perichondrium of the upper lateral cartilage.

SEPTAL MUCOPERICHONDRIAL HINGE FLAP

The anteroinferior blood supply of the septum is derived principally from bilateral septal branches of the superior labial arteries. This robust blood supply is sufficient to nourish a flap composed of unilateral or bilateral septal mucoperichondrium with or without intervening septal cartilage (composite pivotal flap; see later discussion). Septal mucoperichondrial flaps including the entire height of the nasal septum and extending from the caudal septum beyond the bone-cartilage junction may be nourished by a single septal branch of the superior labial artery. We prefer to base ipsilateral septal flaps on the entire height of the caudal septum and then turn the flap laterally as a hinge flap (**Fig. 5**).

Large lining defects (ala and nasal sidewall) often require bilateral septal mucoperichondrial hinge flaps using the contralateral flap to reline the cephalic extent of the defect. The anterior ethmoid artery supplies this mucoperichondrial flap hinged on the dorsal septum. Its dimensions may equal the height and length of the septum, and it is transferred laterally toward the contralateral side as a hinge flap, with the raw surface facing exteriorly. Repair of this type of defect results in the creation of a large septal perforation. This situation results from using bilateral mucoperichondrial flaps for nasal lining and harvesting septal cartilage grafts to provide nasal sidewall structural grafts. In cases of isolated cephalically positioned defects, the contralateral mucoperichondrial flap may be delivered through a superiorly located fenestrum of the contralateral mucoperichondrium. This situation results in a smaller, dorsally located septal perforation and, otherwise intact, ipsilateral mucoperichondrial leaflet.

Although the septal mucoperichondrial hinge flap based on the caudal septum has a sufficient vascular supply in most patients, it is less dependable in patients who use tobacco products, as noted earlier. It has the disadvantage of extending across the nasal airway to reach the lateral aspects of the nasal vestibule and can cause near complete nasal obstruction. Three weeks after initial transfer, the flap is detached from the septum. If an interpolated cheek or forehead flap

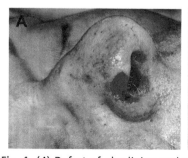 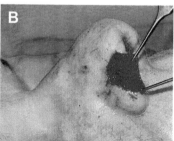 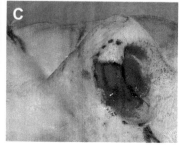

Fig. 4. (*A*) Defect of alar lining and cover. (*B*) Vestibular advancement flap is mobilized to allow tension-free advancement to the nostril margin and (*C*) conchal cartilage is used to secure the flap in position and support the ala.

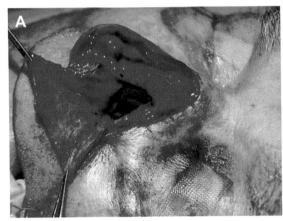
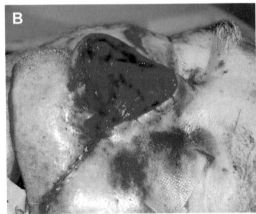

Fig. 5. (*A*) Ipsilateral septal mucoperichondrial flap showed before inset. Entire ala/sidewall defect was repaired with a unilateral hinged mucoperichondrial flap (*B*).

was also performed to reconstruct nasal cover, the septal and cutaneous flaps are detached simultaneously. In contrast, the dorsal septal hinge flap usually does not require detachment because it is draped across the roof and sidewall of the middle vault to reline these areas and does not appreciably constrict the nasal airway.

COMPOSITE SEPTAL PIVOTAL FLAP

The entire septum may be used as a composite chondromucosal flap lined by bilateral mucoperichondrial tissue. This flap can provide lining and structural support for bilateral full-thickness nasal tip and columella defects requiring the composite flap to be pivoted roughly 90° anteriorly from its native position. It is necessary to remove a small amount of bone and cartilage at the nasal spine to allow pivoting of the composite flap into its final position. This procedure requires submucoperichondrial and subperiosteal dissection in the region of the posterior septal angle and nasal spine. During the course of this dissection it is critical to protect the septal vasculature to ensure survival of the composite pivotal flap. Composite pivotal flaps should be designed to provide maximum length (resulting in increased tip projection) and width (providing height of internal nasal lining for bilateral nasal ala and caudal sidewall lining defects). The amount of pivot that the composite flap undergoes also determines the nasal length and rotation of the reconstructed nose. Inadequate pivotal movement results in a foreshortened, overrotated nose. Given the need to provide bilateral septal mucoperichondrial hinge flaps, there is often an excess of septal cartilage and bone that must be trimmed and can then be used for structural grafting. Inadequate projection or insufficient nasal lining interferes with both

the aesthetic and functional result of the nasal reconstruction.

As the composite flap is pivoted out of the nose and into position, its most cephalic aspect is inset and suture-secured to the residual dorsal septal strut (**Fig. 6**). Thus it is important to preserve a dorsal strut of 1 cm or more, but additional width of the dorsal strut borrows from the maximum potential width of the pivotal flap, which should be 1.5 cm wide or greater. For defects involving the nasal tip and dorsum, a composite pivotal flap that encompasses the entire remaining septum is pivoted 90° to 110°, buttressing the flap against the nasal process of the frontal bone.

In either case, the caudal aspect of the pivoted flap becomes the structural support and lining for the missing columella. Cartilage and bone are trimmed to prevent excessive visibility of the columella on profile. The mucoperichondrial leaflets of the composite pivotal flap are dissected free and reflected laterally to provide lining to the tip and nasal alae. Cartilage grafts are obtained from the concha cavum and nasal septum to restore the normal nasal contour of the ala and nasal sidewalls, respectively. Alternatively, costal cartilage can provide both straight and curved cartilage grafts appropriate for nasal sidewall and alar structure but additional warping must be anticipated and countered to ensure stable and predictable results. The mucoperichondrial flaps are suspended to the overlying cartilage grafts with absorbable mattress sutures. Nasal cover is then replaced as described elsewhere.[7]

TURBINATE FLAPS

The inferior turbinate can provide a moderate amount of intranasal mucosa for lining small alar defects. The flap is based on a vascular pedicle

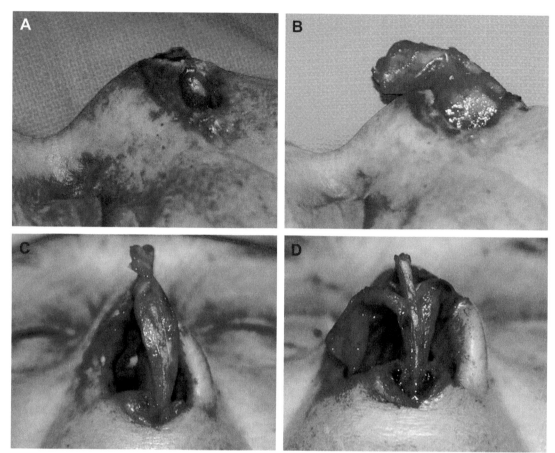

Fig. 6. (*A*) Septal composite pivotal flaps are useful for repair of complex defects of the nasal tip, ala, and columella. The composite flap is freed and pivoted 90° out of the nasal cavity and secured to the dorsal septal strut as viewed from the lateral (*B*) and base view (*C*). Bilateral mucoperichondrial flaps are reflected and inset to the residual alae to replace the lining defect (*D*).

at the head of the turbinate. Thus, a history of turbinate surgery should be investigated because previous turbinectomy could potentially impair not only the size of a turbinate flap but also render its blood supply tenuous. The flap is created by incising the inferior turbinate from posterior to anterior from within the inferior meatus. A Cottle elevator is used to release the posterior and central attachments of the turbinate from the nasal sidewall. The turbinate is delivered out of the nasal passage attached to its mucosal tissue pedicle by pivoting it 180°. The mucoperiosteum is unfurled, and the turbinate bone carefully removed, revealing a thin, pliable mucoperiosteal flap that may be used to line the lateral vestibule (**Fig. 7**). As with the mucoperichondrial flap, the inferior turbinate flap is suspended to overlying framework cartilage grafts with a limited number of mattress sutures. Cautery of the lateral nasal wall donor site is typically adequate for hemostasis but nasal packing is occasionally necessary. The maximum

size of the flap is limited by the size of the inferior turbinate, which in turn limits the usefulness of the flap for large defects.

PARAMEDIAN FOREHEAD FLAP

Although the forehead flap is the workhorse interpolated flap for reconstruction of moderate to large defects of nasal skin cover, attempts at repairing skin cover and nasal lining with a single flap have been problematic. Folding of the forehead flap at the reconstructed nostril margin and use of the distal portion of the flap to recreate the nasal lining results in an overly thick nostril margin and can result in external nasal valve obstruction. Further, folding of the flap on itself can impair the blood supply to the distal flap. Flap necrosis invariably results in contraction of the reconstructed nose with distortion and potential nasal airway obstruction. Even in successful reconstruction of a composite defect with a folded

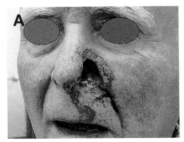
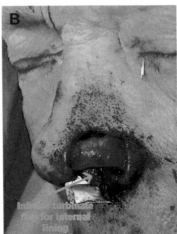
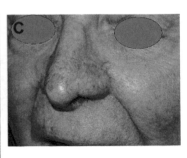

Fig. 7. (*A*) Full-thickness alar defect to be reconstructed via an inferior turbinate flap. (*B*) Inferior turbinate flap inset and buttressed with conchal cartilage graft. (*C*) One-year postoperative result.

forehead flap, it is frequently necessary to debulk the nostril margin as a third procedure 3 months after detachment of the flap pedicle.

Forehead flaps have been successfully used to recreate nasal lining in other ways. The dual blood supply from the supratrochlear artery to the frontalis muscle and forehead skin allows placement of FTSGs on the muscle and insertion of cartilage grafts into precise pockets between the skin and muscle. The limitations of this approach are described earlier. The forehead flap can be tunneled from the glabella. The portion of the forehead flap to be inset to reconstruct the nasal lining is thinned of its frontalis muscle and galea (**Fig. 8**). The flap pedicle is then folded and delivered to the nasal passage by tunneling it under the glabellar skin to reach the lining defect. Alternatively, the flap is inset via the cephalic edge of a full-thickness defect. The flap is suspended to framework grafts of bone and cartilage with mattress sutures. The missing skin cover can be replaced with a second forehead flap, locoregional flap or FTSG.

Reconstruction with the forehead flap[16,17] begins with creation of precise three-dimensional template(s) based on the lining and cutaneous defect(s). The template is created either by outlining the defect with a surgical marker and transferring that image to Telfa gauze or by precise creation of a suture foil template. Care is taken to ensure that the template is properly oriented before marking the forehead incisions. The template is turned 180° to account for the pivotal movement of the forehead flap toward the nasal defect. Adequate pedicle length is confirmed by simulating the pivotal movement of the flap with a heavy suture anchored at the medial brow with

a hemostat. Sufficient pedicle length may require including hair-bearing scalp in a large flap or low hairline. Alternatively, the flap can be turned obliquely along the hairline to gain additional length. The latter maneuver avoids placing hair on the nose. However, obliquely oriented flaps are not advisable when the flap is greater than 3 cm wide because the oblique portion relies on a random pattern vascular supply. The forehead flap is based on the supratrochlear vessels that typically emerge from the orbit between 1.7 and 2.2 cm lateral to the midline (medial extent of the brow). The flap is designed with its vertical axis centered over the supratrochlear vessels. Ipsilateral flaps provide greater effective flap length at the expense of increased pivotal movement about its axis and potential kinking of the pedicle. Conversely, contralateral flaps result in less effective flap length, but require less pivotal movement, reducing the theoretic risk of vessel kinking and flap ischemia. We prefer to use ipsilateral forehead flaps and have not noted any issues resulting from pedicle kinking.

The supratrochlear artery, after emerging from the orbit, pierces the frontalis muscle at the level of the eyebrow and ascends in the subcutaneous tissue plane. Thus, although the flap can be raised in the subcutaneous tissue plane, we prefer to elevate the flap in the subgaleal tissue plane. This dissection is expeditious and bloodless. In the region of the bony supraorbital rim, the flap is dissected bluntly to separate the corrugator muscle fibers from the flap, releasing the pedicle. The flap is thinned at its distal aspect by discarding the frontalis muscle and subcutaneous fat. All but 1 mm of subcutaneous fat is removed centrally and the flap is thinned to the dermis peripherally

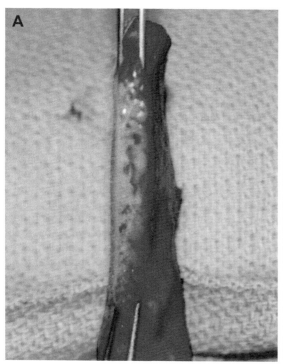
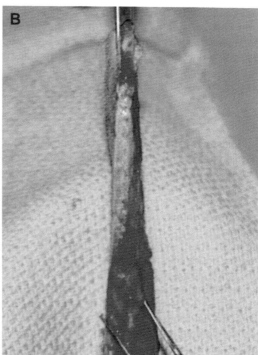

Fig. 8. Paramedian forehead flap before (*A*) and after (*B*) removal of the galea, frontalis muscle, and some subcutaneous fat. This procedure creates a thin, pliable flap suitable for replacement of nasal lining.

to provide a perfect thickness match between flap and the recipient site. The proximal flap, representing the pedicle, is not thinned and is discarded en bloc after pedicle detachment and flap inset. In rare cases, the pedicle can be de-epithelialized and passed through a subcutaneous tunnel into the defect, allowing a single-stage repair.[18]

The forehead donor site is undermined in the subgaleal plane from temporal line to temporal line with blunt dissection. The wound is approximated with interrupted absorbable suture. Regions of the donor site that cannot be closed primarily are left to granulate. After closure of the donor site, the flap is sutured into the defect. The corners are initially secured with 5-0 monofilament absorbable suture placed in a vertical mattress fashion. The skin edges are then accurately reapproximated

with absorbable running stitch. The forehead flap used for nasal lining is detached from the brow after 3 weeks. If a second forehead flap was used for replacing the nasal cover, detachment of the external flap is delayed an additional 3 weeks to maximize revascularization of the framework grafts.

INTERPOLATED CHEEK FLAP

Superiorly based melolabial flaps that are positioned as closely as possible to the site of an alar defect have been used to replace nasal vestibular lining. The flap is hinged on either a subcutaneous (**Fig. 9**) or cutaneous pedicle and turned medially to line lateral alar defects or the entire nasal vestibule. The interpolated cheek flap has the disadvantage of providing a lining with excessive bulk

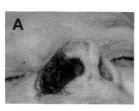
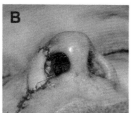
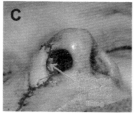
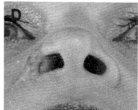

Fig. 9. (*A*) Full-thickness alar defect reconstructed with interpolated cheek flap (lining) and composite conchal cartilage graft (structure and cover). Intraoperative (*B, C*) and 1-year postoperative views (*D*).

that can crowd the airway and camouflage structural cartilage grafts used for nasal framework. As a result, interpolated cheek flaps are used less commonly than vestibular advancement flaps or other pedicled intranasal mucosal flaps for replacing caudal nasal lining.

FREE-TISSUE TRANSFER

Free-tissue transfer is typically reserved for cases in which there is total or near total loss of the nose and adequate mucoperichondrial flaps cannot be developed to replace nasal lining. If there are concurrent hard- or soft-tissue defects of the midface, these should be addressed first to provide a stable platform on which the nose can be reconstructed. The 2 most commonly used free-tissue transfer donor sites to replace nasal lining include the radial forearm and temporoparietal fascia flaps. Although the latter flap is exquisitely thin and pliable, it does require skin grafting to replace the epithelial lining of the nose. The forearm flap has predictable anatomy and provides a moderately sized, pliable skin paddle. This workhorse free flap is familiar to most free-flap surgeons. The flap also has a long vascular pedicle, obviating vein grafting, in most cases. The vascular pedicle is tunneled through the subcutaneous tissues of the cheek to recipient vessels in the neck. The flap is secured to overlying structural grafts with mattress sutures, as described earlier, and the nasal skin is replaced with a forehead flap. Patients are monitored for evidence of vascular compromise for 5 days using a combination of visual inspection and Doppler investigation.

CARTILAGE GRAFTING

Cartilage grafting is required for all cases in which a full-thickness nasal defect is reconstructed.

These grafts resist the contractile forces of wound healing and maintaining a natural nasal contour of the reconstructed nose. For replacement of the nasal ala, cartilage framework grafts are created sufficiently large to span the distance between the pyriform aperture and the nasal soft-tissue facets (see **Figs. 2–4** and **7**). For full-thickness tip and ala defects, alar replacement grafts are secured to the reconstructed columella/anterior septal angle. These grafts are ideally harvested from the concha cavum (**Fig. 10**A) because the shape approximates the convexity of the native ala. Conchal cartilage has adequate structure to resist contraction during wound healing and to resist negative inspiratory pressure during nasal breathing. Grafts are secured with absorbable monofilament suture tied in a horizontal mattress fashion, with the knots placed superficial to the cartilage graft.

Septal cartilage grafts are most often used to support the nasal sidewall after reconstruction of full-thickness defects (see **Fig. 10**B). In addition, septal cartilage is highly useful to support the nasal tip (columella strut graft) or internal nasal valve region (spreader graft). Septal cartilage is suboptimal for use in alar reconstruction given the straight and rigid nature of this source of cartilage. Regardless of the source, grafts are used either to replace the alar cartilage or reinforce the native soft tissue in the reconstructed region. The authors advocate lateral (TDW) or medial (SMW) approaches for harvesting conchal cartilage.[7] The main advantage of the medial approach is the lack of a visible scar. However, this approach is more difficult to perform without an assistant. Regardless of the surgical approach, the antihelical rim is maintained to preserve the appearance of the donor ear. Further, concha cavum harvest should not extend into the cartilaginous ear canal to prevent ear canal stenosis.

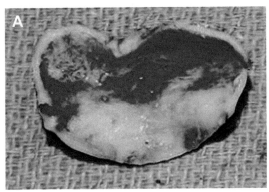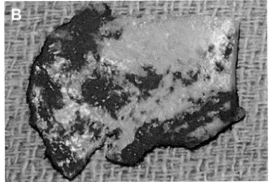

Fig. 10. Both conchal (*A*) and septal (*B*) cartilage grafts are frequently required for reconstruction of composite nasal defects.

REFERENCES

1. Minton TJ. Contemporary Mohs surgery applications. Curr Opin Otolaryngol Head Neck Surg 2008;16:376–80.
2. Johnson TM, Headington JT, Baker SR, et al. Usefulness of the staged excision for lentigo maligna and lentigo maligna melanoma: the "square" procedure. J Am Acad Dermatol 1997;37:758–64.
3. Baker SR, Swanson NA. Management of nasal cutaneous malignant neoplasms. An interdisciplinary approach. Arch Otolaryngol 1983;109:473–9.
4. Baker SR, Swanson NA, Grekin RC. An interdisciplinary approach to the management of basal cell carcinoma of the head and neck. J Dermatol Surg Oncol 1987;13:1095–106.
5. Baker SR. Local flaps in facial reconstruction. St Louis (MO): Mosby Elsevier; 2007.
6. Baker SR, Naficy S, Jewet B. Principles of nasal reconstruction. Philadelphia: Mosby; 2002. p. xii, 301.
7. Weber SM, Baker SR. Management of cutaneous nasal defects. Facial Plast Surg Clin North Am 2009;17:395–417.
8. Goldminz D, Bennett RG. Cigarette smoking and flap and full-thickness graft necrosis. Arch Dermatol 1991;127:1012–5.
9. Kinsella JB, Rassekh CH, Wassmuth ZD, et al. Smoking increases facial skin flap complications. Ann Otol Rhinol Laryngol 1999;108:139–42.
10. Lawrence WT, Murphy RC, Robson MC, et al. The detrimental effect of cigarette smoking on flap survival: an experimental study in the rat. Br J Plast Surg 1984;37:216–9.
11. Nolan J, Jenkins RA, Kurihara K, et al. The acute effects of cigarette smoke exposure on experimental skin flaps. Plast Reconstr Surg 1985;75:544–51.
12. Burget GC, Walton RL. Optimal use of microvascular free flaps, cartilage grafts, and a paramedian forehead flap for aesthetic reconstruction of the nose and adjacent facial units. Plast Reconstr Surg 2007;120:1171–207 [discussion 208–16].
13. Burget GC, Menick FJ. Nasal reconstruction: seeking a fourth dimension. Plast Reconstr Surg 1986;78:145–57.
14. Leibovitch I, Huilgol SC, Richards S, et al. The Australian Mohs database: short-term recipient-site complications in full-thickness skin grafts. Dermatol Surg 2006;32:1364–8.
15. Kuijpers DI, Smeets NW, Lapiere K, et al. Do systemic antibiotics increase the survival of a full thickness graft on the nose? J Eur Acad Dermatol Venereol 2006;20:1296–301.
16. Boyd CM, Baker SR, Fader DJ, et al. The forehead flap for nasal reconstruction. Arch Dermatol 2000;136:1365–70.
17. Driscoll BP, Baker SR. Reconstruction of nasal alar defects. Arch Facial Plast Surg 2001;3:91–9.
18. Park SS. The single-stage forehead flap in nasal reconstruction: an alternative with advantages. Arch Facial Plast Surg 2002;4:32–6.

Cartilage Grafting in Nasal Reconstruction

Sara Immerman, MD[a], W. Matthew White, MD[b],
Minas Constantinides, MD[b],*

KEYWORDS

- Cartilage grafting • Nasal reconstruction • Composite grafts
- Cutaneous malignancy

One of the most common locations for skin cancer is the nose; the unique 3-D structure of the nose poses a challenge for reconstruction. Nasal defects after resections of cutaneous malignancies are frequently disfiguring and distressing to patients. Without proper reconstruction, it is nearly impossible to hide these aesthetic and functional deformities. The goals of nasal reconstruction are twofold. First, the surgeon must restore the functional and breathing capacity of the nose and maintain or regain the structural integrity of the defect site. Second, the surgeon must strive for an aesthetically pleasing result that is in harmony with rest of the face in terms of texture, color, and form.

The nose may be divided into layers for the purpose of planning reconstruction: (1) cover (skin, subcutaneous tissue, and muscle); (2) structure (upper and lower lateral cartilages, septum, nasal bones, and tip-supporting mechanisms); and (3) internal lining (vestibular skin and nasal mucosa). This article focuses on reconstruction of oncologic defects involving the nasal covering and structure, emphasizing the use of cartilage grafting in such repair.

Critical analysis of a defect should precede reconstruction of any wound. The defect's size, including depth, and location have an impact on nasal function. When the depth is such that native structural support has been removed, the defect uniformly requires reconstruction with composite or cartilaginous grafting. During the analysis stage, the location of the defect is also of utmost importance. The alar rim is one of the free margins that represent an immobile landmark. Normal wound healing and contracture tend to pull the alar rim up and create a notch deformity; thus, appropriate planning is necessary.

The patient's age, general health, and aesthetic goals must be included in the decision-making process. A thorough medical history, including prior skin cancer, nasal surgery, and head and neck irradiation, should be completed. Both head and neck irradiation and intervening scars may compromise skin flap vascularity. The use of tobacco products cannot be overlooked because it increases the risk of skin flap and graft failure. Although the mechanism of the harmful effects is multifactorial, the nicotine causes vasoconstriction of cutaneous blood vessels with resultant decreased tissue oxygenation.[1]

After resection of malignancy, often large defects are left where the structural integrity of the nose has been disrupted to get adequate margins. In cases of skin, soft tissue, and cartilage losses, the reconstruction requires a graft that restores the forces of the nasal infrastructure but also withstands the substantial mass of soft tissue that may be transferred.

Grafting materials may be categorized as autogenous tissue, alloplasts, and homografts. The senior author Constantinides, favors the use of autogenous materials for nasal reconstruction. Autogenous material is advantageous for several reasons[1]: it has superior long-term survival,[2] is readily available in the head and neck region, and has flexibility when inside the nose.[3] It has proved

a Department of Otolaryngology, New York University School of Medicine, 550 First Avenue, NB-5EV, New York, NY 10016, USA
b Division of Facial Plastic and Reconstructive Surgery, Department of Otolaryngology, New York University School of Medicine, 530 First Avenue, Skirball Institute, 7, 7U, New York, NY 10016, USA
* Corresponding author.
E-mail address: Minas.Constantinides@nyumc.org

Facial Plast Surg Clin N Am 19 (2011) 175–182
doi:10.1016/j.fsc.2010.10.006

a safe, effective, and reliable grafting material that does not stimulate an immune response. As a result, autogenous grafts have low rates of extrusion. Autogenous tissue can cause donor site morbidity, however, and potentially resorb over time.[2,3] Although most commonly seen with rib grafts, warping remains the most feared complication when using any autogenous graft.[4,5] Situations arise, however, when harvesting such tissue may be deleterious to a patient or is not in sufficient quantity to correct a given defect. Under these circumstances, homografts are a viable alternative. Alloplastic materials also have been used with varying success to augment the nose and serve as a secondary, less acceptable alternative to autografts.[6]

There have been many reconstructive methods described to restore nasal defects after skin tumor excision, including primary repair, healing by secondary intention, skin grafts (split and full thickness), local flaps, composite grafts, free cartilage grafts, and microvascular free flaps.[7,8] Split-thickness and full-thickness skin grafts can be applied in cases where the defects are superficial, but often the defect left by removal of the tumor is too deep to achieve satisfactory results.[7] Local skin flaps serve as another reconstructive option for coverage of a defect of the nose. Not only are they associated with surgical ease and shorter operating time but also they match the color and texture of nasal skin.[9] Donor sites for local flaps for facial skin defects usually provide the best option for reconstruction. Potential drawbacks, however, include additional facial scars, which may be difficult to camouflage, and the possibility of additional procedures (two stages of repair). In addition, dog-ears or a trapdoor phenomenon can result from local flaps requiring a second procedure to create a desired outcome.[9,10] Microvascular free flap reconstruction requires additional training and expertise, long operative time, and substantial effort. Discussion of this type of reconstruction is beyond the scope of this article.

FREE CARTILAGE GRAFTS

Free cartilage to reconstruct the nose after tumor removal can be harvested from the septum, concha, or rib. These cartilage grafts with their overlying perichondrium can provide valuable structural support that may have been lost after tumor removal. Structural grafting is necessary for two reasons. First, it is needed to provide rigidity to the sidewall or dorsum, thus preventing collapse and nasal obstruction. Secondly, it creates or maintains form, especially along the alar rim and tip. Septum and rib grafts are hyaline cartilage, which is strong and stiff yet pliable, and thus can be carved to provide rigid scaffolding for reconstruction.

Septum

Septal cartilage is the graft of choice for reconstructive rhinoplasty surgeons. It is easily accessible during surgery without the morbidity of an additional donor site. It is a relatively straight stiff graft that is more robust than auricular cartilage so is easier to carve and shape precisely. After tumor removal, the straight septal cartilage is ideally used for the middle vault and the nasal sidewall areas. It can also be used, however, for nasal tip grafting, strut grafts, batten grafts, lateral crural grafts, spreader grafts, shield tip grafts, and buttress grafts.[11] Thus, septal cartilage is versatile and valuable for reconstructive surgeons. The thin nature of the quadrangular plate means that stacking of septal grafts may be needed to recreate enough volume; however, the septal cartilage thickens posteriorly. Unlike many investigators, the authors have found that septal cartilage is ideal for all areas of reconstruction, including the tip and alae (**Figs. 1** and **2**). Although it is flat, its strength and resiliency can lend great advantage to restoring various missing components of the tip.

Discussion of the technique for septoplasty harvest is beyond the scope of this article, but regardless of the approach, the amount of septal cartilage to be removed should be dictated by the amount of cartilage required for surgery. It should be remembered that least 1.5 cm of both dorsal and caudal septal cartilage struts should remain in place to adequately support the nose. If more cartilage is needed than can be safely obtained from the nasal septum, alternative sources of autologenous donor cartilage are sought.

Auricular Cartilage Grafts

Auricular cartilage is readily available and can be harvested easily with minimal cosmetic deformity. It gives good support but, despite its similar thickness compared with the upper and lower cartilages of the nose, it is softer and more pliable than septal cartilage.[11,12] Like septal cartilage, auricular cartilage is versatile.[13] It can be used as a substitute for septal cartilage when the septum has been harvested previously. Due to its more brittle nature, however, it can be more difficult to sculpt than septal cartilage.[11] This is especially true in older patients, so extra care should be taken during harvesting and subsequent manipulation.

Conchal grafts can be used as a single layer implant or sutured together to increase girth and

A

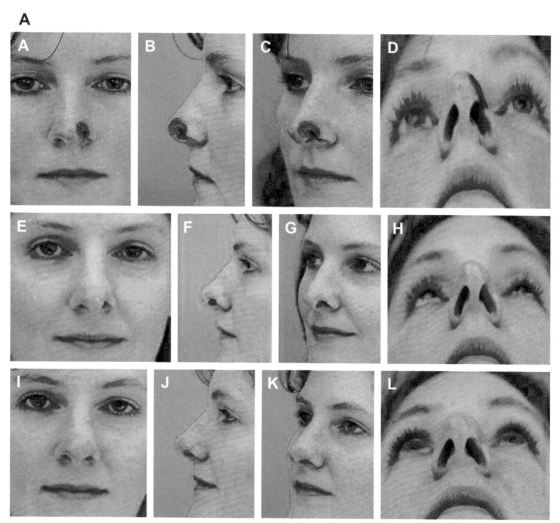

Fig. 1. (*A*) A—D, Full-thickness alar defect. E—H, 14 Months postoperative. I—L, 7 Months post revision.

rigidity. Additionally, because conchal cartilage is curved and less rigid than cartilage harvested from the septum, it is most appropriately used for smaller defects or for contour improvement of the nasal tip. Both concha cavum and cymba can be used. The concha cymba can be divided lengthwise to recreate a missing lower lateral cartilage bilaterally. Structure and support is achieved better with septum or rib cartilage. It has been shown that auricular cartilage frequently does not maintain the structural integrity and rigidity to withstand the contractile forces that follow reconstruction.[3,11] Coverage of a free cartilage graft requires vascularized tissue; local flaps are ideal. Regional melolabial or paramedian forehead flaps are both useful for coverage of free cartilage grafts; both

require a second-stage procedure to divide their pedicles.

Rib Cartilage Grafts

Costal cartilage is an excellent structural graft for large and severe nasal defects due to its ample supply. Although it has historically been used by facial plastic and reconstructive surgeons to address structural defects secondary to congenital deformities, trauma, infection, or previous operations, it is also a valuable graft for reconstruction for malignancy. It is especially useful in patients who have had previous rhinoplasty or septoplasty or who have larger defects. Costal cartilage is strong, abundant, durable, and pliable; it offers

B

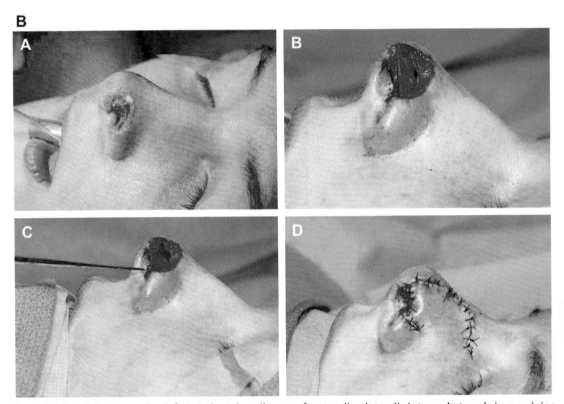

Fig. 1. (*B*) A, Full-thickness alar defect. B, Septal cartilage graft extending laterally into pocket made in remaining lateral ala. C, Bipedicled advancement flap of vestibular mucosa. D, Closure with rotational flap.

the ability to replace or augment missing tissue with similar tissue and recreate the nasal anatomy as close to normal as possible.

Cartilage can be harvested from either the fifth, sixth, seventh, or eighth rib for nasal implantation[14,15] Most rib harvests can be done through skin incisions that are less than 4 cm. The underlying musculature is separated rather than divided by dissecting longitudinal to muscle fibers. Once the rib is encountered, the perichondrium is incised and carefully elevated away from the underlying cartilage. Great care should be taken to avoid penetrating the perichondrium along the undersurface of the rib so that violation of the pleura is avoided. After harvesting sufficient cartilage, the wound is closed in a layered fashion. A drain is not necessary. A straight portion of the rib is harvested and only the central core used because the eccentric portions of the rib graft increase the chance of warping.[5,11,16,17] Proper graft fixation may also reduce the risk of malposition and warping.

Graft resorption and warping are the most common complications that arise. Other disadvantages of using a rib graft include graft displacement, potential iatrogenic pneumothorax, chest

wall scarring, and postoperative pain. In addition, calcification of cartilage in older patients can make carving and shaping nearly impossible.[5,6,11]

Crushed Cartilage

Small defects after malignancy resection may require augmented cartilage grafts to achieve the cosmetic results desired. Solid carved pieces of cartilage often become noticeable with time, especially under thin nasal skin. Crushed autogenous cartilage grafts may offer a wa y to conceal small nasal dorsal and tip irregularities. Many investigators have concluded that crushed cartilage can be used to attain aesthetic goals with a fair degree of predictability.[18–22] Although the viability of crushed cartilage has been questioned,[23] Cakmak and colleagues[24] showed that moderately crushed cartilage still shows good chondrocyte viability and proliferation.

COMPOSITE CARTILAGE GRAFTS

Auricular composite grafts are valuable in nasal reconstruction. They serve as a source of skin, cartilage, and perichondrium and thus they frequently provide sufficient tissue for a simple one-stage

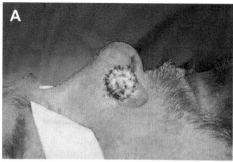
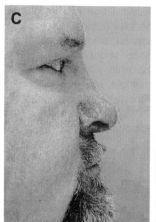
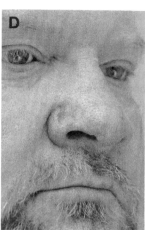
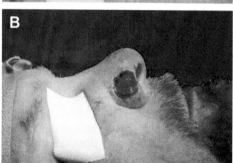

Fig. 2. Nasal alae reconstruction. (*A*) Shallow defect secondary to basal cell carcinoma excision. (*B*) Reconstruction of defect consists of three layers: one, a flap of superficial muscular aponeurotic system (SMAS) of the nose raised through the defect; two, septal cartilage graft tucked beneath it; and three, a full-thickness skin graft from auricular concha. Note that no bolster is used; rather, the graft is quilted with plain gut sutures to maximize take. (*C, D*) Postoperative pictures illustrate that despite the cartilage, full-thickness skin graft heals with shiny, smooth, red surface, ultimately a poor color match for nose.

reconstruction technique that provides excellent aesthetic and functional results.[25] Composite grafts from the ear for reconstruction of nasal defects were first described in 1902 by Konig.[26] They have significantly developed over the past 100 years and have been used for nasal tip reconstruction, repair of alar retraction, and septal perforation repair. Composite cartilage grafts consisting of cartilage, perichondrium, and skin are frequently used to repair defects of the nasal ala and columella. The senior author thinks that a cartilaginous component is almost always necessary to maintain the integrity of the repair. Composite cartilage graft survival can be challenging, and it is limited in its application by the fundamental metabolic needs of the tissues being transplanted. In this case, the cartilage itself is an avascular tissue and thus depends on passive diffusion of oxygen and nutrients through the perichondrium from adjacent vascularized tissue for survival. Composite grafts obtain their nourishment similar to skin grafts, because imbibition occurs during the first 24 hours after transfer. This is followed by vascular inosculation, and then revascularization within these grafts occurs as anastomoses between vessels in the subdermal plexus of the graft and recipient bed. This occurs within 18 hours after transplantation and provides circulation to a limited extent beyond the margin of the

graft.[26,27] From 72 hours onward, there is ingrowth of capillaries from the host tissue bed into the graft providing adequate microcirculation for chondrocyte survival.[26]

Investigators site various diameters as the upper limit of graft size, ranging from 1.0 cm to 2.5 cm.[28] No part of a composite graft should be 0.5 cm from a blood supply; thus, grafts larger than 2 cm are at risk for central necrosis.[27] When using a larger composite graft, however, small perforations (2-mm punch holes) can be created through the cartilage only and leave the overlying skin intact. This allows granulation tissue to penetrate the cartilage and nourish the epithelial lining.

Some investigators advocate composite grafts that contain skin that covers the cutaneous portion of the defect. It is the authors' preference, however, to use cartilage grafts with vascularized local flaps to repair the external nose rather than rely on composite grafts. Composite grafts are more typically used by the authors as structure and lining rather than structure and cover. The exception is in columellar reconstruction, where local flaps are limited.

The ears serve as ideal donor sites for nasal reconstruction for several reasons. They have a wide range of thicknesses and curvatures. They are also an excellent color and texture match for the nose and are readily available. Other advantages of auricular composite graft for nasal reconstruction include its ease of harvest, simplicity of reconstruction, single-stage reconstruction, and availability for use in elderly patients where prolonged hospitalization and multiple stages are undesirable and excellent survival of grafts (**Fig. 3**). Free perichondrium can also be harvested and be used as a camouflaging graft for thin-skinned patients.

Donor Site Considerations

Grafts may be harvested from different areas of the auricle. The helical rim, anterior or posterior concha, antihelix, and fossa traingularis can all serve as possible graft sites. The specific location depends on the defect size, location, and surgeon preference. The dorsal concha and root of the helix provide an excellent source of convex grafts, whereas the ventral concha and fossa triangularis composite grafts provide an excellent source of concave grafts for the nasal wall or columella. Additionally, the concave surface provides a shape similar to the native lower lateral cartilage and can be helpful in reconstruction of the nasal ala. The helical crus can be helpful if a strut graft is necessary and is among the strongest cartilaginous components of the ear.

Auricular Defect Reconstruction

Various techniques have been described in the literature to close the auricular donor site while maintaining an aesthetic match of contour and projection with the contralateral ear. Depending on the size and the location of the defect, auricular defect reconstruction after composite graft harvest may be accomplished using local advancement flaps or by using other local flaps.[28]

A small ventral helix defect can be closed using a preauricular advancement flap. If the defect is too large, however, this type of closure can result in a smaller helical dimension or a cup ear deformity. This is not insignificant because it can impair the use of eyeglasses or hearing aids. For larger defects of the helix, a preauricular advancement flap as a tubed flap plus cartilage from the tragus can be used to best provide stability and 3-D shape for the reconstructed helix.[28] Good results have also been described using full-thickness skin grafts from the postauricular area.[12] Lastly, defects resulting from harvest of convex-shaped grafts from the dorsal concha can be closed by various methods, such as postaricular advancement flaps, V-Y advancement flaps, and postauricular island pedicled flaps (see **Fig. 3**). Postauricular island pedicle flaps are ideal due to color match, ease of application, and convenience. The resulting defect closure heals rapidly and is virtually undectectable.

Limitations to this technique are primarily related to the small size of the graft. Contraindications for conchal cartilage harvesting include collagen vascular diseases, rheumatic diseases, or immunologic disorders involving the auricle, such as lupus, polychondritis, sarcoid, and Wegener granulomatosis; predilection for keloid formation; or previous extensive auricular cartilage harvesting.[6,13] Careful preoperative analysis and

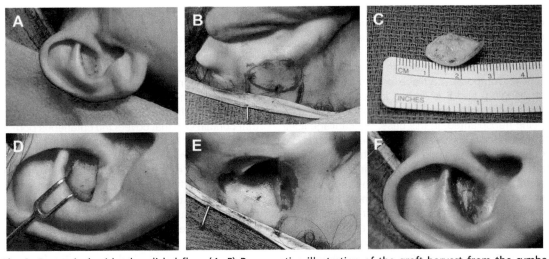

Fig. 3. Postauricular island pedicled flap. (*A, B*) Preoperative illustration of the graft harvest from the cymba conchae and the postauricular incision. (*C*) The auricular composite cartilage. (*D, E*) The flap is completely incised around the periphery but left attached to its base. There is a through and through opening in the ear. (*F*) Postauricular pedicled flap in place at the completion of the case.

questioning guide surgeons as to which ear should be used to harvest cartilage. Complete conchal cartilage removal can result in slight medialization of the pinna. Therefore, the more outstanding ear should be harvested. Additionally, if a patient has a history of sleeping on only one side of the head, the contralateral ear cartilage should be harvested.

POSTOPERATIVE CARE

Postoperative care is important to graft survival. It is crucial that patients do not participate in physical activity and do not use tobacco products. In addition, there is a normal sequence of color changes that should be expected by both the surgeon and the patient as the graft heals. Initially, the graft appears white and then turns pink at approximately 6 hours, a cyanotic bluish occurs by 24 hours, and then areas of pink color progressively appear over the next 3 to 7 days. The graft then turns cherry red color and lastly a normal skin appearance. Preoperative patient education of this pattern is critical.

MORBIDITY

Recipient and donor site morbidity is rare. Early recipient site complications are bleeding, swelling, pain, infection, and necrosis of the graft. Late complications occur infrequently but include extrusion, displacement, or resorption of the graft. These complications, however, are minimized by use of autologous grafts. Donor site problems specific to the ear include but are not limited to asymmetries in size, shape, position, and volume, scarring leading to contractures, banding, webbing, and distortion. Delayed healing, dehiscence, ulceration, and infection, such as chondritis or perichondritis, are also possible **(Fig. 4)**.

SUMMARY

Nasal reconstruction must be approached with a thorough understanding of all three layers of the nose. Cartilage grafting in nasal reconstruction is an essential skill for surgeons to master. It allows the recreation of the structural support system of the nose. Clinical judgment remains the most important determinant in selecting the appropriate graft type to reconstruct nasal deformities secondary to malignancy. Each has advantages and disadvantages that should guide the most appropriate selection to thereby maximize both the functional and cosmetic outcome for patients.

REFERENCES

1. Weber SM, Baker SR. Management of cutaneous nasal defects. Facial Plast Surg Clin North Am 2009;17:395–417.
2. Murakami CS, Cook TA, Guida RA. Nasal reconstruction with articulated irradiated rib cartilage. Arch Otolaryngol Head Neck Surg 1991;117: 327–30.
3. DeFatta RJ, Williams EF. The decision process in choosing costal cartilage for the use in revision rhinoplasty. Facial Plast Sug 2008;24(3):365–71.
4. Toriumi DM. Autogenous grafts are worth the extra time. Arch Otolaryngol Head Neck Surg 2000;126: 562–4.
5. Porter JP. Grafts in rhinoplasty: alloplastic vs autogenous. Arch Otolaryngol Head Neck Surg 2000;126: 558–61.
6. Lovice DB, Mingone MD, Toriumi DM. Grafts and implants in rhinoplasty and nasal reconstruction. Otolaryngol Clin North Am 1999;32:113–41.
7. Van der Erden PA, Verdam FJ, Dennis SC, et al. Free cartilage grafts and healing by secondary intention. Arch Facial Plast Surg 2009;11:18–23.
8. Ozek C, Gurler T, Uekan A, et al. Reconstruction of the distal third of the nose with composite ear-helix free flap. Ann Plast Surg 2007;58:74–7.
9. Jacobs MA, Christenson LJ, Weaver AL, et al. Clinical outcom of cutaneous flap versus full-thickness

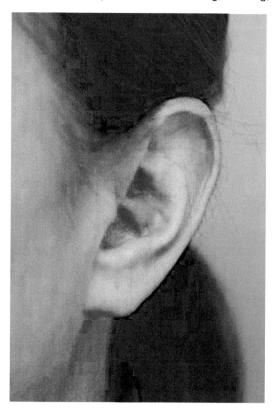

Fig. 4. Keloid at the root of the helix after composite auricular graft.

skin grafts after mohs surgery on the nose. Dermatol Surg 2010;36:23–30.

10. Gurunluoglu R, Shafighi M, Gardetto A, et al. Composite skin grafts for basal cell carcinoma defects of the nose. Aesthetic Plast Surg 2003;27:286–92.

11. Sajjadian A, Rubinstein R, Naghshineh N. Current status of grafts and implants in rhinoplasty: part 1. Autologous grafts. Plast Reconstr Surg 2010; 125(2):40–9.

12. Giberson WG, Freeman JL. Use of free auricular composite graft in nasal alar/vestibular reconstruction. J Otolaryngol 1992;21:153–5.

13. Murrell GL. Auricular cartilage grafts and nasal surgery. Laryngoscope 2004;114:2092–102.

14. Tessier P, Kawamoto H, Matthews D, et al. Taking long rib grafts for facial reconstruction- tools and techniques: III. A 2900-case experience in maxillofacial and craniofacial surgery. Plast Reconstr Surg 2005;116(5):38S–46S.

15. Marin VP, Landecker A, Gunter JP. Harvesting rib cartilage grafts for secondary rhinoplasty. Plast Reconstr Surg 2008;121(4):1442–8.

16. Mashaver A, Gantous A. The use of autogenous costal cartilage graft in septorhinoplasty. Otolaryngol Head Neck Surg 2007;137(6):862–7.

17. Vuyk HD, Adamson PA. Biomaterials in rhinoplasty. Clin Otolaryngol 1998;23:209–17.

18. Breadon GE, Kern EB, Neel BH. Autografts of uncrushed and crushed bone and cartilage: experimental observations and clinical implications. Arch Otolaryngol 1979;105:75–80.

19. Huizing EH. Implantation and transplantation in reconstructive nasal surgery. Rhinology 1974;12:93–106.

20. Guyuron B, Friedman A. The role of preserved autogenous cartilage graft in septorhinoplasty. Ann Plast Surg 1994;32:255–60.

21. Rudderman RH, Guyuron B, Mendelsohn G. The fate of noncrushed and crushed autogenous cartilage in the rabbit model. Ann Plast Surg 1994;32: 250–4.

22. Yilmaz S, Erçöçen AR, Can Z, et al. Viability of diced, crushed cartilage grafts and the effects of surgicel (oxidized regenerated cellulose) on cartilage grafts. Plast Reconstr Surg 2001;108:1054–60.

23. Bujia J. Determination of the viability of crushed cartilage grafts: clinical implications for wound healing in nasal surgery. Ann Plast Surg 1994;32: 261–5.

24. Cakmak O, Buyuklu F, Yilmaz Z, et al. Viability of cultured human nasal septum chondrocytes after crushing. Arch Facial Plast Surg 2005;7:406–9.

25. Singh DJ, Bardett SP. Aesthetic management of the ear as a donor site. Plast Reconstr Surg 2007;120: 899–908.

26. Maves M, Yessenow R. The use of composite auricular grafts in nasal reconstruction. J Dermatol Surg Oncol 1988;14:994–9.

27. Adams C, Ratner D. Composite and free cartilage grafting. Dermatol Clin 2005;23:129–40.

28. Haug MD, Rieger UM, Witt P, et al. Managing the ear as a donor site for composite graft in nasal reconstruction. Ann Plast Surg 2009;63:171–5.

Complex Nasal Reconstruction: A Case Study: Reconstruction of Full-Thickness Nasal Defect

Amit D. Bhrany, MD

KEYWORDS

- Nasal reconstruction • Cartilage graft • Internal lining
- Forehead flap • Aesthetic subunits • Nasolabial isthmus

A 37-year-old-woman presented with a 4-year history of a left alar nasal lesion. The lesion tested positive for an infiltrative basal cell carcinoma. At the initial presentation, her ala was significantly retracted and she had a 4 cm ×2-cm indurated mass centered at the alar-facial sulcus that encompassed her entire left nasal ala and extended superiorly to the inferior nasal sidewall and laterally to the medial cheek. She underwent Mohs micrographic resection that resulted in a composite medial cheek and full-thickness nasal defect that included her left hemitip, dorsum, sidewall, and ala (**Fig. 1**).

FIRST STAGE: NASAL AND CHEEK RECONSTRUCTION

Options for reconstruction included a staged initial reconstruction of the cheek to set a platform for nasal reconstruction followed by a multistage nasal reconstruction of the full-thickness nasal defect. The second option was to perform simultaneous reconstruction of the cheek and nasal defect. Setting the nasal platform by first reconstructing the cheek alone may increase the total number of procedures; however, it decreases the risk of the nasal platform being displaced laterally and inferiorly as the cheek flap heals and contracts.[1] The patient had a strong desire to minimize the number of operative procedures and total time for reconstruction, thus it was decided to perform the first stage full-thickness nasal reconstruction while simultaneously reconstructing the medial cheek defect.

Cheek Defect Reconstruction

The medial cheek defect was reconstructed using a cheek flap that extended from the lateral aspect of the wound just inferior to the medial canthus into a subciliary crease that extended to the lateral orbital rim. After undermining and mobilizing the cheek flap, it was secured medially to the ascending process of the maxilla by passing a 3-0 polydioxanone suture through drilled holes because no periosteum was left after the Mohs procedure. A 5-0 polydioxanone stabilization stitch was also placed at the lateral orbital rim. Once the medial cheek defect was reconstructed, attention was directed at reconstructing the nose.

Intranasal Lining Repair

Repair of the mucosal nasal lining is essential for optimal restoration of nasal function and form. The lining flaps not only help restore nasal airflow but also provide a bed of vascularized tissue to support the integration of cartilage and bone grafts that reconstruct the shape and rigidity of the nose.[2] The patient's mucosal defect comprised the lower middle nasal vault, ala, and hemitip. Options for relining such a defect included the use of a bipedicled lining flap combined with a contralateral septal hinged mucoperichondrial flap, an inferior turbinate flap, or a caudally based ipsilateral septal mucoperichondrial flap.[2–5] The

Department of Otolaryngology—Head and Neck Surgery, University of Washington, Box 356515, Seattle, WA 98195, USA
E-mail address: abhrany@uw.edu

Facial Plast Surg Clin N Am 19 (2011) 183–195
doi:10.1016/j.fsc.2010.10.007
1064-7406/11/$ — see front matter © 2011 Elsevier Inc. All rights reserved.

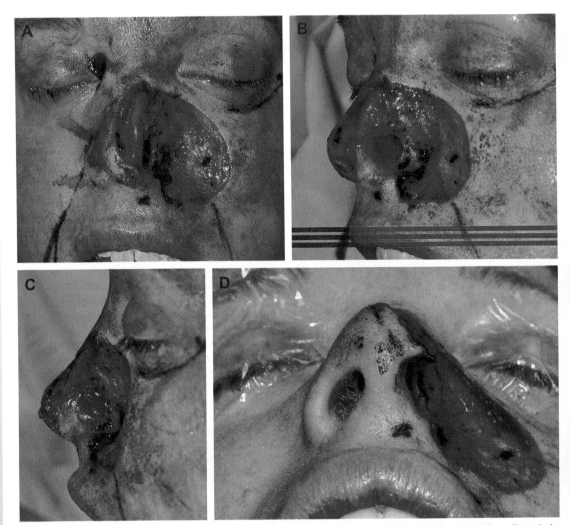

Fig. 1. Composite cheek and full-thickness left nasal defect encompassing left hemitip, dorsum, sidewall, and ala. (*A*) Frontal, (*B*) left oblique, (*C*) profile, and (*D*) base views.

defect size precluded the use of a bipedicled vestibular advancement flap, and a contralateral hinged flap alone would not reach the caudal border of the defect. The lateral wall defect bordered the head of the inferior turbinate, potentially compromising the vascularity of an inferior turbinate flap, thus an ipsilateral septal mucoperichondrial flap was harvested for reconstruction of the nasal lining. The caudally based flap is based on the septal branch of the superior labial artery and is best used to line the defects of the unilateral tip, ala, and lower middle vault. The flap is designed as large as possible typically ranging from 4 to 5 cm in length and 2 to 2.5 cm in width and can be narrowed to 1.3 cm at its base, the caudal septum.[2,5]

After infiltration with local anesthetic containing epinephrine, 2 parallel horizontal incisions were made dorsally and along the nasal floor. The dorsal incision began just posterior to the anterior septal angle, maintaining 1 cm of mucosa for the cartilaginous dorsal strut and extending posteriorly past the bone-cartilage junction. The inferior incision began just posterior to the nasal spine, extending the same distance posteriorly as the dorsal incision, and then a vertical incision was made between the 2. A right-angled blade, such as an otologic round knife or a No. 66 Beaver blade is helpful for the vertical incision.[5] The flap was elevated using standard septoplasty techniques (**Fig. 2**). Once the septal flap was elevated, and before insetting the flap along the lateral nasal wall, septal cartilage was harvested, maintaining a 1-cm dorsal-caudal strut. The flap was then rotated laterally and inferiorly and inset by placing 5-0 chromic gut sutures from the superior border

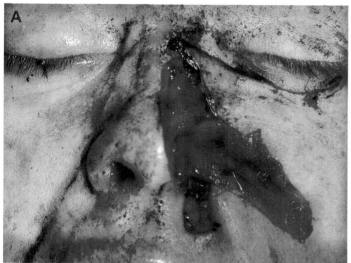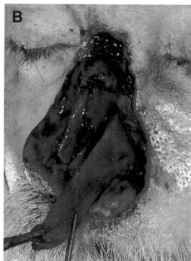

Fig. 2. (*A*) Frontal view after reconstruction of medial cheek defect and harvest of caudally based ipsilateral septal mucoperichondrial internal lining flap. (*B*) Profile view of the same flap harvested in a different patient.

of the mucosal defect to the submucosal surface of the hinged flap (**Fig. 3**).

Nasal Framework Repair

The nasal framework provides external contour to the nose and a patent nasal airway upon inspiration. After portions of the framework are removed, structural grafts are required to reconstruct the shape of the nose, to prevent collapse of the airway upon inspiration, and to prevent cephalic retraction of the alar margin upon healing.[6] Unlike internal lining or cutaneous covering reconstruction, structural grafts of the nose are often nonanatomic, especially when repairing the nasal sidewall and ala. Grafts may span the entire subunit to prevent alar retraction as well as collapse of the middle vault and ala.[2,4,5]

This patient had a defect of the entire cartilaginous nasal sidewall and ala (see **Fig. 1**). The cartilaginous middle nasal vault was reconstructed with a piece of septal cartilage that recreated the upper lateral cartilage, and the ala was reconstructed using a conchal cartilage graft that comprised the entire subunit. The alar conchal cartilage graft was designed to extend to the caudal nasal margin to prevent retraction of the new ala. The medial aspect of the conchal cartilage graft was secured to the remaining medial crura of the left lower lateral cartilage with a 5-0 polydioxanone suture (**Fig. 4**). Both grafts were fixed to the underlying septal lining flap and to each other using a 5-0 polydioxanone suture. A columellar strut graft of septal cartilage was also placed between the remaining medial crura to

provide additional tip support, given the resection of the majority of the left lower lateral cartilage.

Cutaneous Nasal Covering Reconstruction

The cutaneous defect encompassed almost the entire left side of the nose (see **Fig. 1**). A paramedian forehead flap was designed using a template from the contralateral intact side for re-creation of the left hemidorsum, lateral nasal sidewall, ala, and hemitip. Conventional teaching describes that if 50% of a convex nasal subunit is missing, the entire subunit should be reconstructed, but adequate cosmesis can be achieved by reconstructing only half of the tip and dorsal subunits.[5,7]

The supratrochlear artery, on which the paramedian forehead flap is based, is consistently found 1.7 to 2.2 cm lateral to the midline of the glabella. This location correlates closely to the medial aspect of the eyebrow. The flap pedicle is recommended to have a width less than 1.5 cm because a narrower pedicle has less risk of strangulation.[1,8,9] Thus, the flap pedicle with a width of 1.1 cm was based at the medial aspect of the eyebrow. A combination of the patient's low hairline and distal nasal defect required a significant portion of the alar and hemitip subunits of the flap design to include hair-bearing skin (**Fig. 5**). Options to minimize the amount of hair-bearing skin transposed with the flap include angling the flap laterally in an oblique manner or lengthening the inferior incision inferior to the superior orbital rim. For flaps wider than 3 cm (which was the case for this patient), obliquely angling the flap can produce a more unsightly lateral forehead

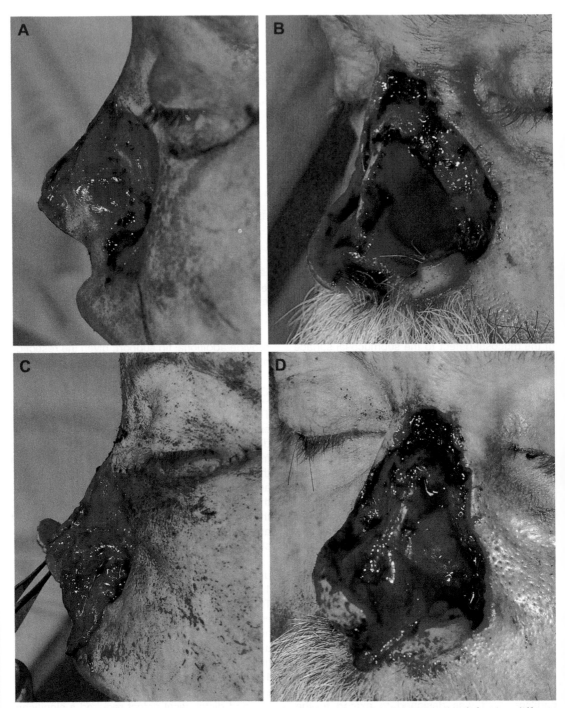

Fig. 3. (*A*) Profile view demonstrating mucosal lining defect of lateral nasal wall. (*B*) A similar defect in a different patient (*C*) Ipsilateral septal mucoperichondrial internal lining flap inset into the lateral nasal sidewall. Excess flap trimmed at the end of the operation. (*D*) Flap inset into the defect shown in Fig. 3B.

scar as well as increase the risk of medial brow elevation as the forehead scar heals by secondary intention.[1,5] Thus, the forehead flap was not angled for this patient.

The flap was incised and elevated in a subcutaneous plane underneath the templated portion of the flap and then transitioned into a subgaleal plane to the base of the flap. Once the flap was

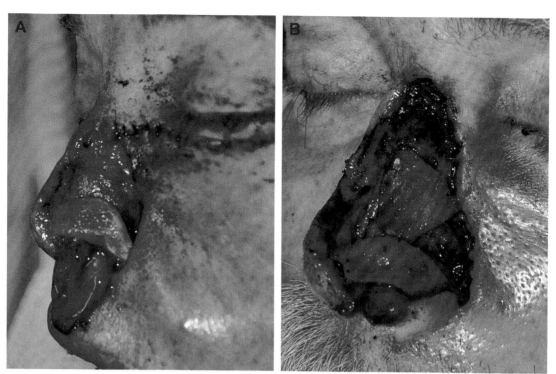

Fig. 4. (*A*) Septal and conchal cartilage grafts in place reconstructing middle nasal vault and alar cartilage, respectively. (*B*) Another example of septal and conchal cartilage grafts reconstructing middle vault and alar cartilages.

elevated, additional thinning of the flap was done briefly to the level of the subdermis to ensure symmetric thickness and to partially depilate the flap. In smokers, the flap is not thinned as aggressively.[1,10] The flap was then transposed to the nasal defect and secured to the recipient nasal skin using a 6-0 nylon suture and a subdermal 5-0 polydioxanone suture along each lateral edge of the flap. Minimal subdermal sutures are required because the flap should not be under any tension. If the flap requires additional length, horizontal releasing cuts can be made through the frontalis muscle to the level of the subcutaneous tissue along 1-cm intervals, which can result in an additional 1.5 cm of length.[1] Additional length can also be achieved by extending the pedicle incision inferior to the medial eyebrow and orbital rim. The distal portion of the flap was wrapped around the margin of the conchal cartilage graft and secured to the septal mucoperichondrial internal lining flap using a 5-0 chromic suture. An additional 2-mm alar marginal septal cartilage graft was placed in a pocket between the forehead and septal flaps just distal to the conchal cartilage graft to provide additional resistance to alar retraction.

The forehead donor site was closed after undermining widely from one border of the anterior temporalis muscle to the other. The muscle and galea were closed using a 3-0 polydioxanone suture followed by a 6-0 nylon suture for the skin. The

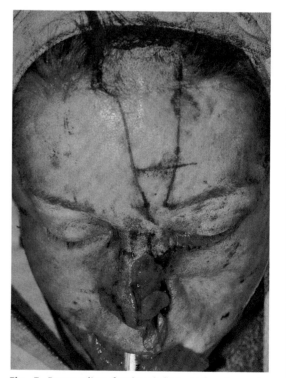

Fig. 5. Paramedian forehead flap design for cutaneous covering reconstruction. A combination of the patient's low hairline and distal nasal defect resulted in a significant portion of the alar and hemitip subunits of the flap design to include hair-bearing skin. The base of the pedicle should have been extended more inferiorly past the superior orbital rim to reduce the amount of hair-bearing skin.

superior portion of the donor site could not be closed and was left to heal by secondary intention (**Fig. 6**). However, the anterior hairline could be reapproximated, and because the flap had been raised in a thin subcutaneous plane at the hair-bearing aspect of the flap, some hair follicles remained at the exposed donor site and regrew through the healed wound (**Fig. 7**). This patient also had thick hair that easily hid the area of alopecia.

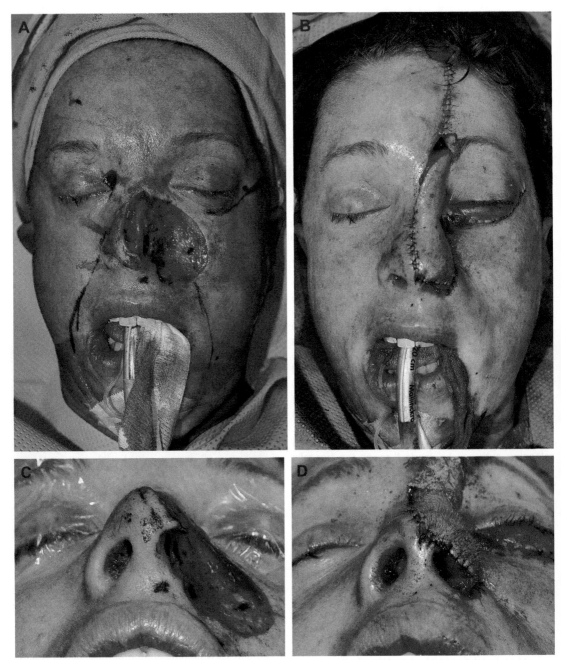

Fig. 6. (*A*) Frontal preoperative cheek and full-thickness left nasal defect. (*B*) Paramedian forehead flap inset and donor site closed, with superior portion of the donor site left to heal by secondary intention. (*C*) Base view of left alar and cheek defect. (*D*) Cheek defect repaired with cheek flap. Left nasal defect completely closed, demonstrating hair on distal aspect of tip and alar reconstruction. Ipsilateral septal lining flap attached to distal tip of the paramedian forehead flap reconstructing nasal vestibule.

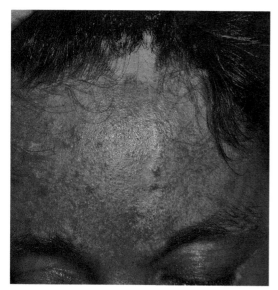

Fig. 7. The 8-month postoperative view of the distal portion of healed paramedian forehead flap donor site demonstrating area of alopecia at hairline and some hair regrowth through wound more distally.

SECOND STAGE: DIVISION OF PARAMEDIAN FOREHEAD AND INTRANASAL LINING FLAPS

After 3 weeks of the first stage procedure, the patient underwent division of the paramedian forehead and intranasal septal mucoperichondrial lining flaps (**Fig. 8**). The paramedian forehead flap was transected just superior to the border of the nasal defect. The incision was extended inferiorly on both sides approximately half way down the flap and elevated just above the cartilage grafts. The elevated portion of the flap was thinned to the subdermis, excess flap pedicle tissue excised, and the flap reinset into the defect using a 6-0 nylon suture.

The base of the flap was returned to the glabellar donor site. The medial aspect of the eyebrow can be displaced inferiorly and medially because of the tension of the flap, especially if the proximal portion of the flap extends below the superior orbital rim. Returning the base of the pedicle to the glabella repositions the eyebrow into its anatomic position. The flap is mobilized superiorly until the brow is repositioned, and only the portion of the base that facilitates repositioning of the eyebrow is replaced, excising excess tissue and converting the proximal pedicle into a triangular flap. Scar tissue that has formed deep at the donor site and on the rolled edges of both the proximal flap and the donor site are removed before reinsetting the base to facilitate the flap lying flat and prevent pincushioning. The wound is closed with

a 5-0 polydioxanone suture for deep dermal repair and a 6-0 nylon suture for skin closure. After pedicle division and returning of the base to the glabella, this patient's medial aspect of the eyebrow should have been elevated more because it is still slightly inferiorly displaced (see **Fig. 8**).

The intranasal flap was incised with a No. 15 blade at the lateral nasal wall, redraping and fixing the proximal portion of the septal flap to the opposite side with a quilting 4-0 chromic gut suture. A rolled piece of Xeroform gauze (Tyco Healthcare, Mansfield, MA, USA) was placed intranasally to help maintain the portion of the nasal flap against the lateral nasal wall. The septal flap often thickens with scar tissue, and thinning of lateral nasal wall may be needed to address vestibular stenosis.

THIRD STAGE: THINNING OF THE NASAL SIDEWALL AND GLABELLAR DONOR SITE, RE-CREATION OF THE CONFLUENCE OF THE NOSE, LIP, AND CHEEK

Four months after division of the paramedian forehead flap, the patient underwent a third operation to revise the thickened glabellar and nasal sidewall scars. She had also developed mild vestibular stenosis but was satisfied with her nasal airway and did not want to undergo revision of her nasal vestibule with thinning of her alar margin (**Fig. 9**). The glabella was pincushioned, and this likely developed by not removing enough subcutaneous tissue of the triangular flap at the initial pedicle division and also insetting too wide of the triangular flap back into the glabella. The glabella was revised by reelevating the entire triangular flap, excising subcutaneous scar tissue, and narrowing the triangular flap. The nasal sidewall was also pincushioned and wide and blunted the nasofacial sulcus. Thus, the sidewall was reelevated, thinned, and narrowed (see **Fig. 9**).

At this same sitting, she underwent a procedure to recreate the confluence of the nose, upper lip, and cheek and re-form an alar crease. The nasal sidewall subunit and the lateral upper lip subunit are connected by a 3- to 4-mm wide channel of tissue termed the nasolabial isthmus.[11] This channel is formed by the hairless apical triangle between the alar base and nasolabial fold. When this isthmus is missing, there is no boundary between the medial cheek and alar lobule, creating an unnatural appearance. Reconstruction of composite cheek and alar defects undoubtedly results in obliteration of the nasolabial isthmus (**Fig. 10**). To recreate this facial landmark, templates were made of the intact contralateral lateral upper lip and alar subunits. The templates were reversed and incisions drawn on the subunit

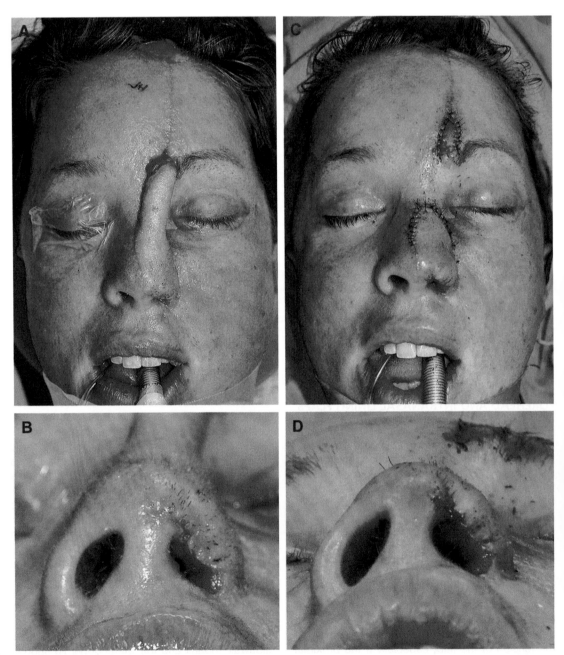

Fig. 8. (*A*, *B*) Paramedian forehead and ipsilateral septal flaps 3 weeks after first stage reconstruction. (*C*) Forehead flap pedicle detached and triangular flap replaced at glabellar donor site. Medial aspect of eyebrow is still displaced slightly inferiorly. (*D*) Septal flap divided demonstrating patent airway but thickened alar margin and nasal vestibule when compared with the nonoperated side.

borders marked by the templates and not in previously placed incisions. After making the incisions, a medially based alar lobule flap, an inferiorly based apical lip triangle flap, and a laterally based nasolabial flap were elevated. The tissue deep to the newly formed apical triangle of the lip was carved such that once tacked back down to the deep tissue with a 5-0 polydioxanone suture, it was in the plane of the upper lip, recessed rather than the plane of the medial cheek.[11] The skin of the nasolabial isthmus was closed with 6-0 and 7-0 nylon sutures (see **Fig. 9**).

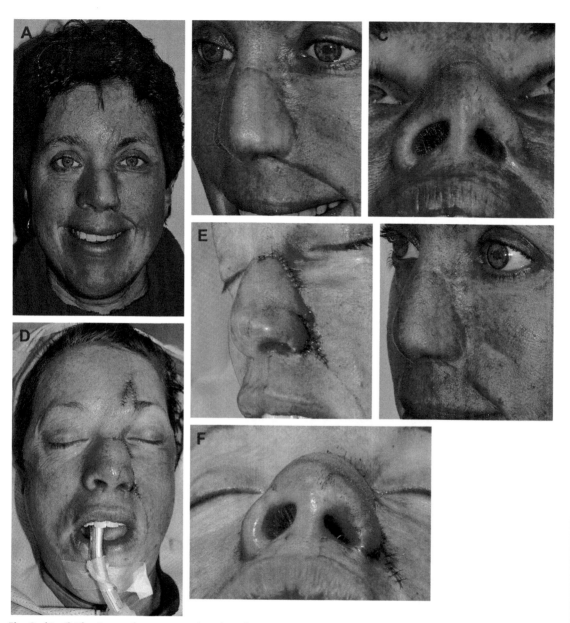

Fig. 9. (*A–C*) The 3-month postoperative view demonstrating pincushioning of glabellar donor site, thickened nasal sidewall, obliteration of nasolabial isthmus, and alar margin thickening with narrowed vestibule. (*D–F*) Glabellar donor site, nasal sidewall, and alar lobule reconstruction revised. Confluence of lip, cheek, and nose at nasolabial isthmus also recreated. (*G*) Nasal sidewall and confluence of lip, cheek, and nose 4 months after revision with decreased sidewall thickness and presence of a nasolabial isthmus. Incisions used to recreate these subunits are based on subunits templated from the intact contralateral nasal subunits and not in previously existing scars.

DISCUSSION

The goals of nasal reconstruction are to produce an aesthetic normal-appearing nose with a functional airway. This patient had a composite cheek and full-thickness nasal defect that required reconstruction of her nasal internal lining, cartilaginous framework, and cutaneous nasal covering. Overall, she has an adequate result, but there are many imperfections.

A better result might have been obtained if the pedicle was extended more inferiorly past the orbital rim, creating less hair-bearing distal flap. Also, her reconstructed nasal sidewall still appears

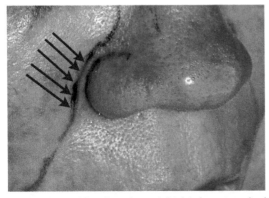

Fig. 10. Lateral border of nasolabial isthmus marked by arrows. The isthmus extends from apical triangle of the upper lip between ala and medial cheek.

slightly too wide at its inferior aspect and her alar lobule needs better definition, even after one revision (**Fig. 11**). The incision to recreate the lateral border of the nasolabial isthmus should have been extended superiorly to create a new inferior nasofacial sulcus medial to the existing scar. In retrospect, the intraoperative photographs of her third procedure demonstrate this omission. The nasofacial incision should have been extended to decrease the width of the inferior aspect of the nasal sidewall, and the incision along the new alar crease should also have been lengthened anteriorly toward the tip to better recreate an alar crease. More deep tissue should have been removed at the crease to better redefine the separate planes of the nasal sidewall and alar lobule (see **Fig. 9**E, G). **Fig. 12** shows another patient who had a more

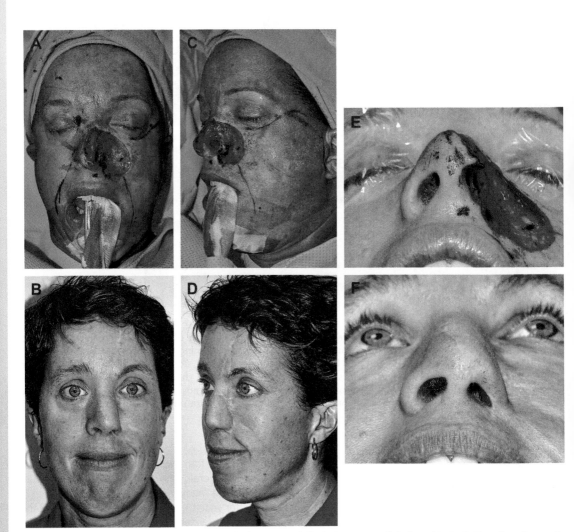

Fig. 11. (*A, C, E*) Preoperative composite left cheek and full-thickness nasal defect. (*B, D, F*) The view 8 months after operation.

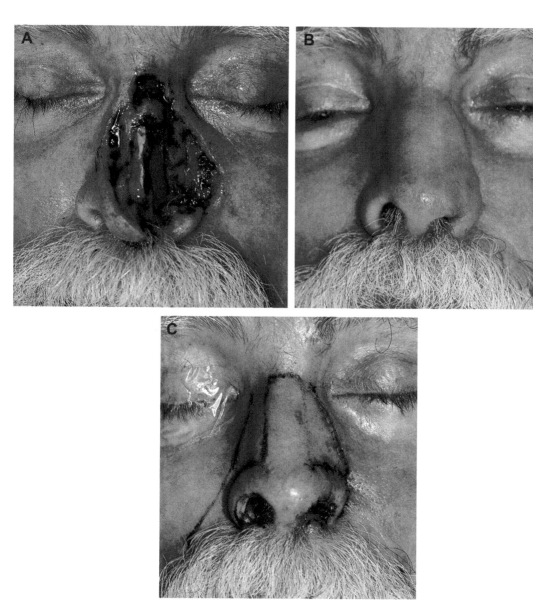

Fig. 12. (*A*) Composite left cheek and full-thickness nasal defect. (*B*) The face 4 months after reconstruction using ipsilateral septal mucoperichondrial internal lining flap, cartilage grafts, and paramedian forehead flap. Nasal sidewall, alar lobule, and alar margin thickened with no alar crease present. Nasolabial isthmus also obliterated. (*C*) Immediate postoperative view after thinning of nasal sidewall, alar lobule, alar margin creation of alar crease, and redefinition of nasofacial sulcus. Purple lines indicate contralateral subunit templates used to redefine reconstructed nasal subunits and alar margin.

defined alar crease re-formation and sidewall re-contouring with extension of the aforementioned incisions and removal of tissue.

In addition to a less defined alar lobule, her alar margin is thick. The recreated alar margin was expectedly thick after the first stage, but scar contracture has further narrowed her reconstructed nasal vestibule, although she denies any airway complaints. Scar contracture from her cheek flap has also resulted in lateralization of her reconstructed left alar base, flattening of her ala, and decreased definition of the alar-facial sulcus (**Fig. 13**). These effects may have been minimized if her cheek defect (ie, the nasal platform) was reconstructed and allowed to heal before reconstructing her nasal defect.[1]

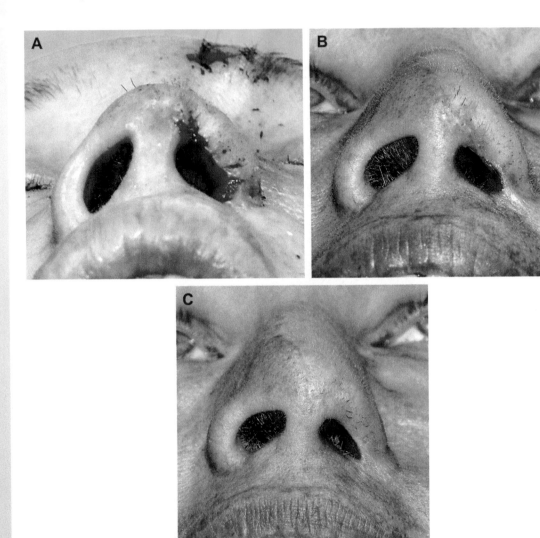

Fig. 13. (*A*) Base view of reconstructed ala 3 weeks after the first operative stage. (*B*) The 3-month postoperative view with mild vestibular stenosis, lateralization of reconstructed alar base, and blunting of alar-facial sulcus. (*C*) The 8-month postoperative view with increased vestibular stenosis, flattening of ala, and blunting of alar-facial sulcus.

The patient was advised to undergo alar margin thinning to enlarge her nasal vestibule, but she preferred not to because she felt no nasal obstruction from a functional standpoint. If she would have consented, her new alar margin would have been modeled on the normal contralateral margin, carving out an ellipse of tissue medial to the cartilage grafts and retacking the flap to the alar margin as was done for the patient in **Fig. 12**. The alar margin thickening is because of thickness of the initial septal lining and forehead flaps and subsequent scar tissue deposition at the distal edges of these flaps. One change in technique that adds an additional procedure but could have potentially decreased the amount of alar margin thickening would have been to use the folded forehead flap technique and intermediate flaying procedure described by Menick.[12] The distal portion of the forehead flap is extended and folded on itself to repair more of the distal portion of the vestibular lining defect compared with this patient in whom the ipsilateral lining flap was used to reconstruct the entire lining defect of the alar margin. At 3 weeks after the initial procedure, the forehead flap is not detached from its pedicle but the cutaneous cover portion of the flap is completely separated from the lining portion and lifted off the nose. This step allows for extensive thinning and depilation that could have also decreased the amount of residual hair left on this patient's reconstruction. The flap is then released from its pedicle as described earlier 3 weeks later.

Despite these limitations, this patient has undergone a complex composite cheek and full-thickness nasal reconstruction with a satisfactory result. She has a well-functioning nasal airway and is content with the appearance of her reconstruction. Patients who acquire such defects should be counseled that multiple stages of reconstruction may be required to provide an adequate nasal airway and recreate the aesthetic landmarks of the nose, upper lip, and cheek.

REFERENCES

1. Burget GC. Aesthetic reconstruction of the nose. In: Mathes SJ, editor. 2nd edition, In: Plastic surgery, vol. II. Philadelphia: Saunders; 2006. p. 573–647.
2. Burget GC, Menick FJ. Nasal support and lining: the marriage of beauty and blood supply. Plast Reconstr Surg 1989;84(2):189–202.
3. Murakami CS, Kriet JD, Ierokomos AP. Nasal reconstruction using the inferior turbinate mucosal flap. Arch Facial Plast Surg 1999;1(2):97–100.
4. Tollefson TT, Kriet JD. Complex nasal defects: structure and internal lining. Facial Plast Surg Clin North Am 2005;13(2):333–43, vii.
5. Baker SR. Local flaps in facial reconstruction. 2nd edition. Philadelphia: Mosby; 2007.
6. Park SS. Reconstruction of nasal defects larger than 1.5 centimeters in diameter. Laryngoscope 2000; 110(8):1241–50.
7. Burget GC, Menick FJ. The subunit principle in nasal reconstruction. Plast Reconstr Surg 1985;76(2): 239–47.
8. Shumrick KA, Smith TL. The anatomic basis for the design of forehead flaps in nasal reconstruction. Arch Otolaryngol Head Neck Surg 1992;118(4): 373–9.
9. Menick FJ. Aesthetic refinements in use of forehead for nasal reconstruction: the paramedian forehead flap. Clin Plast Surg 1990;17(4):607–22.
10. Menick FJ. Nasal reconstruction: forehead flap. Plast Reconstr Surg 2004;113(6):100E–11E.
11. Burget GC, Murrel GL, Toriumi DM. Aesthetic reconstruction of the confluence of the nose, lip, and cheek. Operat Tech Plast Reconstr Surg 1998;5(1): 76–88.
12. Menick FJ. A 10-year experience in nasal reconstruction with the three-stage forehead flap. Plast Reconstr Surg 2002;109(6):1839–55 [discussion: 1856–61].

Complex Nasal Reconstruction: A Case Study: Composite Defect

Frederick J. Menick, MD[a,b,*]

KEYWORDS

- Nasal reconstruction • Facial landmarks • Forehead flap
- Operation

ANALYSIS OF THE DEFECT AND DECISION MAKING

On physical examination (**Fig. 1**), a faint vertical left paramedian forehead scar, which followed the previous reconstruction, is visible. The forehead is otherwise high and expansive.

The left ala appears normal, although it is not. Some years previously, the patient presented with a full-thickness defect of the left entire ala and part of the inferior sidewall. Adjacent lip and cheek were uninjured. The defect had been repaired with a 3-stage folded forehead flap for cover and lining, with a delayed, primary, ear cartilage alar margin buttress graft to support, shape, and brace the left nostril margin.[1,2] Following subunit principles of nasal reconstruction, the normal intact right ala had been used as a guide to design a template with the correct dimension and outline of the contralateral normal ala. The right ala was used to plan the exact replacement of the entire left ala and a few millimeters of the left tip subunit with a vertical forehead flap. A distal extension, about 1.5 cm wide and 7 mm long, was added to the distal covering flap. The extension was folded inward to replace the missing lining. During an intermediate operation 1 month later, the covering flap was elevated completely off the nose with 2 to 3 mm of subcutaneous fat. The distal folded lining was now healed to the adjacent residual nasal lining and was no longer dependent on the supratrochlear pedicle for blood supply. The underlying doubly layered excess of subcutaneous fat and frontalis areolar tissue was excised, exposing thin supple vascular lining. The contralateral normal alar template was then used to design a precise alar margin graft to shape the left nostril margin. The graft was fixed to the restored lining. The thin forehead flap was then returned to the recipient site. One month later, the pedicle of the flap was divided. During a subsequent revision, the left alar crease was further refined through a direct incision to sculpt a flat sidewall, a deep alar crease, and a convex alar contour. The slightly thick rim margin was thinned by excising excess soft tissue between the lining and cartilage graft through the old incision present along the nostril margin.

A short transverse scar is visible within the superior dorsum at the site of a previous skin cancer excision that was closed primarily.

The new defect involves several facial units but is more superficial.

Anatomically, the skin is missing over the entire ala, part of the inferior sidewall, and the adjacent medial cheek and lateral lip. Soft tissue within the cheek over the piriform aperture has been excised. The normal fibrofatty middle layer support of the ala is gone. Nasal lining is intact.

Aesthetically, the complex midface has been destroyed. The expected color and texture, landmark outline, and 3-dimensional shape are abnormal. Because the underlying orbicularis muscle is present, if skin is restored to cover the lip, the lip will function normally.

[a] Private Practice, Tucson, AZ, USA
[b] Division of Plastic Surgery, St Joseph's Hospital, Tucson, AZ 85715, USA
* Corresponding author. 1102 North El Dorado Place, Tucson, AZ 85715.
E-mail address: drmenick@drmenick.com

Facial Plast Surg Clin N Am 19 (2011) 197–211
doi:10.1016/j.fsc.2010.10.008
1064-7406/11/$ – see front matter © 2011 Elsevier Inc. All rights reserved.

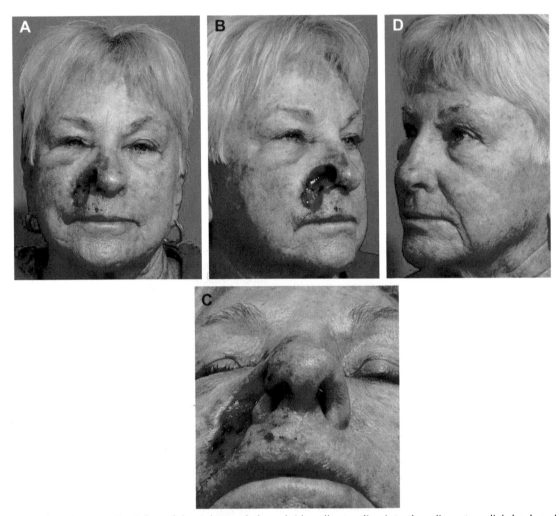

Fig. 1. (*A–D*) Composite defect of the right nasal ala and sidewall extending into the adjacent medial cheek and lateral upper lip. Years before, the patient had undergone a forehead flap reconstruction to repair a full-thickness defect of the left lateral tip, ala, and sidewall. A vertical left paramedian scar is visible.

The face can be divided into geographic areas of characteristic skin quality, border outline, and 3-dimensional contour. The cheek is a peripheral unit, largely flat and expansive with a variable border outline that is not completely seen on frontal view. The nose and upper lip are central units and are exactly contoured and outlined. An abnormality in a part of the lip or cheek is quickly apparent because the contralateral remaining lip or cheek creates a visually disturbing comparison.

The nose sits on a facial platform of the cheek and lip. The nasolabial fold separates the round fullness of the medial cheek and the flat upper lip. The nasolabial fold does not extend into the alar crease but is separated from the crease by a hairless triangle of skin, which lies adjacent to the alar base inset. The nose sits on the facial platform in an exact position and projects with specific angles.[3]

The nose is divided into subunits.[4,5] The flat sidewall is separated from the round convex ala by the alar crease. The alar subunit is outlined by the nostril margin inferiorly, the alar crease superiorly, the slight alteration in contour with the soft triangle and tip subunits medially, and the alar groove laterally where the ala is inset into the lip at the alar base.

Each facial unit must be restored in terms of its own quality, outline, and contour and in relationship to the other facial units. The dimension, volume, position, projection, platform, skin quality, border outline, and 3-dimensional contour of the midface must be reestablished.

PRINCIPLES OF REPAIR

1. Patients wish to look normal.[1,6]
2. The "normal" is defined by visual skin quality, border outline, and 3-dimensional contour.
3. Individual areas of the face can be described in terms of facial units and subunits.
4. The restoration of these visual units defines the surgical result, which looks normal. The wound must be repaired anatomically and aesthetically.
5. Missing tissues must be replaced in exact dimension and border outline to reestablish the normal and prevent distortion of adjacent structures.
6. The contralateral normal or the ideal side should be used as a guide.
7. Exact templates should be used to design covering and lining replacements, cartilage graft dimension and outline, and to determine the position of expected facial landmarks.
8. The nose must be built on a stable platform. If a composite defect of the nose, cheek, and lip is present, the lip and cheek should be rebuild initially. If the new platform is unstable and may shift because of gravity, tension, or resolution of edema, the nasal repair should be delayed to avoid late shifting of the nasal reconstruction into an abnormal position on the face. If the defect is more superficial and the platform base is unlikely to become distorted during wound healing, the nose can be repaired simultaneously with platform restoration.
9. Surgical staging should be used to advantage. The anatomic and aesthetic needs of the repair, priorities, quality of donor tissues, and ideal timing to transfer and modify materials with safety and precision should be designed. Although Gillies and Millard[7] emphasize the use of "like tissue," a flat thick forehead flap, an ear cartilage graft, or a cheek flap have little in common with the delicate outline or contour of the midface.
10. It is often useful to repair a composite defect of the cheek, lip, and nose with individual grafts and flaps to position the final scars in the joins between units and restore 3-dimensional contour.

THE SURGICAL PLAN

The wound is clean, and early reconstruction is appropriate. The defect is debrided, and the wound margins are incised to create clean right-angled skin edges. Templates of the contralateral normal nose and upper lip are used to design the skin replacement and alar margin support and to determine the ideal position, in height and width, of the right alar base after restoration of the cheek and lip platform. The soft tissue deficiency in the medial right cheek is augmented with a Millard flip fat flap. The cheek and lip skin defect is repaired by advancing a cheek flap with a random extension to resurface the upper lip defect. Because this is a relatively superficial defect with intact lining, nasal repair begins simultaneously with the placement of a primary conchal cartilage alar margin cartilage graft and a right paramedian forehead flap to resurface the ala and part of the inferior sidewall. An intermediate operation is planned to allow adjustments and more precise soft tissue contouring before pedicle division. Later, the pedicle is divided and the nasal labial fold recreated. The patient is informed that a late revision some months later may be appropriate to improve the alar crease, revise the forehead scar, thin the nostril margin, and so forth. All surgical procedures are performed under general anesthesia to avoid soft tissue distortion and blanching resulting from the injection of local anesthesia and epinephrine. It is difficult to make precise intraoperative decisions in restoring contour or determining the viability of tissues if they are bloated or chemically constricted.[7-10]

OPERATION 1

The hairline, frown lines, location of the supratrochlear vessels by Doppler, subunits of the nose, nasolabial folds, philtrum, vermilion, old scars within the forehead and nasal dorsum, midline of the lip, and outline of the old forehead flap that resurfaces the left ala and part of the sidewall are marked with ink (**Fig. 2**).

The wound does not represent the true tissue loss and is expanded by edema, gravity, local anesthesia, or tension. If such a wound healed by secondary intention or was previously reconstructed, it may be contracted by scar or inadequate tissue replacement. Templates based on the contralateral normal permit exact replacement of missing tissues and dimension, outline, and position.

Quarter-inch Steri-Strips (3M Corporation, St Paul, MN, USA) are applied to the left nose and upper lip to create a paper pattern of the contralateral ala and hemilip. Collodion is applied externally with a Q-tip to further "glue" the paper tape strips together. Each pattern is then elevated. Because the ink applied to the skin subunit surface adheres to the undersurface of the Steri-Strips, the outline and dimension of the

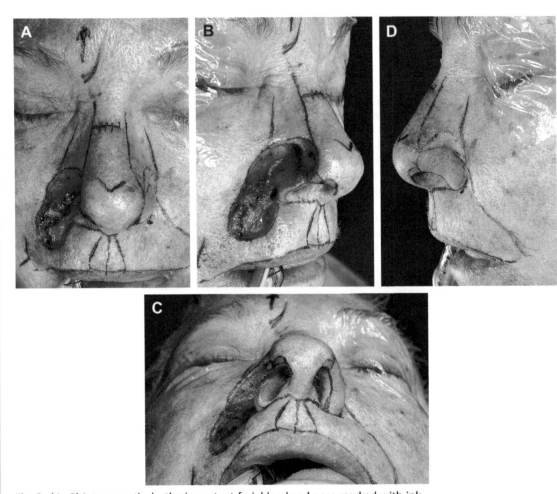

Fig. 2. (A–D) Intraoperatively, the important facial landmarks are marked with ink.

contralateral normal subunits are visible. Excess tape is trimmed, and the contralateral alar and hemilip outlines are transferred to the aluminum foil of a suture pack (**Fig. 3**).

The right cheek skin, with 2 to 3 mm of fat, is undermined laterally for 5 to 8 cm. The medial border of the flap is incised directly in the residual nasolabial fold, inferiorly, and at the junction of the

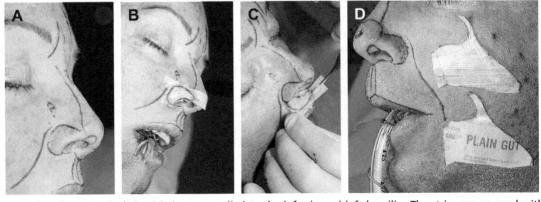

Fig. 3. (A–D) Quarter-inch Steri-Strips are applied to the left ala and left hemilip. The strips are covered with collodion. On tape removal, the exact dimension and outline of the contralateral normal subunits are visible on the deep surface. The excess paper tape is trimmed and the pattern is transferred to the foil of a suture pack (seen in other patient).

cheek and sidewall subunits, superiorly. Residual medial cheek fat, lateral to the piriform soft tissue deficiency, is marked with ink as a medially based hinge-over flap.[7] Subcutaneous fat is hinged over, like a page of a book, and is fixed with absorbable sutures to fill the premaxillary soft tissue loss and reestablish medial cheek fullness in the nasal base platform height (**Fig. 4**). Dog-ears are excised along the side of the nose and lateral to the commissure after advancement of the flap medially to resurface the cheek with a skin extension that replaces missing lateral upper lip skin.[11] The

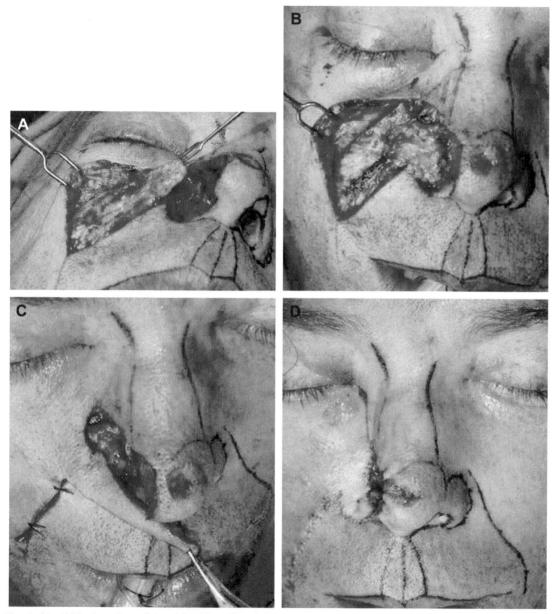

Fig. 4. (A–D) The junction of the right sidewall and cheek units superiorly and the residual nasolabial fold inferiorly are incised. Cheek skin lateral to the defect is elevated superficially for several centimeters. A fat flip flap, based medially, is turned over to fill the premaxillary soft tissue deficiency. The fat donor site is closed by simple advancement of cheek fat. Cheek skin is advanced to resurface the cheek defect. A dog-ear is excised superiorly. Excess skin created by the advancement of the cheek flap within the medial cheek lateral to the nasolabial fold is transposed medially, on a superior-based, randomly based skin extension, to resurface the upper lip defect. Most scars lie within the junction of the sidewall and cheek units and within the nasolabial fold (seen in another patient).

deep surface of the flap is fixed with suture to the deep soft tissues along the nasal facial groove and piriform aperture. Any residual cheek soft tissue deficiency left in the area of the donor fat flap is obliterated with a few sutures by the soft tissues, which advance with the cheek flap. The skin is closed with subcuticular and fine skin sutures.

Residual skin within the right alar subunit is excised, and the wound edges are freshened. Because the alar base inset must be precisely positioned, both vertically and laterally, the contralateral left hemilip template is flipped and positioned on the right upper lip. The ideal position of the alar base and nasolabial fold is marked with ink. The cheek had been overadvanced a few millimeters in the area of the alar base. The excess is trimmed (**Fig. 5**). At this point, the surgeon has repaired the cheek and lip platform, restored soft tissue, and determined exactly where the nose should sit.

The ala normally contains no cartilage, but a reconstructed ala must be supported with a cartilage graft to shape the soft tissues and prevent soft tissue contraction (**Fig. 6**). Although either ear can be used, the contralateral ear often provides ideal donor material. Through a postauricular incision, the left conchal cartilage is excised. The contour of the harvested cartilage is examined. The contralateral alar template is used to design an alar margin batten with the correct length, shape, and nostril margin outline. Although not required in this case, the shape of the cartilage graft can be modified with permanent half-buried mattress sutures to increase or decrease its convexity. The graft is designed about 3 mm too long on its anterior and posterior ends. Small subcutaneous pockets are dissected within the soft triangle at the nostril margin and alar base. A percutaneous suture is passed from the skin into the pocket and out the wound edge. The suture perforates the end of the cartilage graft and then reenters the wound edge, penetrating the external skin surface just within the nostril margin or nostril floor. The distal ends of the cartilage graft are

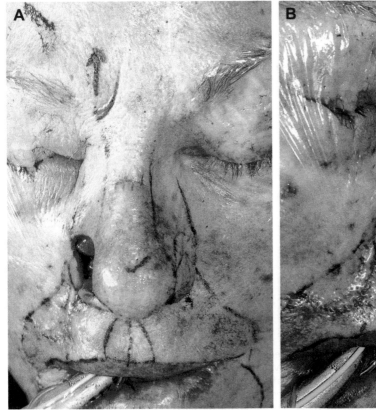
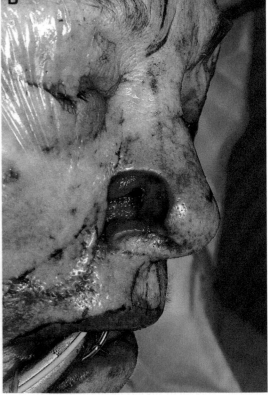

Fig. 5. (A, B) The cheek is advanced with a random skin extension to resurface the upper lip defect. The premaxillary soft tissue deficiency has been filled with a fat flip flap. The ideal position of the right alar base inset and nasolabial fold are marked with ink on the patient based on a template of the contralateral left hemilip.

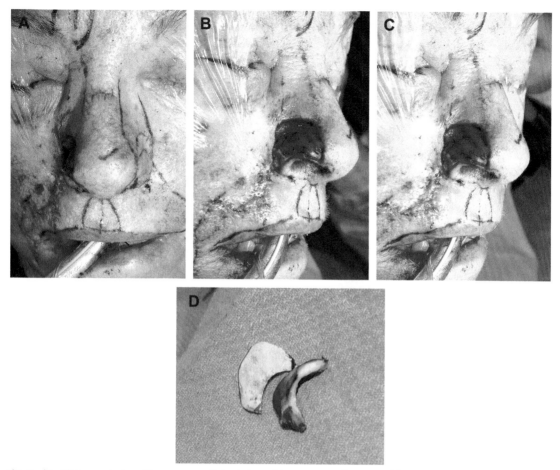

Fig. 6. (*A–D*) A conchal cartilage ear graft is designed to support, shape, and brace the right ala. The graft is designed on the foil template of the contralateral normal ala.

placed within these pockets and securely positioned with these guiding sutures for 1 week. The cartilage graft is also fixed with quilting sutures of 5-0 polypropylene, which pass through the external surface of the cartilage graft into the superficial raw lining surface and back out of the cartilage. The sutures do not pass through the lining into the nasal airway to avoid additional contamination and the possibility of infection.

Several rules should be noted. Although a forehead flap can be designed on either the right or left supratrochlear vessels, a unilateral defect is most easily repaired using an ipsilateral forehead flap because the point of rotation is closer to the defect. A contralateral forehead flap necessitates a longer flap and unnecessarily increases concern about transferring scalp hair to the nose. A midline defect can be resurfaced with a forehead flap based on either pedicle. Paramedian forehead flaps should be designed vertically. Although oblique flaps have been recommended to increase the length of flaps, the blood supply of the forehead

is vertical and an oblique flap transects the axial vessels, creating a random distal extension. Oblique flaps significantly increase the risk of eyebrow distortion on donor closure. Most importantly, these flaps transgress multiple vascular territories, leaving scars within most areas of the forehead and making a second flap harvest much more problematic. Because the previous contralateral forehead flap had been designed vertically, the ipsilateral forehead is easily harvested for a second flap.

The contralateral template is positioned just under the hairline, directly over the supratrochlear vessels (**Fig. 7**). The inferior pedicle of the template is marked inferiorly and passes through the medial eyebrow. The inferior pedicle width is approximately 1.2 cm. Because the inferior pedicle is narrow, the inferior forehead can always be closed without distortion of eyebrow position. Any gap that remains in the superior forehead after flap transfer is allowed to heal secondarily.

The forehead skin is thicker than nasal skin. Traditionally, forehead flaps are transferred in

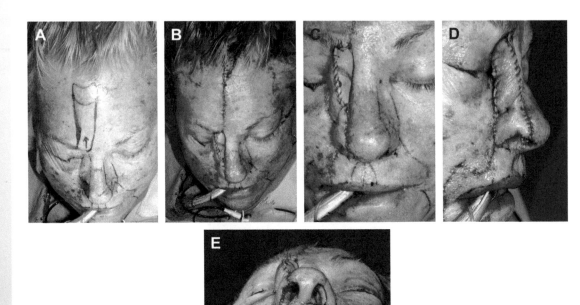

Fig. 7. (*A–E*) The foil template is also placed directly under the hairline above the supratrochlear vessels. The goal is to resurface the entire right alar subunit and part of the inferior sidewall. The left alar template provides the dimensional width of the skin required to resurface the ala and the exact border outline of the nostril margin. The pattern does not have to reflect the superior-inferior dimension of the defect exactly because the dimension can be accurately determined at the time of pedicle division and completion of flap inset. The pedicle is drawn inferiorly through the brow toward the medial canthus. The pedicle is 1.2 cm in width, which allows easy closure of the inferior forehead in almost all circumstances. Despite having already undergone a left alar repair with a forehead flap, the forehead donor site was closed completely in this case. The forehead flap was elevated with all layers; the frontalis muscle or subcutaneous fat was not excised distally. The flap was inset with a single layer of fine sutures. A quilting suture fixes the flap gently to the recipient site in the vicinity of the future alar crease.

2 stages. During the first stage, frontalis muscle and subcutaneous fat are excised distally from the deep surface of the flap to remove unneeded bulk. The thinned flap is inset at the recipient site. Several weeks later, once healed to the nose, the proximal pedicle, which provided blood supply initially, can be divided and partially reelevated superiorly and additional debulking can be performed, before the completion of skin inset. Although quite safe and satisfactory for smaller, less-contoured defects, the author prefers to resurface the nose with a full-thickness forehead flap in 3 stages when the defect is large, complexly contoured, or of full thickness. The flap is transferred without thinning. After 4 weeks, the flap skin is effectively "surgically delayed." The vascularity of the flap was not diminished by initial frontalis excision and is now augmented by physiologic delay. At the intermediate operation, forehead skin with 2 to 3 mm of subcutaneous fat is completely reelevated off the defect. This operation exposes the underlying excess subcutaneous fat and frontalis muscle, which is now adherent to

previously placed cartilage grafts and underlying lining. These soft tissues are directly excised, sculpting fat, frontalis, and cartilage graft, as necessary, into a nasal shape. The alar crease can be better defined. An old cartilage graft could be repositioned if poorly designed initially or distorted by scar. An additional cartilage graft can be added (eg, tip graft) depending on the defect. If the defect is of full thickness, the 3-stage modified fold forehead flap technique is used to provide lining (previously used for a left alar defect).

A full-thickness right paramedian forehead flap is incised and elevated inferiorly over the periosteum. The inferior pedicle of the flap passes through the medial brow, which effectively lengthens the flap, lowers the pivot point, and brings the flap closer to the defect. Most foreheads do not require preexpansion to avoid transferring hair to the nose.

The supratrochlear vessels are not directly visualized (see **Fig. 7**). The flap is rotated medially toward the nose and released until it reaches the

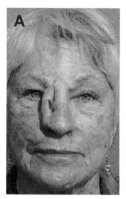
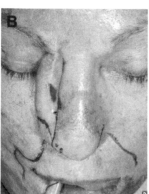
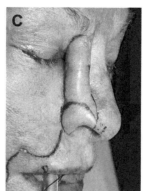
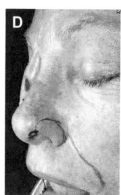

Fig. 8. (A–D) One month later, an intermediate operation is performed. The alar subunits and the borders of the forehead and cheek flap are outlined with ink.

defect without tension. Fibrous bands and corrugator muscle fibers are spread and clipped. The skin excision is extended inferiorly toward the medial canthus as necessary. The flap was then inset with a single layer of fine skin sutures. One or two percutaneous quilting sutures of 5-0 polypropylene can be used to apply the superior aspect of the flap to the side of the nose for 48 hours. The raw surface of the pedicle is covered with a full-thickness skin graft, harvested from the groin crease, to minimize oozing and establish a cleaner wound. The forehead is undermined bluntly into both temples, advanced, and closed in layers with an occasional 4-0 polypropylene tension suture through all layers, 4-0 slowly dissolving suture for the frontalis, 5-0 subcuticular, and 6-0 sutures for the skin. Despite a previous forehead flap, the patient's forehead was closed primarily. The dog-ear, within the hairline, was excised and closed with a running 4-0 polypropylene suture.

I have most patients stay overnight. The patients may shampoo and shower the following day, and their pedicle is often covered with a small dressing.

OPERATION 2

After 4 weeks, the wounds are healed. Landmarks are marked with ink, the left nasolabial fold; right residual nasolabial fold and border of the advancing cheek flap, which resurfaced part of the upper lip; borders of the forehead flap; and, based on the contralateral normal alar template, the general vicinity of the desired future right alar crease. The medial extension of the ear cartilage graft is visible as a small bulge within the soft triangle. This distortion is dotted with ink. The skin of the soft triangle is undermined and the external surface of the cartilage graft shaved to decrease its bulk (**Fig. 8**).

The border edges of the forehead flap are incised, and it is completely reelevated with 2 to 3 mm of subcutaneous fat. The flap is temporarily placed on the forehead within a wet 4 × 4 gauze. All tissue layers have now healed together and can be carved "like a bar of soap." The underlying excess subcutaneous fat and frontalis muscle are completely exposed, which are excised, with a knife, to create the round convex fullness of

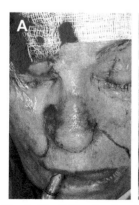
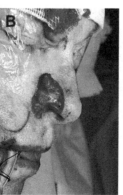
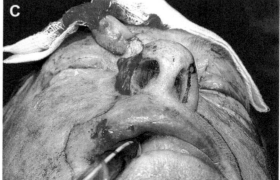

Fig. 9. (A–C) The forehead flap is completely reelevated with 2 to 3 mm of subcutaneous fat. The underlying excess of subcutaneous fat and frontalis muscle are exposed completely.

the alar lobule, a defined alar crease, and a flat sidewall subunit contour symmetric to the contralateral normal. The underlying cartilage graft is also reshaped by direct excision, if appropriate (**Fig. 9**). Now forehead skin of nasal "thinness" is reapplied to the contoured recipient site with a few quilting sutures of 5-0 polypropylene, which fix the skin flap to the underlying recipient bed but do not pass into the airway, and a single layer of fine skin sutures (**Fig. 10**).

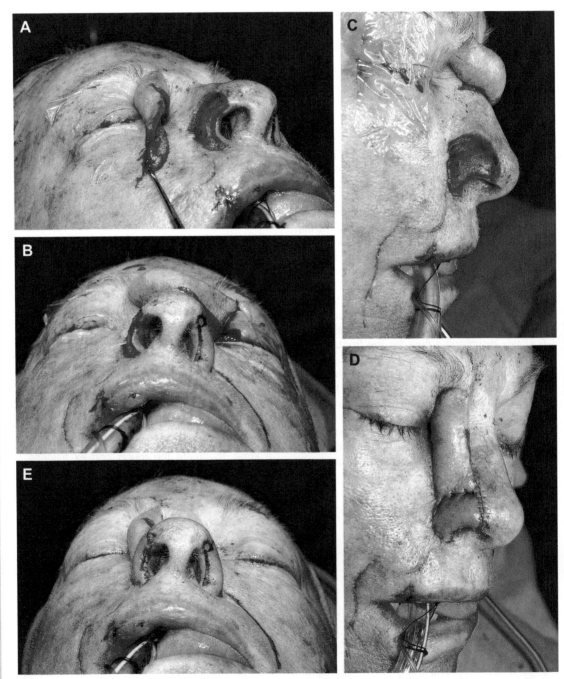

Fig. 10. (*A–E*) Excess subcutaneous bulk and the underlying skin graft, now healed to lining, are excised to sculpt a flap sidewall, distinct alar crease, and alar shape. The uniformly thin forehead flap is returned to the recipient site with several quilting sutures in a single layer of peripheral sutures.

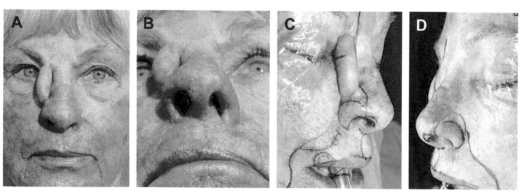

Fig. 11. (*A–D*) One month later (2 months after initiating repair), the patient returns to the operating room for pedicle division and recreation of the right nasal labial fold. Although the cheek skin that was advanced into the lip defect has the correct skin quality, the right nasolabial fold was obliterated by its transposition across the cheek-lip junction and the border scar of the flap is visible as a curvilinear scar under the right alar base. The inferior forehead scar, the peripheral outline of the forehead flap, the position of the ideal alar crease and nasal labial fold, the lip units, and a planned excision of a recently diagnosed basal cell carcinoma above the right lip vermilion is marked with ink. The scar of the cheek extension within the lip is crosshatched. The ideal alar crease and nasolabial fold positions were determined by templates based on the contralateral normal.

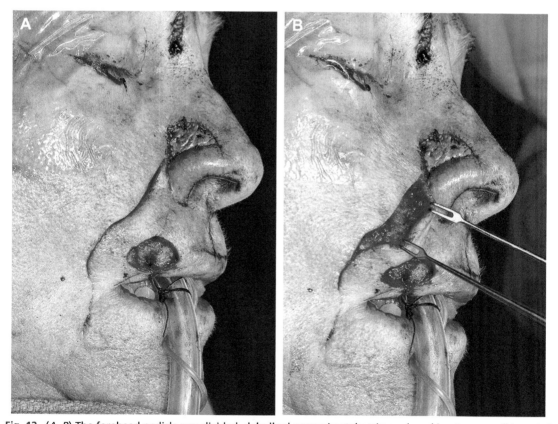

Fig. 12. (*A, B*) The forehead pedicle was divided, debulked approximately, trimmed, and inset as a small inverted "V" within the medial brow. Distally, forehead skin was elevated with a few millimeters of subcutaneous fat below the ideal alar crease position. Excess soft tissue and scar were excised to create a defined alar crease, a round superior ala, and a flap sidewall. Skin was reapproximated to the recipient site with quilting sutures. A direct incision was made at the location of the ideal nasolabial fold. Skin was elevated medially with a few millimeters of subcutaneous fat. Excess subcutaneous bulk was excised over the underlying orbicularis oris muscle to sculpt a flat upper lip and hairless triangle. Skin was then reapproximated to the lip recipient site with quilting sutures and the nasolabial fold incision closed in layers. The fullness of the lateral cheek was maintained.

OPERATION 3

The essential facial landmarks are largely restored (**Fig. 11**). The right nostril margin is pulled a millimeter or two superiorly and the medial brow inferiorly by the contraction on the undersurface of the forehead pedicle. The right nasal labial fold has been obliterated by the extension of the advanced cheek flap. The border scar of the fold is visible within the right upper lip subunit.

The inferior forehead scar, borders of the old left and new right forehead and cheek flaps, and nasal and lip subunits are marked with ink. The advanced cheek flap scar within the right upper lip is crosshatched. The ideal right alar crease and nasolabial folds are marked based on templates of the contralateral left normal subunits. A newly diagnosed basal cell carcinoma just above the right vermilion of the upper lip is marked for excision.

The forehead pedicle is transected. Superiorly, the skin graft on the proximal pedicle is excised and the inferior forehead reopened. The medial brow is repositioned after excision of excess subcutaneous soft tissue and inset of the proximal pedicle of a small inverted "V." The excess skin graft, soft tissue, and proximal skin are discarded. The inferior distal flap inset is elevated with 2 to 3 mm of subcutaneous fat inferior to the new ideal alar crease. The underlying soft tissue excess is excised to create a flat sidewall contour, deeper alar crease, and full convex superior ala. The skin is reapproximated to the newly established recipient contour with quilting sutures and sutured peripherally with a single layer of 5-0 sutures.

To better define the nasolabial fold, a direct incision was made within the advanced cheek skin at the position of the ideal nasal labial fold, disregarding old scars (**Fig. 12**). The skin was elevated medially over the lip with 2 to 3 mm of subcutaneous fat. Excess soft tissue was excised to create a flat upper lip surface, while maintaining the fullness of the cheek. The cheek flap was fixed to the underlying tissues with quilting sutures and

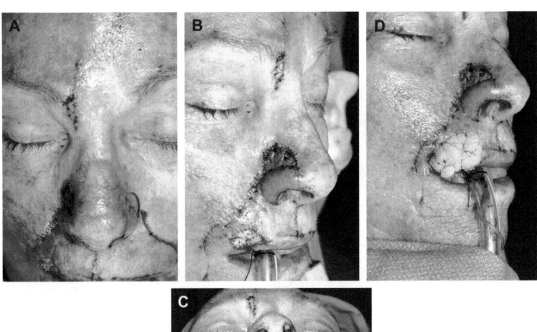

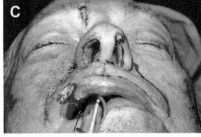

Fig. 13. (*A–D*) After closure, the medial eyebrow has been returned to its normal position and the inferior forehead scar appears as a small inverted "V," simulating the frown line. The contour of a flat sidewall and convex ala, separated by the alar crease, and the full cheek and flat upper lip, separated by the nasolabial fold, had been restored in symmetry to the contralateral normal. Full-thickness forehead skin, harvested from the residual pedicle, was applied as a graft to the upper lip defect, which followed the lip basal cell excision.

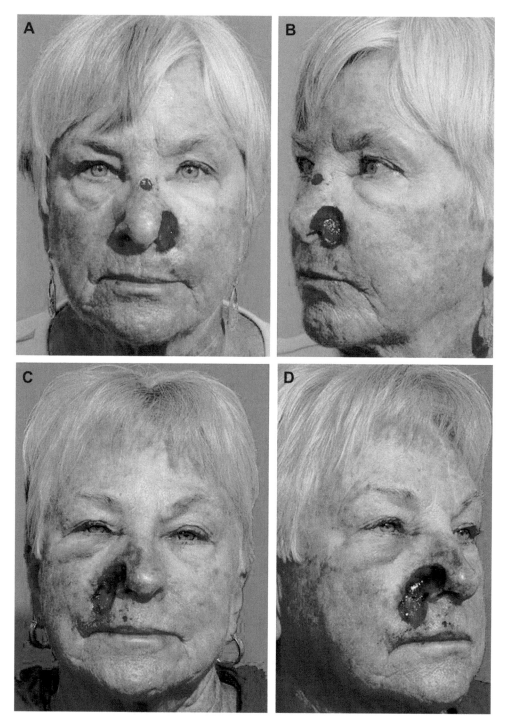

Fig. 14. (A–D) Nonsynchronous defects of the left ala with missing lining and composite defect of the right ala, cheek, and lip.

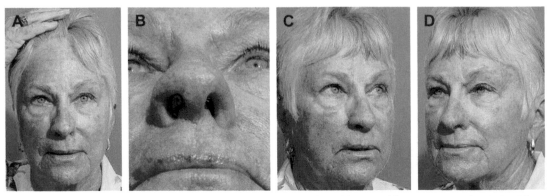

Fig. 15. (A–D) Postoperatively, the patient's appearance is normal, and her nasal function is good. Despite 2 forehead flaps, there is minimal scarring visible within the forehead donor site. The dimension, volume, position, projection, quality, outline, and contour of the nose, lid, and cheek are good. Also, multiple facial scars are largely invisible.

the new nasal labial fold was repaired with subcuticular and fine skin sutures. The basal cell carcinoma of the lip was excised, and its margins verified by frozen sections. The defect was repaired with a nonsubunit full-thickness forehead skin graft that was available from the discarded forehead pedicle. The graft was fixed to the lip recipient site with quilting sutures and peripheral sutures and covered with a foam bolus for 1 week (**Fig. 13**).

After 6 months or more, the patient's second forehead flap nasal reconstruction of bilateral nasal defects (**Fig. 14**), appearance, and function were very good. Forehead scarring is minimal.

Her left eyebrow is minimally elevated compared with the right, its natural position before either reconstruction. The inset of the pedicle into each medial brow simulates a frown crease. The patient's facial and nasal scars are virtually invisible (**Fig. 15**). Although a direct incision was made within the advanced cheek flap to re-create the right nasolabial fold, it cannot be seen. Because the cheek and lip contours are correct, the scar created by the advancement of the cheek flap into the lip subunit has disappeared. The complex contours of the nose, cheek, and lip are restored (**Fig. 16**). The patient looks normal, after 2 significant nasal defects and

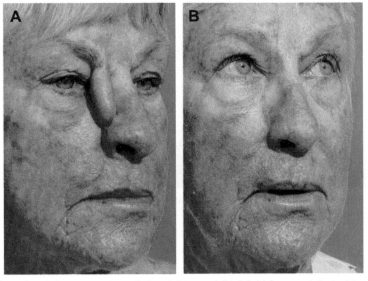

Fig. 16. (A, B) Although subtle, re-creation of the right nasolabial fold has contributed to the restoration of normal facial landmarks. The curvilinear scar, which followed the nonsubunit advancement of cheek skin into the lip, is much less apparent because the contour of the upper lip has been restored.

2 forehead flaps! If ever necessary, a third forehead flap can be harvested with or without preexpansion.

This reconstruction was successful because

- Both the patient and the surgeon wished to restore the normal.
- Time was taken to analyze the defect, establish priorities, formulate a plan to solve each clinical problem, and perform careful intraoperative steps.
- The best technique, not the easiest or quickest, was chosen.
- Principles and techniques were applied to reestablish the facial units, rather than close the wound or fill "the hole."
- Tissues were transferred or modified to recreate "like" tissue, whether quality, contour, or outline.

REFERENCES

1. Menick FJ. Nasal reconstruction: art and practice. Philadelphia: Saunders-Elsevier; 2008.
2. Menick FJ. "The modified folded forehead flap for nasal lining-the Menick method" in reconstructive surgery in oncology for surgical oncology seminars. In: Cordiero P, editor. Journal of Surgical Oncology, 94. Pennsylvania: John Wiley & Sons; 2006. p. 509–14.
3. Menick FJ. "Defects of the nose, lip, and cheek: rebuilding the composite defect". Plast Reconstr Surg 2007;120:887.
4. Burget GC, Menick FJ. "Subunit principle in nasal reconstruction". Plast Reconstr Surg 1985;76:239.
5. Menick FJ. Artistry in facial surgery: aesthetic perceptions and the subunit principle. In: Furnas D, editor. Clinics in plastic surgery, vol. 14. Philadelphia: WB Saunders; 1987. p. 723.
6. Burget GC, Menick FJ. Aesthetic reconstruction of the nose Mosby. St Louis (MO): Mosby; 1993.
7. Menick FJ. Ten-year experience in nasal reconstruction with the three-stage forehead flap. Plast Reconstr Surg 2002;109:1839.
8. Menick F. Nasal reconstruction CME. Plast Reconstr Surg 2010;125:135e–50e.
9. Menick F. Nasal reconstruction: forehead flap. Plast Reconstr Surg 2004;113:100e–11e.
10. Gillies HD, Millard DR. The principles and art of plastic surgery. Boston: Little Brown; 1957.
11. Menick F. Reconstruction of the cheek. Plast Reconstr Surg 2001;108:496–505.

Index

Facial Plast Surg Clin N Am 19 (2011) 213–227
doi:10.1016/S1064-7406(10)00173-2
1064-7406/11/$ – see front matter © 2011 Elsevier Inc. All rights reserved.

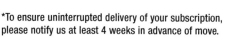
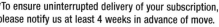

Printed and bound by CPI Group (UK) Ltd, Croydon, CR0 4YY

03/10/2024

01040357-0001